Index

S.S.Patel , M.D.

Anatomy – Head & Neck

* **Pharyngeal Arches:** Mesoderm + Neural crest
- **1st arch:** formed muscles of mastication, tensor tympani, tensor palatine, incus, malleus, maxilla, mandible and mandibular nerve (CN-5-III)
- **2nd arch:** formed muscles of facial expression, stapedius, stapes, styloid process, lesser horn & upper body of hyoid and facial nerve (CN-7)
- **3rd arch:** formed stylopharengeus muscle, greater horn & lower body of hyoid and glossopharyngeal nerve (CN-9)
- **4th arch:** formed cricothyroid muscles, right subclavian artery, laryngeal cartilage and superior laryngeal nerve [a branch of Vagus nerve (CN-10)]
- 5th arch is obliterated normally
- **6th arch:** All laryngeal muscles <u>except</u> cricothyroid muscle, laryngeal cartilage and recurrent laryngeal nerve [a branch of Vagus nerve (CN-10)]
- Very easy to remember **nerve supply of different derivatives of all arch. The cranial nerve derived from particular arch is responsible to supply them**!

* **Pharyngeal Pouches:** Endoderm
  1. Epithelial lining of auditory tube & middle ear cavity
  2. Epithelial lining of crypts of palatine tonsil
  3. **Thymus, Inferior parathyroid gland** (<u>absent in DiGeorge</u>)
  4. Ultimobracheal body, superior parathyroid gland

  - Neural crest cells migrate into the ultimobrachial body to form parafollicular cells of thyroid gland (secrete Calcitonin)

* **Pharyngeal grooves:** Ectoderm
  1. Epithelial lining of external auditory meatus
  All others grooves are obliterated

* **Paranasal Sinuses:**
- Sphenoidal – in Superior meatus
- Maxillary, Frontal, Ant & Middle Ethmoidal – in Middle meatus
- Post Ethmoidal – in Sup meatus
- Hiatus semilunaris (in middle meatus) – frontal, maxillary & Ant ethmoidal sinus
- Bulla Ethmoidalis (in middle meatus) – Middle ethmoidal sinus

* **Ansa cervicalis (C1,2,3):**
- Supply 3 strap muscles – sternohyoid, omohyoid (both bellies), sternothyroid
- Remaining 2 strap muscles – thyrohyoid, giniohyoid (supplied by C1 fiber)

- Post belly of digastric & stylohyoid – supplied by CN-7 (facial N)
- Ant belly of digastric & mylohyoid – supplied by CN-5-III (Mandibular N)

- **Tongue:** Anterior 2/3 – General sensation – CN-5-III (Mandibular N)
  Taste sensation – CN-7 (Facial N)
  Posterior 1/3 – General and Taste sensation – CN-9
- **All the muscles of tongue** innervated by CN-12 **except** palatoglossus
- Palatoglossus is innervated by CN-10
- **Test for CN-12 lesion:** On protrusion of tongue, tongue deviates **towards** the site of lesion
- Protrusion of tongue – Genioglossus muscle

- **All muscles of mastication** are innervated by Mandibular N

- **All muscles of Pharynx** supplied by CN-10 **except** tensor palatine
- Tensor palatine (Mandibular N) elevate soft palate to avoid regurgitation of food/liquid in nasopharynx during swallowing

* **Muscles of larynx:**
- Lat cricoarytenoid – Adduct vocal cord
- Post cricoarytenoid – Abduct vocal cord
- Thyroarytenoid – sphincter of vestibule, narrowing the laryngeal inlet
- Cricothyroid – lengthen and stretch the vocal cord
- Paired laryngeal cartilage – Arytenoid, corniculate & cuneiforms
- Single laryngeal cartilage – Cricoid, thyroid & epiglottis
- **All muscles of larynx** are supplied by recurrent laryngeal nerve **except** cricothyroid (Superior laryngeal nerve)

* **Important points about Cranial Nerve lesions:**
- **CN-1 (Olfactory N):** loss of smell
- **CN-2 (Optic N):** different sign & symptoms according to the site of the lesion (see neuroscience notes)
- **CN-3 (Occulomotor N):** loss of accommodation, ptosis, outward deviation (LR)
- **CN-4 (Trochlear N):** weakness of downward and inward eye movement (SO)
- **CN-6 (Abducent N):** Inability to look laterally (weak LR) (inward deviation)
- **CN-5 (Trigeminal N):** the jaw deviates to the weak side when the mouth is opened, loss of corneal reflex, loss of sensation on face
- **CN-7 (Facial N):** Ipsilateral paralysis of <u>all</u> facial muscles (Bell's palsy)
- **CN-8 (Vestibulocochlear N):** unilateral sensorineural deafness, vestibular symptoms (balance and postural problem)
- **CN-9 (Glossopharyngeal N):** loss of sensation on posterior 1/3 of tongue, loss of gag reflex [Gag reflex – sensory (CN-9); Motor (CN-10)]
- **CN-10 (Vagus N):** uvula deviates **opposite** side of lesion
- **CN-11 (Accessory N):** loss of shoulder shrugging (trapezius) and weakness of sternocleidomastoid
- **CN-12 (Hypoglossal N):** tongue deviates **towards** the site of lesion on protrusion
- All cranial nerve lesion produce defect on the same side **except** CN-10 (Vagus N)
- Pupillary Reflex: Sensory (CN-2); Motor (CN-3)
- Corneal Reflex: Sensory (CN-5) (ophthalmic division); Motor (CN-3)

Anatomy - THORAX

- Breast – Lateral ½ - Axillary lymphnode
  - Medial ½ - Parasternal lymphnode
- 1-7: true ribs
- 8-10: false ribs – attached to the costal cartilage of the rib
- 11-12: false ribs – no anterior attachment ["floating ribs"]

- Intercostal Muscles Blood supply:

Anterior Intercostal Arteries	Posterior Intercostal Arteries
12 pairs – 11 intercostal & 1 subcostal	12 pairs – 11 intercostal & 1 subcostal
- Pairs 1-6: Internal thoracic - Pairs 7-9: Musculophrenic - No anterior intercostal artery in 11 & 12 space. It is supplied by branches of posterior intercostal arteries	- Pairs 1-2: Superior intercostal artery (branch of subclavian) - Pairs 3-12: Branch of Thoracic aorta
- Drain into internal Thoracic & Musculophrenic veins	- Drain into Azygos system of veins

- Collateral b/w internal thoracic & aorta produce rib notching in coarctation of the Aorta
- Bottom of the pleura is 2 ribs lower than bottom of the lung

	Bottom of Lung	Bottom of Pleura
Midclavicular line	6th rib	8th rib
Midaxillary line	8th rib	10th rib
Paravertebral line	10th rib	12th rib

- Any penetrating injury below 4th intercostal space on Rt side can injure Liver
- Roots of phrenic nerve – C3,4,5
- Broncho pulmonary segments – 10 on the Rt, 8 on the Lt

Borders of Heart:
- **Rt** – Rt Atrium [3rd to 6th ribs]
- **Lt** – Lt Ventricle [2nd to 5th rib]
- Superior – Rt & Lt auricles + conus arteriosus of Rt ventricle
- Apex – tip of the Lt ventricle
- **Ant wall** – Rt ventricle
- **Post wall** – Lt atrium
- **Diaphragmatic wall** – Lt ventricle

- **Pericardial space** – space b/w epicardium & parietal pericardium

Rt & Lt Atrium:
- Auricle: pectinate muscles (rough part)
- Crista terminalis: ventricle ridge which separate smooth & rough parts
- Sinus venerum: smooth walled (formed by SVC & IVC)

- **Rt & Lt Ventricle:**
  - Trabaculae carneae (same as pectinate muscle)
  - Papillary muscles
  - Chordea tendinae
  - Infundibulum (Rt ventricle)
  - Aortic vestibule (Lt ventricle)

- **Rt Coronary artery:**
  - SA node, AV node
  - Rt atrium, Rt ventricle
  - Part of Lt atrium & ventricle
  - Post part of the Interventricular septum [In Lt dominant, it is supplied by Lt circumflex artery]

- **Lt Coronary artery:**
  - Lt Ant Descending: most part of interventricular septum, Apex of the Lt ventricle
  - Circumflex: Lt Atrium, Lt Ventricle, Lateral wall

- **Venous drainage of the Heart:**
  - Great cardiac vein: travel with Ant interventricular artery
  - Middle cardiac vein: travel with Post interventricular artery
    [Both open in Coronary sinus]
  - Venae Cordis minimae (Thebesian vein) & Ant cardiac vein directly open in the chambers of heart
  - Coronary sinus travel in Post coronary sulcus & open in Rt atrium

- **Thoracic duct:** starts in the abdomen from cisterna chyli [L2,3 level]
  - Drain: Lt upper limb (UL)
    Lt thorax, Lt H&N [head & neck]
    Pelvis, abdomen & lower limb (LL)
  - Empty in Lt Brachiocephalic vein
  - Found in posterior & superior mediastinum

- **Rt Lymphatic duct:**
  - Drain: Rt thorax & Rt H&N, Rt UL
  - Empty in Rt Brachiocephalic vein
- **Azygos System of Veins:**
  - Rt side – Azygos
  - Lt side – Hemiazygos & Accessory Hemiazygos [both drain to Azygos vein]
  - Posterior thoracic & Abd wall are drain by the azygos system of veins
  - Azygos – arise from the posterior aspect of IVC (Inferior venacava)
  - Hemiazygos – arise from the Left renal vein
  - Azygos vein empty into Superior venacava
  - **Openings in Diaphragm:** Caval (T8) [plus Rt phrenic nerves]
    Esophageal (T10) [plus Vegus nerve]
    Aortic (T12) [[plus Azygos vein & thoracic duct]

Anatomy - UPPER LIMB

- Musculocutaneous N (C5 to C7): All the muscles of the anterior compartment of arm [Biceps, Brachialis, Coracobrachi]

- Long thoracic N (C5 to C7): Serratus anterior

- Axillary N (C5, C6): Deltoid & teres major muscle [Deltoid – origin: clavicle & acromion]

* **Median N (C5 to T1):** Supracondylar region of humerous
- All muscles of Ant compartment of forearm except 1½ muscles [flexor carpi ulnaris & ulnar ½ of the flexor digitorum profundas]
- 3 Thenar muscles and 1st & 2nd lumbricals
- **If injured:** ulnar deviation of hand on flexion

* **Ulnar N (C7 to T1):** Medial epicondyle of humerus
- Flexor carpi ulnaris
- Ulnar ½ of flexor digitorum profundas
- 3rd & 4th lumbricals
- All introssei muscles

* **Radial N (C5 to T1):** Shaft of the humerus
- The posterior muscles of Arm & Forearm (there are no muscles in Post hand)

- Upper trunk (C5, C6): Axillary N, Musculocutaneous N
  Erb's palsy – muscles of **shoulder & Ant arm** ["waiter's tip"]
  Arm – medially rotated & adducted
  Forearm – extended & pronated

- Lower trunk (C8, T1):
  Klumpke's palsy – loss of the muscles of forearm & **hand**

- Lumbricals (4): flex metacarpophalangeal joint & extend interphalangeal joint
- Introssei (7): 4 dorsal (abduct fingers) & 3 palmar (adduct fingers)

Thenar muscles	Hypothenar muscles
- Abd. Pollicis bravis	- Abd. digiti minimi
- Flex. Pollicis bravis	- Flex. digiti minimi
- Opponens pollicis	- Opponens digiti minimi

* **Abductors of Thumb:**
- Abd pollicis bravis – Median N
- Abd pollicis longus – Radial N (Post interosseous nerve)
  So, Patient can abduct his hand in Median N injury

S.S.Patel , M.D.

* **Flexors of Thumb:**
  ▪ Flex pollicis bravis – Median N
  ▪ Flex pollicis longus – Median N (Ant interosseous nerve)
* **Adductors of Thumb:**
  ▪ Adductor pollicis – Ulnar N

  ▪ Therefore Muscles of thumb get nerve supply from all three nerves [Radial, Median & Ulnar]

* **<u>Test for injury of different Nerves:</u>**
  ▪ <u>Axillary N</u>: loss of abduction of the arm to the horizontal level
  ▪ <u>Radial N</u>: loss of extensors; "wrist drop"
  ▪ <u>Median N</u>: loss of opponens; pt can't oppose thumb (can't count with fingers)
  ▪ <u>Ulnar N</u>: loss of Abd & Add of fingers (introssei); ask pt to hold paper in b/w two fingers
  ▪ <u>Long thoracic N</u>: winging of the scapula

Anatomy - ABDOMEN

- **Layers of the Abdominal wall:** From outside to inside
    1. Skin
    2. Superficial fascia
    3. Deep fascia
    4. External (Ext) oblique
    5. Internal (Int) oblique
    6. Transversus abdominis
    7. Transversalis fascia
    8. Parietal Peritoneum

- **Superficial fascia:** There are two types of superficial fascia. One is Camper's fascia which mainly composed of fat and another is Scarpa's fascia which is membranous. Scarpa's fascia is continuous with fascialata of thigh, Dartos fascia of scrotum and Colle's fascia of perineum
- **Muscles of abdominal wall:** All three muscles of abdomen consist of its covering fascia, muscles and its apponurosis
- Free border of External oblique apponurosis form inguinal ligament
- Superficial inguinal ring is an opening in Ext oblique apponurosis
- Int oblique & transversus apponurosis muscles fibers join to form Conjoint tendon
- Deep inguinal ring begin as an out pouching of transversalis fascia
- Arcualte line: b/w umbilicus & pubis
- Above arcuate line: rectus sheath is covered by all three muscles apponurosis, both Anteriorly & Posteriorly
- Below arcuate line: covers only anteriorly by three muscles apponurosis; Posteriorly it is covered by transversalis fascia only

* **Boundaries of Inguinal Canal:**
- Roof: Int oblique & transversus abdominis
- Ant wall: Apponurosis of Ext oblique & Int oblique
- Floor: Inguinal ligament
- Post wall: Transversalis fascia (weaker part) & Conjoint tendon (reinforce medial part)

* **Boundaries of Femoral Canal:**
- Ant – Inguinal ligament
- Post – Pubis
- Med – Lacunar ligament
- Lat – Femoral vein

- **Direct Inguinal Hernia** – abdominal contents herniate through a weak point in the fascia of the abdominal wall and into the inguinal canal
- **Indirect Inguinal Hernia** – abdominal contents protrude through the deep inguinal ring [failure of closure of processus vaginalis]
- **Femoral hernia** – Inferior & Lateral to the pubic tubercle

S.S.Patel , M.D.

- **Processus Vaginalis** – developmental outpouching of the peritoneum – it precedes the testis in their descent down within the gubernaculum, and closes – the remaining portion around the testis becomes **tunica vaginalis**
- Psoas major – chief flexor of hip

- Foregut: up to 1st part of Duodenum
- Midgut: up to proximal 2/3 of transverse colon
- Spleen is **not** a derivative of foregut, but it is **supplied by foregut artery** [branch of Celiac artery]

- **Greater omentum:** gastrophrenic, gastrocolic & gastrosplenic ligaments
- **Lesser omentum:** hepatoduodenal & hepatogastric ligaments
- **Greater & Lesser peritoneal sacs** are separated by Hepatogastric ligament on Rt (surgical access to lesser sac) & by gastrosplenic ligament on Lt
- **Epiploic Foramen:** An opening into Omental bursa (lesser sac); finger in epiploic foramen touch Hepatoduodenal ligament anteriorly & IVC posteriorly
- Free edge of lesser omentum (**Hepatoduodenal ligament**) contain 3 structures: hepatic portal vein, common bile duct and hepatic artery
- **Spleenorenal ligament** contain splenic artery & vein
- **Gastrosplenic ligament** contain short gastric vessels and left gastro-epiploic vessels
- **Hepatogastric ligament** contain Rt & Lt gastric artery **near** the stomach
- **Retroperitoneal organs:** Duodenum, ascending colon, descending colon, kidneys & adrenal glands

- **Branches of Celiac trunk:** Lt gastric artery (lesser curvature), Common Hepatic artery & Splenic artery
- **Hepatic artery:** Proper hepatic artery, Cystic artery, Gastroduodenal artery, Rt gastric artery (lesser curvature)
- **Splenic artery:** Lt gastroepiploic artery, Dorsal pancreatic artery, Short gastric artery

* **Blood Supply of Stomach:**
- Lt gastric: proximal lesser curvature
- Rt gastric: distal lesser curvature
- Lt gastroepiploic: proximal greater curvature
- Rt gastroepiploic: distal lesser curvature
- Short gastric: short greater curvature above splenic artery

* **Portosystemic Anastomoses:** [Branch of Portal vein + Branch of Systemic vein]
    1. Lower Esophagus: Esophageal branch of Lt gastric (Portal) & Azygos vein (systemic)
    2. Upper Anal Canal: Sup rectal vein (Portal) & Middle / Inf rectal veins (systemic)
    3. Umbilicus: Vein of ligamentum teres (Portal) & Sup / Inf epigastric vein (systemic)
    4. Bare area of Liver: Hepatic / Portal vein (Portal) & Inf Phrenic vein (systemic)
    5. Patent ductus venosus (rare): Lt branch of portal vein (Portal) & IVC (systemic)
    6. Retroperitoneal: colonic veins (Portal) & Body wall veins (systemic)

* **Kidney:**
- Pronephros – cervical intermediate mesoderm (4th week of gestation)
- Mesonephros – thoracic & lumbar intermediate mesoderm (5th week)
- Metanephros – lumbar & sacral intermediate mesoderm (5th week)
- **Tubule regress & Duct persists**
- Pronephros – nonfunctional
- **Mesonephric duct forms (Wolffian duct)** – epididymidis, ductus (vas) deferens, ejaculatory duct, seminal vesicle
- Metanephros – <u>Ureteric bud</u> (also known as <u>metanephric duct</u>) (diverticulum of metanephric duct) & metanephrogenic blastema
- **Ureteric bud forms:** ureters, renal pelvis, collecting ducts, major & minor calyces
- **Metanephrogenic blastema (Lumbar & Sacral mesoderm) forms** – renal tubules [PCT, DCT, loop of Henle, Bowman's capsule] & definitive glomerulus

- Upper & largest part of urogenital sinus becomes **urinary bladder**

- **Male urethra:** Prostatic, membranous & proximal penile derived from urogenital sinus; Distal penile derived from glans of penis
- **Female urethra:** upper 2/3 derived from mesonephric duct; lower 1/3 derived from urogenital sinus

- **Prostate gland** in male is also derived from urogenital sinus

* **Relationship of Ureters:**
- Lies on Ant surface of Psoas major
- Crossing Ext iliac as they pass over the pelvic brim
- <u>Posterior to the uterine artery in female</u>

* **Blood supply of Kidney:**
- Interlobar arteries
- Arcuate artery
- Interlobular artery [branch of Arcuate artery]
- Afferent arterioles leads to capillary tuft of glomeruli

- **Blood supply of urinary bladder:** Internal iliac artery

* **Content of Sup Perineal pouch:**
- Bartholin's gland (<u>in female</u>)
- Cura of penis or clitoris
- Bulb of penis or bulb of vestibule
- Ischiocavernous muscle
- Bulbospongious muscle

* **Content of Deep Perineal pouch:**
- Bulbourethral gland (<u>in male</u>)
- Sphincter urethrae muscle

S.S.Patel , M.D.   10

- Deep transverse perineal muscle

- **Descend of Testis:** Testis develop in extraperitoneal layer (b/w layer 7 & 8) and descends from abdomen into scrotum. When it starts descending from abdomen into the Scrotum, it covers by fascia comes in its way. Three fascias [Internal spermatic fascia, Cremasteric fascia & External spermatic fascia] cover it from <u>inside to outside</u> respectively. These three fascias derived from transversalis, internal oblique and external oblique fascias respectively. Skin & Scarpa's fascia make scrotum. When testis starts decent, it brings part of peritoneum with it (processus vaginalis) which obliterated after birth.

* **Testis:** seminiferous tubule + Stroma [contain interstitial cells (<u>Leyding cells</u>)]
- <u>Seminiferous tubule</u>: site of spermatogenesis
- <u>Sertoli cells</u>: irregular columnar cells extend from the basal lamina to the lumen
    - Provide blood-testes barrier
    - Tight junction b/w Sertoli cells divide seminiferous tubule in two compartment: Basal compartment (Spermatogonia) & Adluminal compartment (Spermatocytes & Spermatids)
- Spermatogonia are near basal lamina & b/w two sertoli cells (all germ cells are between two sertoli cells)
- Sperm undergoes maturation in epididymis
- Seminal vesicles secrete fluid which contain fructose & sever as an energy source for the sperm

* **Ovary:** Cortex: ovarian follicles
           Medulla: nerves & blood vessels
- **Ovarian follicles:** composed of oocytes surrounded by follicular (granulosa) cells
    - <u>Primordial follicle</u>: primary oocytes surrounded by single layer of flattened follicular cells
    - <u>Primary follicle</u>: Primary oocytes + one/more layers of cuboidal like follicular cells
    - <u>Secondary follicle</u>: follicular cavity (antrum), cumulus oophorus, corona radiata, thica interna (secrete androgens which convert into estradiol by granulosa cells), thica externa, Zona pellucida around the oocyte (zona pellucida is PAS positive)
    - <u>Graafian follicle</u>: mature follicle extends through cortex
    - <u>Ovulation</u>: Increase in antral fluid causes rupture of follicle & ovum along with corona radiata passes out of the ovary
    - Follicular cavity changes occur leads to formation of <u>corpus lutem</u>
    - Thica interna – <u>thica lutin interna</u> (in Corpus lutem) – secrete Estrogen
    - Thica externa – <u>granulosa lutin cells</u> (in Corpus lutem) – secrete Progesterone
    - Corpus lutem persists until 3-months by hCG secreted by embryo. After 40th day, placenta produces progesterone necessary to maintain pregnancy

- **Spermatogenesis:** primordial germ cells <u>arrive in the indifferent gonad at week 4</u> and **remain dormant until puberty**

- **At puberty**, primordial germ cells differentiate into Type-A Spermatogonia, which serve as stem cells throughout adult life

- **Oogenesis:** primordial germ cells <u>arrive in the indifferent gonad at week 4</u> and **differentiate into Oogonia**
  - Oogonia enter Miosis-I to form primary oocytes. <u>All primary oocytes formed by 5th month of fetal life</u>, **remain arrested in prophase (diplotene) of Miosis-I until puberty**
  - **At puberty**, complete Miosis-I & become secondary oocyte & polar body
  - Secondary oocyte <u>arrested in metaphase of miosis-II & is Ovulated</u>
  - **At fertilization**, secondary oocyte complete miosis-II to form mature oocyte & polar body

  - **Miosis-I:** Synapsis (pairing), crossing over, disjunction (**without** centromere splitting)
  - **Miosis-II:** <u>No</u> synapsis, <u>No</u> crossing over, disjunction **with** centromere splitting

Anatomy - LOWER LIMB

* <u>Femoral N (L2,3,4):</u> Posterior division
- Ant compartment of thigh [quadriceps femoris, sartorius, pectineus]
- **Injury:** weakened hip flexion, loss of knee extension, sensory loss occur on Ant thigh, Medial leg & foot

* <u>Obturator N (L2,3,4):</u> Anterior division
- Medial compartment of thigh [Gracillis, Add longus, Add bravis, Ant portion of Add magnus]
- **Injury:** loss of adduction of thigh, sensory loss occur on Medial thigh

* <u>Tibial N (L4,5,S1,2,3):</u> Anterior division
- Post compartment of thigh [semimembranous, semitendinous, long head of biceps, Post portion of Add magnus]
- Post compartment of leg [gastrocnemius, soleus, Flex digitorum longus, Flex hallucis longus, tibialis posterior]
- Planter muscles of foot
- **Injury:** loss of flexion of the knee & digits, loss of palter flexion, weakened inversion; sensory loss on the leg (**<u>except</u>** medial side) & planter foot

* <u>Common Peroneal N (L4,5,S1,2):</u> Posterior division
- Short head of biceps
- <u>Superficial Peroneal N:</u>
- Lat compartment of leg [Peroneus longus, Peroneus bravis]
- <u>Deep Peroneal N:</u>
- Ant compartment of leg [tibialis anterior, Ext hallucis, Ext digitorum, Peroneus tertius]
- **Injury:** "foot drop"
- <u>Sup Peroneal N:</u> loss of eversion; sensory loss on dorsum of foot **<u>except</u>** 1st web space
- <u>Deep Peroneal N:</u> sensory loss on Anterolateral leg & 1st web space; weakened inversion, loss of extension of digits, loss of dorsiflexion of foot (foot drop)

* <u>Sciatic N:</u> Tibial N + Common Peroneal N
- **Injury:** weakened extension of thigh, loss of flexion of knee & loss of function below knee; sensory loss on Post thigh, leg (**<u>except</u>** medial side) & foot

* <u>Superior Gluteal N (L4,5,S1):</u> Posterior division
- Gluteus medius, gluteus minimus, tensor fascialata
- Injury: loss of Abd of limb, "**Trendelenburg gait**"

* <u>Inferior Gluteal N (L5,S1,2):</u> Posterior division
- Gluteus maximus
- **Injury:** weakened hop extension; pt has difficulty rising from sitting position <u>or</u> climbing stairs
- Medial sural N – Branch of Tibial N
- Lateral sural N – Branch of Common Peroneal N

- Sural N = Medial sural N + Lateral sural N

* **Knee joint:**
- Medial collateral ligament: resist abduction
- Lateral collateral ligament: resist adduction
- Ant & Post Cruciate ligaments – prevent Ant & Post displacement of tibia on femur respectively; test for injury – "Drawer's sign"
- **"Triad" Knee injury:** Medial collateral ligament, Medial meniscus, Ant Cruciate ligament

- DEP = Dorsiflexion & Eversion – Peroneal N
- PIT = Planter flexion & Inversion – Tibial N

Anatomy - SPINE

- Herniation of nucleus pulposus is almost always occur in Posterolateral direction [L_4 - L_5 most common location]
- Intervertebral foramen contains spinal nerve
- Inferior limit of the dural sac and the subarachnoid space is at S_2
- Inferior limit of the spinal cord is at L_1 & L_2

Anatomy - Miscellaneous

- **Remnants in Adults:**
- Rt & Lt Umbilical artery – Medial umbilical ligaments
- Urachus – Median umbilicus ligaments
- Umbilical vein – ligamentum teres
- Ductus venosus – Ligamentum venosum
- Ductus arteriosus – Ligamentum arteriosum
- Ventral mesentery – Falciform ligament

- Ductus Arteriosus – Lt Pulmonary artery to Aorta
- After birth, it reverse – Aorta to Lt pulmonary artery

S.S.Patel , M.D.

Basic Concepts

- Our cerebral cortex has an ultimate control on over body!
- Our body send sensation to our cortex so sensory fibers are always afferent (goes toward brain)
- Our cortex send information to different part of body to do their function so motor fibers are always efferent (goes away from brain)
- No matter which fibers [afferent or efferent], both cross midline so our brain control opposite side of our body! Right side of brain control left side of body! So any lesion to our brain produce Contralateral (opposite side) defect. Exception to this rule is cerebellum. Cerebellar fibers cross midline twice so cerebellar lesion produce Ipsilateral (same side) defect.
- For Cranial Nerves (CN), most of the CN nuclei are located in brain stem so these nuclei work as LMN for those CN and their control (cerebral cortex) work as UMN for them.
- UMN lesion – spastic paralysis, usually contralateral
- LMN lesion – flaccid paralysis, usually ipsilateral
- As I mentioned above cerebral cortex control opposite side of our body, involvement of CN in cerebral cortex lesion is contralateral and ipsilateral in brainstem lesion.
- Important parts of our brain – Cerebral cortex, Brain stem (Mid brain, Pons and Medulla) and Cerebellum. Other small parts are Basal ganglia, Thalamus, Hypothalamus, and Internal Capsule. Spinal Cord is also a part of CNS!

- **Forebrain** – Telencephalon [Cerebral cortex, basal ganglia, Lateral ventricles & Olfactory bulb] & Diencephalon [prethalamus, thalamus, hypothalamus, subthalamus, epithalamus, pretectum and the posterior pituitary gland]

- **Midbrain** – Mesencephalon [Midbrain, Cerebral aqueduct]

- **Hindbrain** – Metencephalon [Pons & Cerebellum] & Myelencephalon [Medulla] [4th ventricle forms from both metencephalon & myelencephalon]

- **Anterior Pituitary gland** – is an outgrowth of oral **ectoderm** [**Rathke's pouch**]. Remnant of Rathke's pouch forms **Craniopharyngioma** that compress Optic chiasm and produce bitemporal heteronymous hemianopsia

- **Neural Crest form** – Adrenal medulla, Primary sensory neurons & Post-ganglionic autonomic neurons [Cell bodies in ganglia (Peripheral Nervous System (PNS)]
- **Neural tube form** – skeletal motor neurons & Pre-ganglionic autonomic neurons [Cell bodies in SC (Central nervous system (CNS)]

- **Schwann cells make myelin for PNS**
- **Oligodendrocytes make myelin for CNS**

- Optic N (CN-2) is an outgrowth of brain so its myelin is formed by oligodendrocytes. CN-2 is affected in Multiple Sclerosis

- **Sympathetic Outflow** – T1 to L2 [Descending hypothalamic fibers drive all Pre-ganglionic sympathetic nerve fibers]

- **Parasympathetic Outflow** – **CN-3,7,9,10** and S-2,3,4

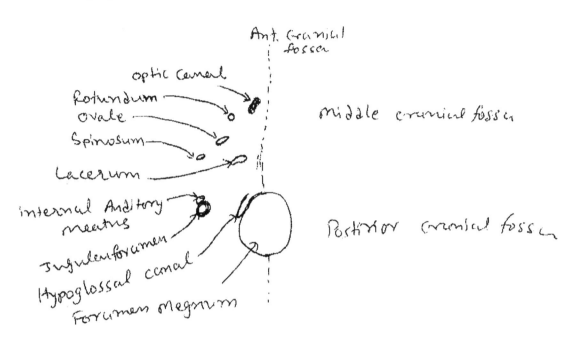

- Optic canal – CN-2 (optic N) & ophthalmic artery
- Rotundum – Maxillary N (CN-5 second division) (V2)
- Ovale – Mandibular N (V3) [Ophthalmic division V1 pass through Superior orbital fissure]
- Spinosum – Middle meningeal artery [epidural hematoma]
- Lacerum – **nothing**
- Internal auditory meatus – CN-7,8
- Jugular foramen – CN-9,10,11, sigmoid sinus
- Hypoglossal canal – CN-12
- Foramen magnum – CN-11, Vertebral artery, spinal cord – brain stem junction

* **Spinal Cord (SC):**

- **Cell bodies** of **Sensory fibers** – **Dorsal root ganglion (so not in SC)**
- **Cell bodies** of **Motor fibers** – **Ventral horn of gray matter of SC**

- **Dorsal root of Spinal Cord** – sensory fibers
- **Ventral root of Spinal Cord** – motor fibers

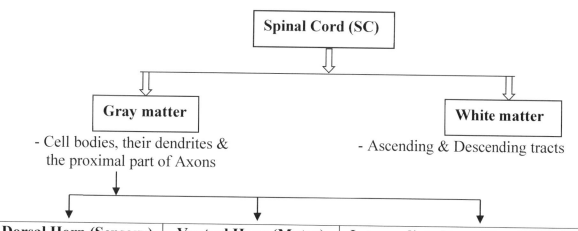

Spinal Cord (SC)

Gray matter

- Cell bodies, their dendrites & the proximal part of Axons

White matter

- Ascending & Descending tracts

Dorsal Horn (Sensory)	Ventral Horn (Motor)	Intermediate Horn (Cerebellar tract)
All incoming sensory fibers enter in dorsal horn [dorsolateral part of the SC]	α & γ motorneurons	**Present b/w T1 to L2 only**
	α innervate extrafusal fibers of skeletal muscles	**Clarke's** nucleus send **unconscious proprioception** to the **cerebellum**
	γ innervate intrafusal fibers of muscle spindles	
	Both neurons **leave the SC by way of ventral root**	

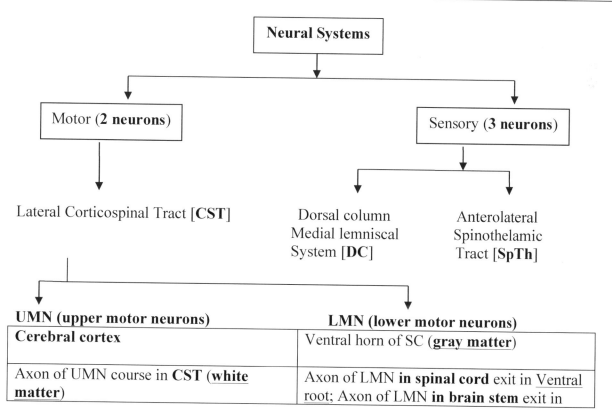

Neural Systems

Motor (**2 neurons**)

Sensory (**3 neurons**)

Lateral Corticospinal Tract [**CST**]

Dorsal column Medial lemniscal System [**DC**]

Anterolateral Spinothelamic Tract [**SpTh**]

UMN (upper motor neurons)	LMN (lower motor neurons)
Cerebral cortex	Ventral horn of SC (**gray matter**)
Axon of UMN course in **CST** (**white matter**)	Axon of LMN **in spinal cord** exit in <u>Ventral root</u>; Axon of LMN **in brain stem** exit in

S.S.Patel , M.D.

	cranial nerves (CN)
Occupy venteromedial position during their course	Play roles in reflexes (α & γ) α – contraction of muscles γ – carry stretch sensation to SC
Cross at lower medulla (Pyramidal Decussation)	UMN & LMN lesions are opposite to each other. See below signs of UMN

- UMN has <u>**net inhibitory effect**</u> on reflex **therefore in UMN lesion,** there is **hyperreflexia, spastic paralysis** & Babinski sign present (**extension of toes**)

- ■ <u>**Dorsal Column – Medial Lemniscal System (DC): (3 neurons)**</u>

- Discriminative touch, joint position sense, vibratory and pressure sensation from the trunk & limbs

- **Fasciculus Gracillis (LL):** found at all level of SC   [LL = lower limb]
- **Fasciculus Cuneatus (UL):** found only at upper thoracic & cervical level of SC

- Cell bodies of 1ˢᵗ neuron – DRG [DRG = dorsal root ganglion]
- Cell bodies of 2ⁿᵈ neuron – lower medulla
- Cell bodies of 3ʳᵈ neuron – Thalamus (VPL) [VPL = ventral posterolateral nucleus of thalamus]
- Fibers of <u>**2ⁿᵈ neuron cross at lower part of medulla**</u>
- From VPL, it goes to somatosensory cortex in to the post-central gyrus

- **Lesion of the Dorsal Column:** loss of two point discrimination, joint position sense, vibratory & pressure sensation; Astereognosis – loss of ability to identify the characteristic of an objects; Dx: Romberg's sign [patients sway when they close their eyes] & vibratory sensation by 128 Hz tuning fork [If patient have **cerebellar damage,** patient will **sway even with their eyes open**]

- Fibers of 2ⁿᵈ neurons <u>**MUST**</u> cross midline **in** <u>**both**</u> **(DC & SpTh) sensory systems**

- ■ <u>**Anterolateral Spinothelamic Tract System: (3 neurons)**</u>

- Pain, temperature (temp) & crude touch sensation from the extremities and trunk

- Cell bodies of 1ˢᵗ neuron – DRG
- Cell bodies of 2ⁿᵈ neuron – Dorsal Horn Gray matter
- Cell bodies of 3ʳᵈ neuron – Thalamus (VPL)
- Fibers of <u>**2ⁿᵈ neuron cross at Spinal Cord**</u>

- Because the pain & temp information crosses almost as soon as it enters the SC, **any unilateral lesion of the SpTh in the SC or Brain stem will result in a Contralateral loss of pain & temp**

- SpTh fibers run closely to the SC and can affect 1st in SC cavitations (**Syringomyelia**). Cavitations usually occur at cervical level so bilateral loss of Pain & Temp in UL occurs first.

- Descending Hypothalamic fibers **run with SpTh without** crossing at brain stem therefore **any lesion of SC above T2 produce Hornor's syndrome (Ipsilateral)**

- **Amyotrophic Lateral Sclerosis (ALS) (Lou Gehrig's disease)** – is a pure motor system disease & **affect both UMN & LMN** and typically **begin at cervical level** of spinal cord – occurs due to mutation in superoxide dismutase gene; increase level of glutamate is seen in patient with ALS – Rulizole is currently the only FDA approved drug for ALS [see figure below]

■ **Brain Stem:** Home of 9 cranial nerves

- **Midbrain** – 3rd & 4th [4th is the only CN which exit from Dorsal brain stem]
- **Pons** – 5th, 6th, 7th, 8th
- **Medulla** – 9th, 10th, 12th
- **M**otor nuclei of CN situated **M**edially & Sensory nuclei situated lateral to motor nuclei
- Pure Motor CN – 3,4,6,11,12
- Pure Sensory CN – 1,2,8
- Mixed CN (both motor & sensory function) – 5,7,9,10

- **Lesion in Brain Stem:** loss occur on Contralateral side of any 3 long track (1 motor & 2 sensory), Hornor's syndrome (always Ipsilateral) & Ipsilateral CN lesion

- **Medial longitudinal Fasciculus (MLF)** fiber bundle is a center for **Horizontal gaze** connect vestibular nuclei & nuclei of CN-3,4,6
- Lesion of MLF leads to disrupt vestibule-occular reflex
- **M**LF is located in Pons & Midbrain in **m**idline

- Solitary Nucleus (7,9,10) – taste & visceral sensation
- Nucleus Ambiguus (9,10) – motorneurons [muscles of soft palate, larynx, pharynx & upper esophagus)
- Dorsal Motor nucleus of CN-10 – Visceral motorneurons [major parasympathetic nucleus of the brain stem; viscera of thorax, foregut & midgut]

- **Midbrain:** Superior colliculus (**Vertical gaze**) & Inferior colliculus (Auditory information – lateral lemniscus)

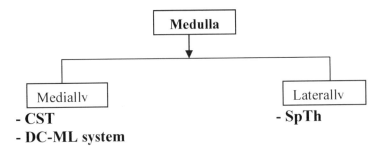

- **CST**
- **DC-ML system**

- **SpTh**

- **Blood Supply of Brain Stem:**

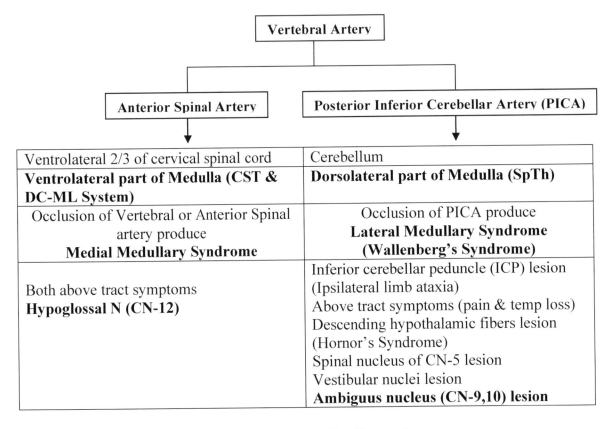

Ventrolateral 2/3 of cervical spinal cord	Cerebellum
Ventrolateral part of Medulla (CST & DC-ML System)	**Dorsolateral part of Medulla (SpTh)**
Occlusion of Vertebral or Anterior Spinal artery produce **Medial Medullary Syndrome**	Occlusion of PICA produce **Lateral Medullary Syndrome (Wallenberg's Syndrome)**
Both above tract symptoms **Hypoglossal N (CN-12)**	Inferior cerebellar peduncle (ICP) lesion (Ipsilateral limb ataxia) Above tract symptoms (pain & temp loss) Descending hypothalamic fibers lesion (Hornor's Syndrome) Spinal nucleus of CN-5 lesion Vestibular nuclei lesion **Ambiguus nucleus (CN-9,10) lesion**

- **Two Vertebral arteries joined to form Basilary artery**
- **Labyrinthine artery – a branch of Basilar artery, supply inner ear**

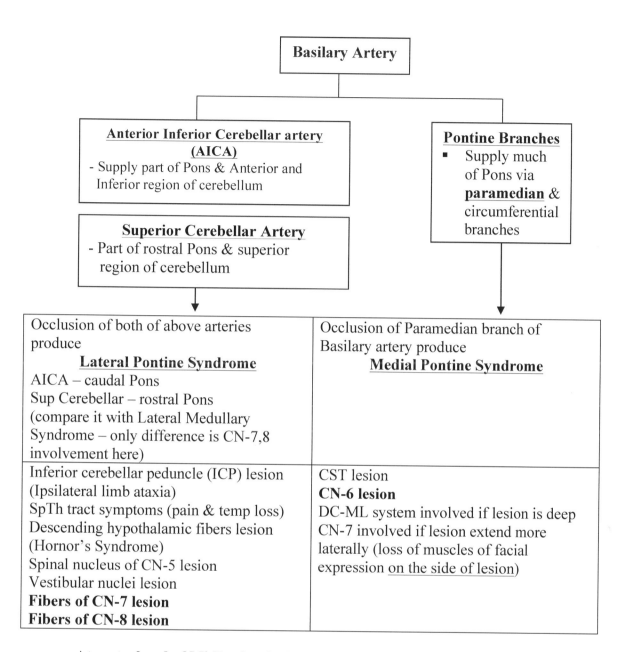

Basilary Artery

Anterior Inferior Cerebellar artery (AICA)
- Supply part of Pons & Anterior and Inferior region of cerebellum

Superior Cerebellar Artery
- Part of rostral Pons & superior region of cerebellum

Pontine Branches
- Supply much of Pons via **paramedian** & circumferential branches

Occlusion of both of above arteries produce **Lateral Pontine Syndrome** AICA – caudal Pons Sup Cerebellar – rostral Pons (compare it with Lateral Medullary Syndrome – only difference is CN-7,8 involvement here)	Occlusion of Paramedian branch of Basilary artery produce **Medial Pontine Syndrome**
Inferior cerebellar peduncle (ICP) lesion (Ipsilateral limb ataxia) SpTh tract symptoms (pain & temp loss) Descending hypothalamic fibers lesion (Hornor's Syndrome) Spinal nucleus of CN-5 lesion Vestibular nuclei lesion **Fibers of CN-7 lesion** **Fibers of CN-8 lesion**	CST lesion **CN-6 lesion** DC-ML system involved if lesion is deep CN-7 involved if lesion extend more laterally (loss of muscles of facial expression <u>on the side of lesion</u>)

- **At rostral end of Midbrain, the Basilary artery divides into pair of Posterior Cerebral artery**
- <u>How will you identify all different syndromes on exam?</u> – <u>By looking at involvement of different cranial nerves.</u> Involvement of CN-12 (Medial Medullary Syndrome), CN-9,10 (Lateral Medullary Syndrome), CN-7,8 (Lateral Pontine Syndrome), CN-6 (Medial Pontine Syndrome) and CN-3 (Medial Midbrain Syndrome)

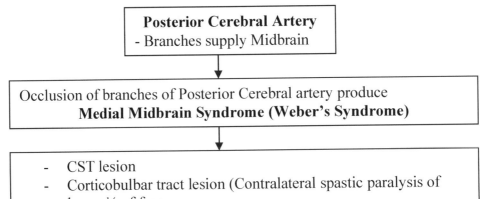

Posterior Cerebral Artery
- Branches supply Midbrain

Occlusion of branches of Posterior Cerebral artery produce
Medial Midbrain Syndrome (Weber's Syndrome)

- CST lesion
- Corticobulbar tract lesion (Contralateral spastic paralysis of lower ½ of face
- **Fibers of CN-3** – Ipsilateral oculomotor nerve palsy (dilated pupils, ptosis, Lateral strabismus

* **Pontocerebellar Angle Syndrome:** caused by Acoustic neuroma (Schwannoma) of CN-8 – **absence of long tracts signs** indicates that the lesion must be outside of brain

* **Parinaud Syndrome: Pineal gland tumor** compressing superior colliculus – the most common sign is **paralysis of upward (vertical) gaze** ["sun set sign"] combined with bilateral pupillary abnormality

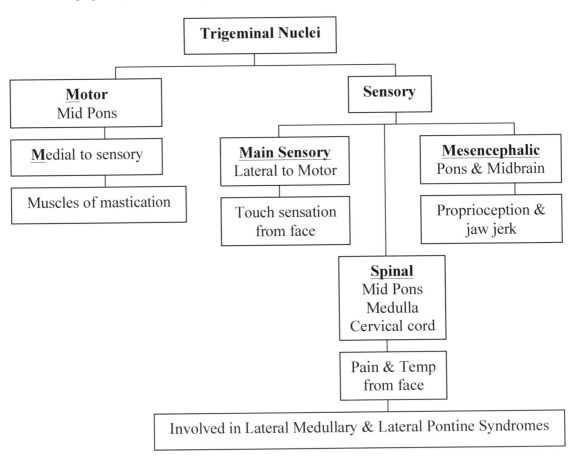

Trigeminal Nuclei

Motor
Mid Pons

Sensory

Medial to sensory

Muscles of mastication

Main Sensory
Lateral to Motor

Mesencephalic
Pons & Midbrain

Touch sensation
from face

Proprioception &
jaw jerk

Spinal
Mid Pons
Medulla
Cervical cord

Pain & Temp
from face

Involved in Lateral Medullary & Lateral Pontine Syndromes

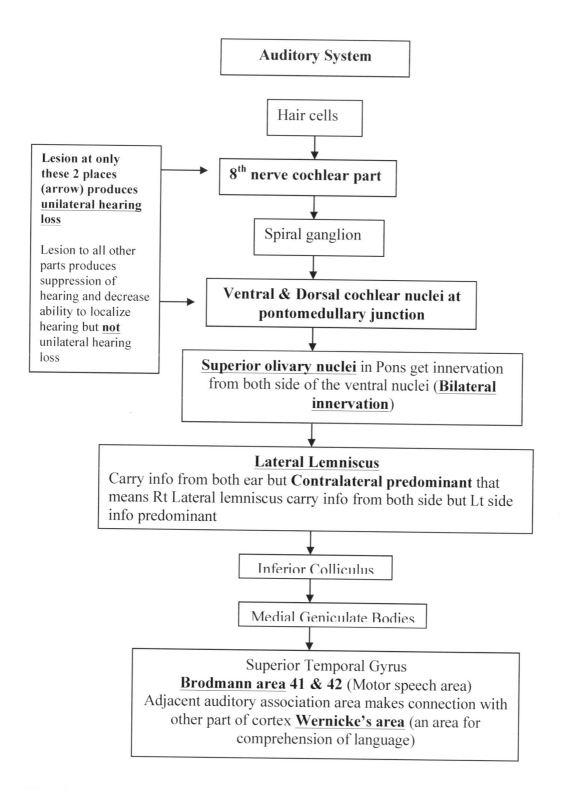

Auditory System

Hair cells

8th nerve cochlear part

Spiral ganglion

Ventral & Dorsal cochlear nuclei at pontomedullary junction

Superior olivary nuclei in Pons get innervation from both side of the ventral nuclei (**Bilateral innervation**)

Lateral Lemniscus
Carry info from both ear but **Contralateral predominant** that means Rt Lateral lemniscus carry info from both side but Lt side info predominant

Inferior Colliculus

Medial Geniculate Bodies

Superior Temporal Gyrus
Brodmann area 41 & 42 (Motor speech area)
Adjacent auditory association area makes connection with other part of cortex **Wernicke's area** (an area for comprehension of language)

Lesion at only these 2 places (arrow) produces **unilateral hearing loss**

Lesion to all other parts produces suppression of hearing and decrease ability to localize hearing but **not** unilateral hearing loss

- **High** frequency sounds – **base** of cochlea
- **Low** frequency sounds – **Apex** of cochlea

S.S.Patel , M.D.

* **Vestibular System:**

- Urticle & Saccule: linear acceleration – positional changes in the head relative to gravity
- Ampullary Crest: Angular acceleration – results from circular movement of head

- **Head** turns **right** leads to **Both** **eyes** move **left**

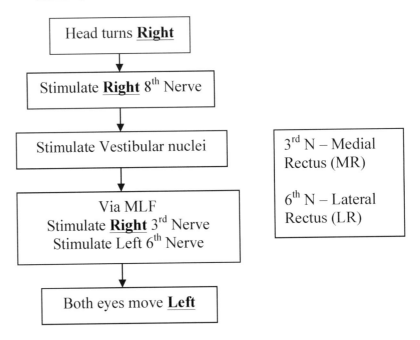

* **Nystagmus:** unilateral vestibular nerve <u>or</u> nuclei lesion produce nystagmus

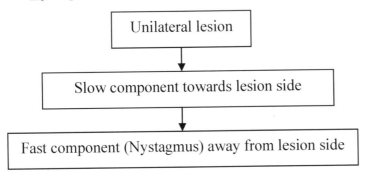

* **Caloric Test:**

- Pouring **Cool water** (mimic nerve lesion) into ear – Nystagmus **Opposite side**
- Pouring **Warm water** (mimic nerve stimulation) into ear – Nystagmus **Same side**

* **Horizontal Gaze:**

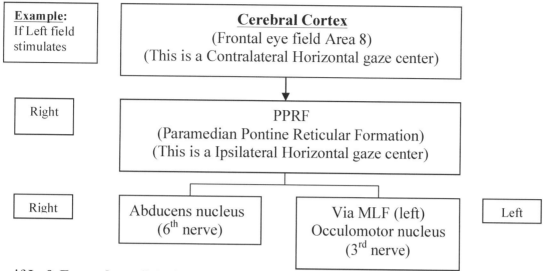

So, if **Left Frontal eye field is stimulated**, activation of Pontine gaze center occur on Right and saccadic **Horizontal eye movements of Both** eyes occur to the **Right**

- **Left frontal eye field lesion** – Both eyes can't look to the Right (but slow drift occur to the Left)
- **Left MLF lesion** – Left eye can't look to the Right and therefore Right eye exhibits nystagmus
- **Right Abducens nucleus or Right PPRF lesion** – Both eyes can't look to the Right (but slow drift to the Left)
- **Right 6ᵗʰ Nerve lesion** – Right eye can't look to the Right

* **Visual System:**

- **Pathway:** Retina → Optic nerve (nasal & temporal fibers) → Optic chiasm → Optic tract → LGB (lateral geniculate body) → Optic radiation (**lateral fibers & medial fibers**) → Cerebral cortex (Occipital lobe – Cuneus & Lingual)

- Nasal field projects on temporal fibers & Temporal field projects on nasal fibers
- Nasal fibers cross at optic chiasm, but temporal fibers doesn't cross

- Upper field projects on lower retina & lower field projects on upper retina
- Image from **L**ower retina → **L**ateral fiber → make Mayer's **L**oop (Temporal lobe)
- Image from Upper retina → Medial fiber (pass through Parietal lobe)
- Calcarine sulcus (occipital lobe) – Cuneus (**up** – **u**pper retina – medial fiber) & Lingual (below cuneus – lower retina – lateral fiber)

- All lesions **past the chiasm** produce Contralateral defect (**Homonymous**)
- **Only optic chiasm lesion** produce **heteronymous**
- Destruction of macula produce **central scotoma**

- Hemianopsia = loss of half visual field
- Anopsia = loss of total visual field
- Homonymous =

  L   R

- Heteronymous =

  L   R

Examples	Lesion of Visual System pathway	Defect
Right	Optic N (nasal + temporal fibers)	Rt eye anopsia
Right	Temporal fiber	Rt nasal hemianopsia
	Optic chiasm	Bitemporal heteronymous hemianopsia
Right	Optic tract	Lt homonymous hemianopsia
Right	Optic radiation (Medial + Lateral)	Lt homonymous hemianopsia
Left	Lateral fibers of optic radiation	Rt homonymous Superior quadrantanopsia
Left	Medial fibers of optic radiation	Rt homonymous Inferior quadrantanopsia
Left	Cerebral cortex (Visual)	Rt homonymous hemianopsia with macular sparing

- Lesion of Optic N produce blindness (anopsia) but lesion of Visual cortex (occlusion of Posterior cerebral artery) leads to Contralateral Homonymous Hemianopsia with **macular (central) vision spared** (Macula has collateral blood supply from Middle Cerebral artery)
- Macular atrophy (elderly people) leads to loss of central vision

* **Important point about Facial N (CN-7) lesion:** <u>Upper face muscles</u> (which wrinkles forehead & shut eyes) get <u>bilateral cortical innervation</u> where as lower face has unilateral cortical innervation therefore **Cortical lesion** leads to <u>**only**</u> **drooping of angle of mouth** on Contralateral side whereas **Facial nerve lesion** leads to **Ipsilateral paralysis of <u>all</u> facial muscles** (Bell's palsy)

- Most people (80%) are Right-handed so Left hemisphere is more highly developed. Speech & language functions are also predominantly organize in the left hemisphere therefore left middle artery occlusion produce Aphasia [Broca's, Wernicke's or Both]

■ **Middle Cerebral Artery (MCA):**
- Bulk of **Lateral surface** of hemisphere
- **Genu & Posterior limb of internal capsule**
- Basal ganglia
- **Occlusion of MCA:** Contralateral spastic paralysis and anesthesia of <u>lower face & UL</u>, Aphasia (in left MCA occlusion), Left side neglect (in right MCA occlusion), Contralateral superior quadrantanopsia (occlusion of branches that supply Mayer's loop of visual radiation)

- **Anterior Cerebral Artery (ACA):**
- <u>Medial surface</u> of frontal and parietal lobes which include **motor & sensory** areas for the <u>pelvis & lower limb</u>
- **Anterior 4/5 of Corpus callosum**
- **Anterior limb of internal capsule**
- **Occlusion of ACA:** Contralateral spastic paralysis & anesthesia of LL, **urinary incontinence, Transcortical apraxia** (patient can not move left arm in response to verbal command. This is because left hemisphere (language dominant) has been disconnected from the motor cortex of right hemisphere. Both of which are connected through corpus callosum)

- **Posterior Cerebral Artery (PCA):**
- Occipital lobe & posterior 2/3 of temporal lobe on <u>Medial surface</u> of hemisphere
- Thalamus, **Splenium of corpus callosum**
- Subthalamic nucleus
- **Occlusion of PCA:** Homonymous hemianopsia of the Contralateral visual field with macular sparing, Left PCA occlusion produce **Alexia <u>without</u> Agraphia** (Can't read but can write) [This is because involvement of Splenium of corpus callosum prevents visual information from intact right occipital cortex to language comprehension cortex in the left hemisphere therefore patient can see word in the left visual field but can't understand what word mean]

- **Frontal lobe:**
- Primary motor cortex (area 4)
- Premotor cortex (area 6)
- Frontal eye field (area 8)
- Motor speech areas of Broca (areas 44, 45) (inferior frontal lobe)
- Precentral gyrus – primary motor cortex contain motor homunculus
- **Frontal lobe syndrome:** lesion in the frontal area – can't concentrate, **apathy** (severe emotional indifference), abullia (slowing of intellectual faculties, slow speech, decrease participation in social interaction), **emergence of infantile suckling or grasp reflex in adult, personality change, expressive aphasia,** inability to make voluntary eye movements towards Contralateral side (frontal eye field – Contralateral horizontal gaze center)

- **Parietal lobe:**
- Primary somatosensory cortex (Postcentral gyrus) (areas 3,1&2)
- Posterior parietal association cortex (area 5&7)
- Wernicke's area (area 39&40) [Area 22 is in temporal lobe]
- Area 22 – spoken word; Area 39 – written word
- **Parietal lobe lesion: Receptive aphasia,** Transcortical apraxia, **Asomatognosia (left side neglect)** (lesion in area 7, 39 & 40), **Conductive aphasia** (Arcuate fasciculus – large fiber bundle which connect areas 22,39&40 to Broca's area)
- **Gerstmann's syndrome:** lesion to angular gyrus (area 39) – Alexia with Agraphia (can't read and can't write) but patient can understand spoken words

- **Temporal lobe:**
- Auditory cortex (area 41 & 42)
- Wernicke's area 22
- **Temporal lobe lesion:** Unilateral lesion to auditory cortex leads to **only little loss** of auditory sensitivity but have some difficulty in localizing sound, **problem with memory, receptive aphasia** (area 22)

- **Occipital lobe:**
- Primary visual cortex (area 17)
- Visual association cortex
- Bilateral visual cortex lesion produce cortical blindness means the patient can't see but pupillary reflexes are intact (center for pupillary reflex is in Pretectal area in Midbrain) [Pupillary reflex – Sensory (CN-2) & Motor (CN-3)]
- **Visual association cortex → forms & color** → parvocellular-blob system → "cone stream" project on blob zone of primary visual cortex → **Temporal lobe (area 20 & 21)**
- **Unilateral lesion to areas 20 & 21:** Achromatopsia (complete loss of color vision in contralateral hemifield. Patient see everything is shades of gray), Prosopagnosia (inability to recognize face), Visual agnosia (inability to recognize visual pattern including object)
- Visual association cortex → **Motion & Depth** → Magnocellular system → "Rod stream" project on the stripe zone of primary visual cortex → **Parietal lobe (area 18 & 19)**
- **Unilateral lesion to areas 18 & 19:** deficit in perceiving visual motion (visual field, color vision & reading are unaffected)

- **Olfactory System:** central projection of olfactory structures reach parts of the temporal lobe & Amygdala [Pyriform cortex is a primary olfactory cortex]
  - Fracture of the cribriform plate (occur in head injury) can tear the olfactory nerve fibers. As olfactory nerve is an outgrowth of the CNS, it is covered by meninges, and tear of olfactory nerve fiber may tear meninges causing CSF leaking through cribriform plate into nasal cavity

- **Limbic System: Hippocampal formation** on the **medial aspect of temporal lobe** (include hippocampus, dentate gyrus, subiculum & adjacent entorhinal cortex), **Amygdala** (located rostral to hippocampus) and **Septal nuclei**

* **Cerebellum:**
  - Major input – ICP & MCP [Inferior & Middle cerebellar peduncle]
  - Major output – SCP [superior cerebellar peduncle]
  - Granule cells are the only excitatory cells within the cerebellar cortex
  - Purkinje cells are the only outflow from the cerebellar cortex. It sends fibers to deep cerebellar nuclei
  - Climbing fibers from inferior olivary nucleus of Contralateral medulla provide direct excitatory input to the Purkinje cells
  - Mossy fibers provide an indirect excitatory input to the Purkinje cells
* **Spinocerebellar Pathway:** send unconscious proprioception

* Fibers of spinocerebellar tract <u>**cross two times in central nervous system**</u> therefore cerebellar injury produce loss of function on Ipsilateral (same side). As these fibers are involved in unconscious proprioception, **patient tends to fall on same side of cerebellar lesion** (Cerebellar injury always produce Ipsilateral loss of function)

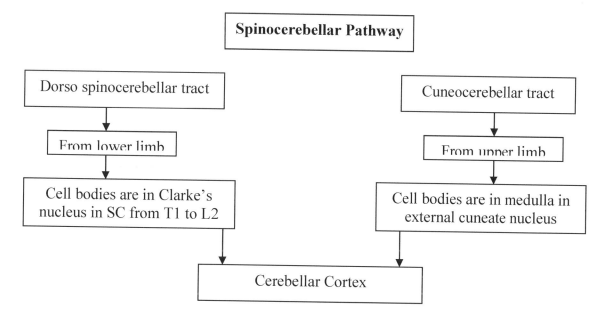

- **Deep Cerebellar Nuclei & Cerebellar Area:**
- **Flocculo nodular lobe** → <u>Fastigeal nucleus</u> → Vestibular nucleus → Elicit positional changes of eyes & trunk in response to movement of Head
- **Intermediate Hemisphere** → <u>Interpositus nucleus</u> → Red nucleus & Reticular formation → influence LMN via Rubrospinal & Reticulospinal tracts to adjust posture & affect movements
- **Lateral Hemisphere** → <u>Dentate nucleus</u> → Thalamus (VL), then Cortex → influence LMN via CST which affect voluntary movements, especially, sequence & precision

* **Cerebellum** is involved in planning & fine tuning of skeletal muscles contraction therefore cerebellar lesion produce **Intention Tremor** [tremor occur during voluntary movements]

* **Basal ganglia** initiate & provide gross control over skeletal muscles movements therefore basal ganglia lesion produce Dyskinesia (movement disorder) and slow initiation of movement. **Tremor at rest**

* <u>**Basal ganglia:**</u> Striatum (Caudate nucleus & Putamen), Globus palidus, Substantia nigra (Substantia nigra is in Midbrain)

- Disinhibition: one population of inhibitory neurons inhibit second population of inhibitory neurons
- <u>Direct Pathway</u>: net effect is excitation of cortex & promotion of movement
- <u>Indirect Pathway</u>: net effect is inhibition [decrease cortex excitation]

- ACh – stimulate indirect pathway [ACh found within striatum]
- Dopamine – stimulate direct pathway & inhibits indirect pathway

* **Indirect pathway lesion:** Chorea, Athetosis, Hamiballismus
* **Direct pathway lesion:** Parkinsonism
* **Hamiballismus:** wild flinging movement (violent projectile movements) of half of the body – typically observed in upper limb – usually seen in **hypertensive patient**
* **Tourett's Syndrome:** also a basal ganglia disease involves facial and vocal ticks that progress to jerking movements of the limb – frequently associated with **explosive, vulgar speech** – <u>Tx</u>**:** Pimozide

■ **Thalamus:** process and relay sensory information selectively to various parts of the cerebral cortex

- Involvement of Thalamus in CV stroke identified by contralateral painful anesthesia means burning <u>or</u> aching on one half of the body. It often accompanied by mood swing.

■ **Hypothalamus:** One of the most important functions of the hypothalamus is to link the nervous system to the endocrine system via the pituitary gland. It synthesizes and secretes neurohormones (hypothalamic-releasing hormones), and these in turn stimulate or inhibit the secretion of pituitary hormones.

▪ **Hypothalamic nuclei:**
  - Medial preoptic nucleus [urinary bladder contraction, decrease heart rate and decrease blood pressure]
  - **Paraventricular & Supraoptic nuclei** [synthesize ADH & Oxytocin]
  - Anterior hypothalamic nucleus [thermoregulation, sweating, thyrotropin inhibition]
  - Lateral nucleus [thirst and hunger]
  - **Suprachiasmatic nucleus** [visual input from retina; plays role in circadian rhythm (24-hrs light-dark cycle)]
  - Arcuate nucleus [produce LH & FSH releasing hormones]
  - Venteromedial nucleus [satiety center & regulate food intake, neuroendocrine control; lesion to this produce Obesity]
  - Dorsomedial hypothalamic nucleus [GI stimulation]
  - Mammillary bodies – memory
  - Posterior nucleus – increase blood pressure, pupillary dilation and shivering [lesion to this produce hypothermia]
  - **Preoptic area** – responsive to androgens & estrogen; influence the production of sex hormone by anterior pituitary – lesion to preoptic area Before puberty (arrest sexual development) After puberty (Amenorrhea <u>or</u> Impotence)
  - Ventrolateral preoptic nucleus – They are primarily active during Non-REM sleep, and inhibit other neurons that are involved in wakefulness.

▪ Epithalamus: **Pineal body** – synthesize melatonin, serotonin, cholecystokinin – environmental **light regulates the activity** of the Pineal gland

* **Internal Capsule:** Anterior limb, Genu & Posterior limb – course taken by all fibers those are leaving <u>or</u> entering cortex – Thalamocortical (limbic system) in Anterior limb; Corticobulbar (Cranial nerve sign) in Genu; CST & all somatosensory thalamocortical projections in Posterior limb

- Six layers of Cerebral cortex:
    1. Molecular layer
    2. External Granular layer
    3. External Pyramidal layer
    4. Internal Granular layer
    5. Internal Pyramidal layer
    6. Multiform layer
- Internal pyramidal layer gives rise to axons that form CST & Corticobulbar tract
- Pyramidal layer well developed in Frontal lobe
- Granular layer well developed in Parietal, occipital & temporal lobes. It is a site for termination of major sensory neurons

- **Reticular Formation:** is a poorly-differentiated area of the brain stem, centered roughly in the Pons. The ascending reticular activating system connects to areas in the thalamus, hypothalamus, and cortex, while the descending reticular activating system connects to the cerebellum and sensory nerves.
- It controls respiration, cardiovascular responses, behavior arousal & <u>sleep</u> – lesion to this produce coma & death
- Three nuclei [Raphe, Locus Cerulus & Periaqueductal Gray]
- **Raphe nuclei:** synthesize Serotonin (5-HT) – Serotonin seems to be the culprit in many of our modern psycho-pharmaceutical problems, such as anorexia, depression, and sleep disorders – SSRI works here
- **Locus Cerulus:** located within the dorsal wall of the rostral Pons in the lateral floor of the fourth ventricle – synthesize Norepinephrine – involved with physiological responses to stress & panic and in arousal – decrease NE level in REM sleep
  Both of above nuclei are degenerate in Alzheimer

- **Periaqueductal Gary:** opioid receptors

* **Wernicke–Korsakoff syndrome:** combined manifestation of two disorders, Korsakoff's Psychosis and Wernicke's encephalopathy – **Wernicke's encephalopathy** is characterized by confusion, nystagmus, ophthalmoplegia, ataxia, coma & death – **Korasakoff's psychosis** is characterized by anterograde & retrograde amnesia, hallucination and confabulation – Wernicke's encephalopathy results from severe **acute deficiency of thiamine** (Vitamin B_1), whilst Korsakoff's psychosis is a chronic neurologic sequel after Wernicke's encephalopathy – **In the United States**, it is usually found in malnourished **chronic alcoholics** who undergo **prolonged intravenous (IV) therapy without Vitamin B_1** supplementation – lesion is believe to be found in **mamillary body** & the medial dorsal thalamus

* **Klüver–Bucy Syndrome:** occurs when both the right and left medial temporal lobes of the brain malfunction – **Amygdala** (main site for the pathogenesis of this syndrome) – placidity (Docility) (↓↓ aggressive behavior), Hyperorality (put everything in mouth), dietary changes, hypersexuality, Hypermetamorphosis (an irresistible impulse to notice and react to everything within sight), memory loss

Anatomy- HISTOLOGY

- **Skin** – stratified squamous keratinized
  <u>Layers of epidermis</u> (**deep to superficial**)
  Stratum basale
  Stratum spinosum
  Stratum granulosum   • Epidermis is devoid of blood vessels
  Stratum lucidum
  Stratum corneum

- **RS** – Pseudostratified
- <u>Nasopharynx</u> – Respiratory epithelium
  <u>Oropharynx</u> – striated squamous non-keratinized
- <u>Alveolar sac</u> – simple squamous
  <u>Alveoli</u> → Type –1 pneumocytes – simple squamous (thin)
        → Type –2 pneumocytes – cuboidal like

- **GIT** – Esophagus – upper 2/3   - Pseudostratified
               lower 1/3   - Squamous non-keratinized

  - (SI) Small Intestine – columnar Absorptive (villi present)
  - Large Intestine – Villi absent (Paneth cells unique to SI secrete bactericidal Enzymes)
  - Duodenum – Brunner's gland
  - Ileum - Payer's patches
  - Liver - Sinusoids – lined by fenestrated endothelial cells & scattered kupffer cells
  - <u>Bile canaliculi</u> – (lined by Hepatocytes)
    ↓
    Hering's canal
    ↓
    Hepatic duct (Right & Left)
    ↓
    Common Hepatic duct.

- **Kidney** – PCT, DCT - cuboidal
- PCT is the **only** site in kidney which has "**brush border**" (like small intestine, brush border help in reabsorption of substances like glucose, etc.)

- **Bladder & Ureter** – transitional epithelium
- **Urethra** – Prostatic – transitional epithelium
                  Penile – stratified epithelium
- **Epididymis** – Pseudostratified epithelium **with stereo cilia**
- **Vagina** – stratified squamous
- **Uterus** – simple columnar
- **Fallopion tube – Ciliated columnar**

Physiology - Cardiovascular System

- CO = HR x SV   [CO = cardiac output]

  $CO = \dfrac{MAP}{TPR}$

- Fick's **Principle** involves calculating the oxygen consumed over a given period of time from measurement of the oxygen concentration of the venous blood and the arterial blood.

  Q = (VO2/CA - CV)*100

  CA = Oxygen concentration of arterial blood and CV = Oxygen concentration of venous blood

  VO2 = Oxygen consumption

- PP [pulse pressure] = SP – DP
- Mean Pressure (MAP) = diastolic + $\dfrac{1}{3}$ PP

  =2/3 DP + 1/3 SP

  (MAP is always near DP but MAP>DP)

* SV = EDV – ESV
* Ejection Fraction = $\dfrac{SV}{EDV}$ = $\dfrac{EDV – ESV}{EDV}$

* **Cross sectional Area:** single vessel with large diameter has small cross-sectional area than more vessels with small diameter.
  - Velocity is **inversely** proportional to cross-sectional area
  - Aorta has small cross sectional area therefore velocity in Aorta is high
  - In Respiratory System, velocity decreases as air moves from trachea to alveoli because cross-sectional area increases due to severe branching of trachea

* **Vascular resistance:** is the resistance to flow that must be overcome to push blood through the circulatory system. **Total peripheral resistance** (TPR) is the sum of the resistance of all peripheral vasculature in the systemic circulation.

- **R** = ΔP / Q = $\dfrac{mmHg}{ml / min}$ = $\dfrac{\textbf{Pressure}}{\textbf{volume / time}}$

- Resistance is **inversely** proportional to radius^4 [r^4] that means a decreased radius will greatly increase the resistance – eg. Vasoconstriction
- It also depends on the capacitance of the blood vessel
- The amount of pressure lost in a particular segment is proportional to the resistance of that segment. E.g. In capillary bed resistance is high (small diameter) so pressure loss is high therefore Pressure loss **from** 120/80 in aorta **to** 30-50 in capillary bed. **Highest**

S.S.Patel , M.D.   34

pressure Loss occurs in arterioles [capillary bed is made by joining of arterioles and venules].

- **Series circuits:** $R = R_1 + R_2 + R_3 + \text{-----}$
  - Adding a resister in series **increases the resistance of the system**
  - Flow is **equal at all points** in series system.
- **Parallel circuits:** $1/R = 1/R_1 + 1/R_2 + 1/R_3 + \text{-------}$
  - Therefore **adding** a resister in parallel system **decreases the resistance of the system** and **removal of resistor** from parallel system **increase total resistance** and tends to increase in BP.
    - **Total resistance is always less than any individual resistance in parallel circuits.** (Contrast to series system)
    - **Flow is regulated independently**
- **CVS** is connected in **series** circuit whereas **different organs** are connected in **parallel** circuit
- **Increase Flow → decrease Resistance [R = $\triangle$P / Q]**
  Therefore pulmonary circuit is the least resistance circuit in the body. (100% of blood flow from right ventricle)
  Renal circuit has low resistance (25% of blood flow)
  Coronary circuit has **highest** resistance (only 5% of blood flow)

* **Vessel compliance (C):**
  $C = \triangle V / \triangle P$
  Veins have a much higher compliance than arteries
  Decrease C means stiffer vessel
  Decrease C leads to increase SP but decrease DP therefore increase PP

- **Causes of $\uparrow$ SP** – $\uparrow$ SV, $\downarrow$ **Compliance**, $\downarrow$ HR
- **Causes of $\uparrow$ DP** – $\uparrow$ SV, $\uparrow$ **TPR**, $\uparrow$ HR

* **Wall Tension (T):**
  T $\propto$ PR   P = pressure
          R = radius
  In aneurysm, **R** increases; as aneurysm enlarge → increase R → increase T → more likely to burst

* **Effect of GRAVITY:**
  Gravity reduces the rate of blood return from the body veins <u>below</u> the heart back to the heart, thus **reduce stroke volume and cardiac output.** – **Compensation:** the veins below the heart quickly constrict (**increase TPR**) and the **heart rate increases.**

* **Characteristics of Auto-regulating Tissues (No involvement of nervous system):**
- Keep blood flow constant when blood pressure varies
- Seen in the kidney, the heart, and the brain; **Skeletal muscles during exercise**

- Blood flow α tissue metabolism [**increase metabolism → increase blood flow**]
- **In the kidneys:** maintain renal blood flow and glomerular filtration rate – <u>Myogenic mechanism</u>: as blood flow increases, the afferent arterioles are stretched, they contract, and subsequently reduce blood flow – <u>Tubuloglomerular feedback</u>: the macula densa "senses" the low blood pressure and causes vasoconstriction to maintain GFR
- **In the heart:** state of **high metabolic activity [increase metabolism – increase blood flow]** – mediated by the equilibrium of ATP, ADP, AMP, and Adenosine in the myocardial cell – lack of oxygen, the equilibrium is shifted toward Adenosine. Adenosine causes vasodilation and therefore increases the supply of oxygen [**Adenosine:** formed in the myocardial cells during hypoxia, ischemia, or vigorous work, due to the breakdown of high-energy phosphate compounds – causes vasodilation in the small and medium sized resistance arterioles – it can cause a **coronary steal phenomenon,** where the vessels in healthy tissue dilate as much as the ischemic tissue and more blood is shunted away from the ischemic tissue that needs it most. This is the principle behind adenosine stress testing]
- **In the brain:** flow α arterial PCO_2 [**CO_2 = Vasodilator**] [↑ Arterial PCO_2 (Hypoventilation) → ↑ cerebral blood flow; ↓ Arterial PCO_2 (Hyperventilation) → ↓ cerebral blood flow] – **Large ↓ in PO_2 → ↑ Cerebral blood flow** [In these conditions low art PO_2 determine cerebral blood flow, **not** PCO_2]

- As already mentioned above that the heart has high metabolic activity, the tissue **extracts almost all the O_2** they can from the blood, even under **"basal" condition.** Therefore, the **lowest** venous PO_2 in a resting individual is in **coronary sinus** – **Highest** venous PO_2 is in **Renal veins**

Left coronary artery	Right coronary artery
* **Very little** if any blood flow can occur **during systole** [due to **mechanical compression which is more prominent in subendocardium**]	* **Significant flow** can occur during **systole** due to less mechanical compression
* **Most** blood flow occur during **diastole [phase-1]**	

- **Pulmonary circuit:**
  High flow, **Low** resistance [**R** = ΔP / **Q**], **Low** pressure
  Very compliant circuit – Both Arteries & veins
- **Hypoxic vasoconstriction** (exception)
  (↓ O_2 → ↑ CO_2, **normally CO_2 acts as a vasodilator but in lung it acts as vasoconstrictor**)
- ↑ Cardiac Output α ↑ pressure & flow in pulmonary circuit means ↓ resistance
  ↓ CO α ↓ pressure & flow in pulmonary circuit means ↑ resistance
  ↓ CO α ↑ Pulmonary Vascular resistance

2. **Carotid sinus** (dilatation of the **wall of internal carotid artery**) → **Baroreceptors** (medulla) (provides a **negative** feedback loop to increase blood pressure) → Sensory [CN – 9, 10] & Motor [CN – 10 (Vegas nerve)] → **Medulla only interprets Afferent** (Aff.) activity **as an index of BP** [↑ BP → ↑ Aff. Activity; ↓ BP → **no** Aff. Activity] → [↑ **Aff. Activity** → ↑ Efferent activity (CN-10) → ↓ **CO & ↓ TPR**]   [CO = cardiac out put, TPR = total peripheral resistance]
3. **Carotid body** (at the origin of external & internal carotid arteries) – chemoreceptor (see in Respiratory System)

■ **Cardiac Action Potential: Automaticity** – the ability of the cardiac muscles to depolarize spontaneously, i.e. without external electrical stimulation from the nervous system. It is most often demonstrated in the sinoatrial (SA) node, ["Pacemaker of the Heart."] Abnormalities in automaticity result in rhythm changes – During a cardiac cycle, once an action potential is initiated, there is a period of time that a new action potential cannot be initiated. This is called the **effective refractory period (ERP)** of the tissue – ERP acts as a protective mechanism and keeps the heart rate in check and prevents arrhythmias and coordinates muscle contraction – **Conduction system of heart** [SA node – AV node – Bundle of His – Purkinje fibers – Ventricular wall] – The AV node delays impulses by approximately 0.12 seconds before allowing the impulses through to the His-Purkinje conduction system. This delay in the cardiac pulse is extremely important: It ensures that the atria have ejected their blood into the ventricles first before the ventricles contract

■ **AP of Ventricles:**

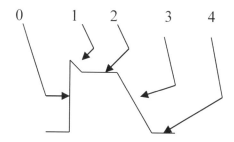

- **Phase-0:** ↑ Na^+ influx causes depolarization
- **Phase-1:** slight repolarization due to K^+ current & closing of Na^+
- **Phase-2:** Ca^{++} channel open (↑ influx of Ca^{++}), voltage gated K^+ closed (plateau depend on this), K^+ efflux continue through unvoltage gated channel
- **Phase-3:** Ca^{++} channel closed and voltage gated K^+ channel open
- Under resting condition voltage gated K^+ channel is open. Depolarization is a signal for closing them.

- **AP of SA node:**

Threshold

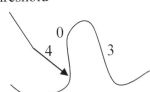

Phase-0: mainly Ca^{++} spike rather than Na^+
Phase-1: K^+ efflux (rapid)
Phase-4: gradual depolarization towards threshold
mainly due to $\downarrow K^+$ conductance

Once threshold reach, AP generate

- **Sympathetic:** Beta-1 receptors are present here which work through Gs protein so when it stimulates it increases heart rate by increasing Ca^{++} conductance → threshold reach sooner

- **Parasympathetic:** M2 receptors are present here which work through Gi protein so when it stimulates it decreases heart rate by increasing K^+ conductance → take long time to reach threshold

- **Preload:** the pressure stretching the ventricle of the heart
- Heart muscle at the end of diastole is **below Lo** therefore ↑ **in preload in normal heart** – ↑ **force of contraction**
- **Afterload:** the tension produced by a left ventricle in order to contract – increase Afterload is seen in aortic stenosis, hypertension.
- **Frank-Starling law of the heart:** under **normal physiologic state**, the greater the volume of blood entering the heart during diastole (end-diastolic volume), the greater the volume of blood ejected during systolic contraction (stroke volume). [The law is true for normal physiologic condition because, for example, in CHF, end-diastolic volume is increase but SV is not increased.

- ↑ Contractility → ↓ Systolic interval
  ↑ Heart Rate → ↓ Diastolic interval
- Isovolumatric → Both valve closed

- **Pathophysiology of main valvular heart diseases:**

* **Aortic stenosis (AS):**
  - Increase Ventricular systolic pressure – systolic murmur
  - Stenosis means small opening so pressure gradient b/w LV & Aorta during ejection
  - Concentric hypertrophy due to increased after load

* **Mitral insufficiency (MI):**
  - Systolic murmur
  - No pressure gradient b/w atrium & ventricle
  - Left atrium & ventricle, both enlarge

– Increase Atrial pressure in systole in MI

* **Aortic insufficiency (AI):**
– ↑ Preload (↑ in force of contraction → slight ↑ in ventricular systolic pressure
– ↑ PP (↑ SP & ↓ DP)
– Eccentric hypertrophy due to increase volume load in LV
– Diastolic murmur

* **Mitral stenosis (MS):**
– Stenosis means small opening so pressure gradient b/w atrium & ventricle
– Only left atrium is enlarged
– Diastolic murmur
– Increase Atrial pressure in diastole is seen in MS

- **Pressure-volume loop:**

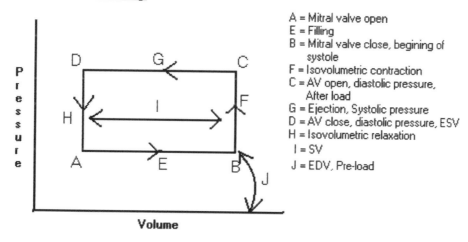

A = Mitral valve open
E = Filling
B = Mitral valve close, begining of systole
F = Isovolumetric contraction
C = AV open, diastolic pressure, After load
G = Ejection, Systolic pressure
D = AV close, diastolic pressure, ESV
H = Isovolumetric relaxation
I = SV
J = EDV, Pre-load

Think of two parameters
- Preload If ↑ → Loop shift to Rt
           If ↓ → Loop shift to Lt
- Ventricular systolic pressure (peak pressure)
• J = **Pre-load**
• G = **Systolic pressure**
• B = beginning of systole
• D = beginning of diastole
• C = diastolic pressure

[Remember & understand landmarks in figure very well, most likely to get on exam]

- It always a **pressure difference** which **causes the valves to open & close**.
  E.g. what causes MV to open? (Open in ventricular diastole)
  → MV open b/c pressure in Lt Ventricle goes below than pressure in Lt Atrium
- Opening of AV → terminates Isovolumatric contraction & begins ejection phase

- **<u>Jugulovenous pulse:</u>**

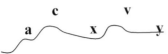

- ▪ **a wave:** Right atrium contraction
- ▪ **c wave:** Bulging of tricuspid valve (occurs in early ejection so occurs after Aortic valve open)
- ▪ **v wave:** occurs when Mitral valve open

* <u>Arterial – Venous (A-V) difference</u>**:**

$\downarrow$ Venous PO2 $\rightarrow$ $\uparrow$ A-V difference

Cell & Muscle Physiology

- **Diffusion:** transport of molecules from a region of higher concentration to one of lower concentration. It is proportional to concentration gradient across the membrane, surface area and solubility of substance in the medium. It **inversely** depends on thickness of membrane.

- **Osmosis: water diffuses from <u>High concentration To Low concentration</u>**
  - Higher water conc. means low solute conc. means low Osmolarity
  - High water conc. = Low solute conc. = Low Osm
  - Low water conc. = High solute conc. = High Osm
  - Therefore **water diffuse from <u>Low Osm to High Osm</u>**

  - Isotonic solution = 300 mOsm = 150 mM NaCl = 300 mM glucose

- **Protein (carrier) mediated transport:**
  - First transportation increases as concentration [conc.] increases but once saturation occurs it becomes steady, even though conc. increases and **show plateau.**
  - **Plateau is a characteristic of all protein-mediated transport**

- In **simple diffusion** graph **show straight line** relationship i.e. as concentration increases rate of diffusion is increased   [i.e. = that means]
  - **<u>No</u> carrier** in simple diffusion

- **Facilitated transport: <u>passive</u>** process, **carrier mediated** transport
  - Require **<u>no</u> ATP**
  - Always down a concentration gradient **like simple diffusion but require carrier.**

- **Active Transport:** require ATP
  - **Against** concentration gradient
  - **Primary active transport:** directly use ATP
  - **Secondary active transport:** indirectly depends on ATP, two main forms
  - **Counter-transport:** In counter-transport two species of ion or other solutes are pumped in opposite directions across a membrane. One of these species is allowed to flow from high to low concentration which yields the entropic energy to drive the transport of the other solute from a low concentration region to a high one. An **example** is the sodium-calcium exchanger or antiporter, which allows three sodium ions into the cell to transport one calcium out.
  - **Co-transport:** uses the downhill movement of one solute species from high to low concentration to move another molecule uphill from low concentration to high

concentration (against its electrochemical gradient). An **example** is the glucose symporter, which co-transports one glucose molecule into the cell for every two sodium ions it imports into the cell.

- **Endocytosis** is the proccess by which cells ingest materials. The cellular membrane folds around the desired materials outside the cell. The ingested particle is trapped within a pouch, vacuole or inside the cytoplasm. Often enzymes from lysosomes are then used to digest the molecules absorbed by this process.
- Endocyctosis can be split up into two main types: pinocytosis and phagocytosis.
- In **pinocytosis**, cells engulf liquid particles
- In **phagocytosis**, cells engulf solid particles.
- **Exocytosis** is the process by which cells excrete waste and other large molecules from the protoplasm

- Body Compartments:

Total body water (60% of body weight) → 2/3 ICF / 1/3 ECF → 2/3 interstitial / 1/3 vascular

- Concentration of NA^+ determines the effective Osm b/w ICF & ECF
- Conc. of plasma protein determines the effective Osm b/w interstitial & vascular fluid
- If you give fluid by any route i.e. infusion <u>or</u> orally, ECF volume enlarge
- If you loose fluid by any route, ECF volume decrease

Therefore in **any question, first determine Osm of ECF** [i.e. increase <u>or</u> decrease] then think of water movement accordingly [remember water always move from Low Osm to High Osm]

- Movement of sodium b/w blood & interstitial fluid is via diffusion through channel b/w endothelial cells.

- Vol^m measurement: V x C = A
  V - Volume of the compartment
  C - Conc. of tracer in that compartment
  A - Amount of tracer

- Blood vol^m **vs** Plasma vol^m:
  Blood vol^m = $\dfrac{\text{Plasma vol}^m}{1 - \text{HCT}}$ [HCT = hematocrit]

- **CHANGES IN RBC VOLUME:**
  - In **isotonic saline** (300 m0sm = 150 mM NaCl) – <u>**No**</u> change in volume.
  - In **hypotonic saline** – RBC swells
  - In **hypertonic saline** – RBC shrinks

- The presence of a substance such as **UREA** that penetrates the cell membrane quickly does **not** affect osmotic movement of water.
- Osmotic movement of water **depends on presence of any salt** like NaCl which affect osmolarity.
- There is **no** osmotic effect **at equilibrium**.
- When there are NaCl <u>or</u> any salt + slowly penetrating substance (like glycerol) present in solution then consider both of its Osm as total Osm so **initially** there is **increase** in Osm of solution but as slowly penetrating substance penetrate membrane slowly & reach at equilibrium there is decrease in Osm.
- **Sweating** → **loss of hypotonic fluid** → **Increase** ECF Osm
- **Drinking tape water** (very few solute) (same as infusing hypotonic fluid) → **dilute ECF** → **decrease** ECF Osm
- **Infusing isotonic Saline** → <u>**no**</u> change in ECF 0sm but **increase** ECF volume therefore <u>**no**</u> osmotic movement b/w ECF & ICF therefore **ICF volume <u>not</u> change**

- **Concentration force:** determined by conc. difference across the membrane
    - Nernst equation convent conc. force into mV.(Ex)
    - If there are 10 fold conc. differences across the membrane, then the conc. force has a magnitude of <u>60 MV</u>.
- **Electrical force:** electrical difference across the membrane.
    - In vivo magnitude is determine by membrane potential.(Em)
    - The direction of force is based on facts that LIKE CHARGES REPEL AND OPPOSITE CHARGERS ATTRACT.
    e.g. If Em -70mv; then force of 70mv that attract all positive ions and repel all negative ions

- If Em & Ex both are in same direction then net force is Em + Ex.
- If Em & Ex are in opposite direction then net force is difference b/w Em & Ex & directed along the Axis of the larger force
- If Em & Ex both are equal & opposite direction then net force is zero & ion is in the state of equilibrium. So An **equilibrium = Em=Ex**

- All cells have ungated K^+ channels

- **■ Action Potential:** a self-regenerating wave of electrochemical activity that allows nerve cells to carry a signal over a distance.
- A typical action potential is initiated at the axon hillock when the membrane is depolarized sufficiently (i.e. when its voltage is increased sufficiently). As the membrane potential is increased, both the sodium and potassium ion channels begin to open up. This increases both the inward sodium current and the balancing outward potassium current. For small voltage increases, the potassium current triumphs over the sodium current and

the voltage returns to its normal **resting** value, typically **−70 mV**. However, if the voltage increases **past a critical threshold**, typically 15 mV higher than the resting value, the sodium current dominates. This results in a runaway condition whereby the positive feedback from the sodium current activates even more sodium channels. Thus, the cell "fires", producing an action potential

- Action potentials that do reach the ends of the axon generally cause the **release of a neurotransmitter (ACh)** into the synaptic cleft. This may combine with other inputs to provoke a new action potential in the post-synaptic neuron or muscle cell.

- The principal ions involved in an action potential are sodium and potassium cations; sodium ions enter the cell, and potassium ions leave, restoring equilibrium

- **Hyperpolarization:** Sometimes more potassium channels open than usual which leads to membrane potential reach close to the potassium equilibrium voltage. This is called a hyperpolarization which persists until the membrane potassium permeability returns to its usual value

- **Refractory period:** The opening and closing of the sodium and potassium channels during an action potential may leave some of them in a "refractory" state, in which they are unable to open again until they have recovered

- **Absolute refractory period:** so many ion channels are refractory that no new action potential can be fired. Significant recovery requires that the membrane potential remain hyperpolarized for a certain length of time

- **Relative refractory period:** enough channels have recovered that an action potential can be provoked, but **only with a stimulus much stronger than usual**

- Refractory period ensure that the action potential travels in only one direction along the axon

- A cell's resting membrane Potential is very sensitive to changes in the **Extracellular potassium (K^+) ion conc. <u>not</u>** to Na^+ conc.
  Hypokalamia → ↑ efflux of k+ → Hyperpolarize the cell
  Hyperkalemia → ↓ efflux of k+ → Depolarization of the cell

- Preventing the opening of voltage gated Na^+ channel in response to depolarization will prevent the depolarization of AP.

- Preventing the opening of **voltage** gated K+ channel slows repolarization as **k^+ efflux continue <u>via ungated K^+ channel</u>**

- **Conduction Velocity of AP:**
1. <u>Cell diameter</u>: increase diameter – increase conduction velocity
2. <u>Myelin</u>: increase myelin – increase conduction velocity
3. Large myelinated fibers = fast conduction
4. Small unmyelinated fibers = slow conduction

- **Synaptic Transmission:** As mentioned above, AP travels down the axon and release ACh in the pre-synaptic cleft which open sodium – potassium channels in the post-synaptic neurons or muscle cells. Their opening causes the initiation of **AP** that **spread across the surface of the skeletal muscles.**

- **ACh:** enzymatic degradation by AChE (acetylcholine esterase) is the major factor in terminating Ach action
- **NE → E** by PNMT [Phenylethanolamine N-methyltransferase]
- **Reuptake** of NE is a major factor in terminating NE action
- Some of NE is converted to Deaminated derivatives by MAO

* **Skeletal Muscles Contraction:**
- **A band** – **No** change during contraction
- **H band** – shortens
- **I band** – shortens
- **A band** contains most of **myosin filaments** and some actin filaments [**H band is inside A band**]
- **Actin** – Troponin (binding site for Ca^{+2}) & Tropomysin (covers the attachment site of the cross-bridge in **resting muscle**)
- Overlap of actin & myosin is required for maximum achievable force during contraction but if both actin filaments are overlap in resting stage then it decrease maximum achievable force during contraction. If muscles are overstretched in resting stage then also very few actin-myosin coupling occur & decrease force during contraction.
- Pre-load align actin-myosin overlap in resting condition.
- As already mentioned above, AP spread across the surface of the skeletal muscles, it then travels through T-tubular membranes (an extension of the surface membrane) and activate dihydropyridine receptors in T-tubular membrane which pull the junctional foot process away from the calcium releasing channels in sarcoplasmic reticulum and release calcium into intracellular environment
- **As long as calcium is attached to Troponin, cross-bridge cycles continue. Contraction is terminated as calcium is sequestered by the sarcoplasmic reticulum. [Contraction is the** continuous cycling of cross-bridges. Intracellular release of calcium attach to Troponin which leads to bonds formation between actin & myosin. However bonds are **NOT** maintained; rather there is continuous cycling of those cross-bridges.]
- ATP is used to power the mechanical aspect of contraction in the form of active tension and/or active shortening of muscles

- ■ **Red Muscles (Type-I, Slow Oxidative, Slow twitch):** utilize for long term
- Small muscle mass (less powerful)
- Low ATPase activity

- maintain aerobic glycolysis (**mitochondria**)
- Has **myoglobin** (red color) [myoglobin store O2 and speed up delivery of O2 to mitochondria]

- ■ **White Muscles (Type-II, fast twitch):** utilized for short term
- Large mass per motor unit (more powerful)
- High ATPase activity
- High capacity of anaerobic glycolysis
- **No** myoglobin
- Ex: ocular muscles of eye (not large but fast)

Skeletal	Cardiac	Smooth
No gap junction so AP doesn't move from cell to cell so **each fibers are innervated**	Gap junction present so AP can move from cell to cell electrical syncytium	Gap junction present so AP can move from cell to cell electrical syncytium
Troponin, to bind Calcium	Troponin, to bind Calcium	**Calmodulin**, to bind Calcium
High ATPase activity	Intermediate ATPase activity	Low ATPase activity

Physiology - Endocrinology

- **Important Concepts:** hormone synthesis, positive and negative feedback system to regulate hormones level, Other factors that regulate hormones, M/A of hormones, Effect of hormones in our body, Primary, Secondary and Tertiary Hyper- and Hypo- status of the gland

- **Hypothalamus:** Secrete releasing hormones that stimulate pituitary gland to secrete stimulating hormones; GnRH [LHRH, FSHRH], TRH, CRH, GHRH, PIH, Somatostatin [GHIH]

- **Pituitary Gland:** Secrete all stimulating hormones that stimulate secretion of hormones from different glands; LH, FSH, TSH, ACTH, GH, Prolactin [Anterior], Oxytocin & ADH [Posterior]

- **Positive and Negative Feedbacks:** When level of **free** hormone is decrease in blood stream, hypothalamus stimulates pituitary gland to secrete stimulating hormones to increase **free** level of decreased hormone. This is called positive feedback. When **free** level of hormone is increased in blood stream, the hormone itself inhibits release of releasing hormone from hypothalamus or inhibits release of stimulating hormones from pituitary gland. This is called negative feedback. Most of the hormones in our body remain attached to the plasma protein or remain stored in the gland and release into blood stream when need arise.

- Hormones which are **not** regulated by pituitary: Aldosterone, Epinephrine, Insulin, Glucagon

- <u>Concepts:</u> It is a **free** hormone level which plays important role in positive and negative feedback. Example: Estrogen can <u>increase the circulating level of binding proteins</u>. Therefore transient decrease in level of free hormones occur which stimulate positive feedback loop leads to increase in free hormone level back to normal. **Therefore in pregnancy, <u>total</u> plasma hormone <u>increase</u> but <u>free</u> plasma hormone remains constant.** Same thing happen when person is on OCP.

- <u>Concept:</u> Damage to pituitary stalk (connection b/w hypothalamus and pituitary) leads to decrease in all Ant. Pituitary hormones <u>except</u> Prolactin which level is increased because decrease level of PIF (Prolactin inhibiting factor).

- **Mechanism of action of hormones:** (see pharmacology notes for details)
- <u>Lipid-soluble hormones:</u> (steroids, thyroid hormones)
  $t_{1/2}$ is proportional to affinity of hormone to plasma protein carrier. Receptors are **inside the cell**, stimulates the synthesis of specific proteins to exert their action. [$t_{1/2}$ – **long** (hrs, day)]
- <u>Water-soluble hormones:</u> (peptides, proteins)
  Receptors are on **outer surface of the cell membrane**; production of second messenger which modify action of intracellular proteins. [$t_{1/2}$ – **short** (minutes)]
- All hormones in the hypothalamic-anterior pituitary system are **water** soluble.

- Chronic high circulating levels of a hormone can cause the number of receptors on a hormone target cells to decrease.
- Permissive action: one type of hormone **must** be present before another hormone can act.
- In the hypothalamic pituitary system, hormonal release is pulsatile **except** thyroid system.

Metabolism	Insulin	Glucagon	Epinephrine	Cortisol	GH
Glycogen synthesis	**Increase** by stimulating glucokinase & glycogen synthase	**Decrease** by inhibiting glucokinase & glycogen synthase	Decrease	Decrease	Decrease
Glycogen degradation in liver for **gluconeogenesis**	**Decrease** by inhibiting Phosphorylase & glucose-6-Phosphatase	**Increase** by stimulating Phosphorylase & glucose-6-Phosphatase	**Increase** by stimulating Phosphorylase & glucose-6-Phosphatase	Increase gluconeogenesis by providing more substrate in form of **AA, free FA & Glycerol**	Increase gluconeogenesis by providing more substrate in **free FA & Glycerol**
Fat synthesis by adipose tissue	**Increase** by stimulating lipoprotein lipase (endothelium of capillary)	**Decrease** by inhibiting lipoprotein lipase	Decrease	Decrease	Decrease
Fat degradation for **gluconeogenesis**	**Decrease** by inhibiting hormone sensitive lipase	**Increase** by stimulating hormone sensitive lipase [It **does not** increase lipolysis in adipose tissues]	**Increase** lipolysis in adipose tissue leads to increase delivery of free FA & Glycerol to liver	**Increase** lipolysis in adipose tissue leads to increase delivery of free FA & Glycerol to liver	**Increase** lipolysis in adipose tissue leads to increase delivery of free FA & Glycerol to liver
Protein synthesis	**Increase** by increasing AA uptake by muscles	Decrease	Decrease	Decrease	**Increase** [anabolic hormone]
Protein degradation for **gluconeogenesis**	Decrease	Increase	Increase	**Increase delivery of AA to liver**	

S.S.Patel , M.D.

Hormone secretion	Stimulated by	Inhibited by	Other comments
Epinephrine (80% of Adrenal Medulla)	Exercise, Emergency, Exposure to cold		
Norepinephrine (20% of Adrenal Medulla)	When one goes from a lying to a standing position		Most circulating norepinephrine arises from post-ganglionic sympathetic neurons
Cortisol	ACTH	Negative feedback	Peak Cortisol secretion occurs in the **early morning**
Adrenal Androgens	ACTH	Negative feedback	
Insulin	Glucose (increase ATP in B-cells), GIP (gastric inhibitory peptide), CCK, Secretin, Gastrin, Glucagon, AA (Arginine)	Somatostatin, alpha-2 agonist	
Glucagon	Hypoglycemia, AA (Arginine)	Somatostatin, Insulin	
Aldosterone	Angiotensin-II, Elevated plasma K^+	Weightlessness	See Renin-Angiotensin system below
ADH (Vasopressin)	Increase serum Osm	Weightlessness	
ANP (Atrial Natriuretic Peptide)	In response to Rt atrium stretching, increase salt intake, Weightlessness		
Thyroid hormone	TSH	Negative feedback (regulated by **free T$_4$**)	
GH	Deep sleep, Exercise, AA (Arginine), Hypoglycemia	Somatostatin, IGF-1 [Somatomedin-C], Elevated Glucose	Secreted in pulses & mainly **at night; Requires the presence of normal plasma levels of thyroid hormones**
PTH	Hypocalcemia	Negative feedback (regulated by **free Ca^{+2}**)	
LH	LHRH	Testosterone (male), Increase estrogen in follicular phase, Increase progesterone in luteal phase (female) Suckling of	

		the baby (inhibits GnRH)	
FSH		Inhibin (male), Increase estrogen in follicular phase, Increase progesterone in luteal phase (female) Suckling of the baby (inhibits GnRH)	
Oxytocin	Suckling of the baby		
Prolactin	Suckling of the baby	PIH from hypothalamus	

- **Adrenal Hormones:**
- Zona Glomerulosa : Aldosterone; Controlled by Angiotensin-II, K^+
- Zona Fesciculata : Cortisol; controlled by ACTH
- Zona Reticularis : Androgen; controlled by ACTH
- Medulla : Epinephrine; controlled by ANS

- If **problems** develop **with Ant. pituitary secretion**, glucocorticoids secretion may be affected but **mineralocorticoid** system **remains intact** which are controlled by Angiotensin-II, K^+.

- **Urinary 17-OH steroids** are usually an index of **cortisol secretion**.
- **Urinary 17-ketosteriods** are an index of all androgens, **adrenal & testicular**.

- **Desmolase** is a **rate limiting enzymes in all steroid hormone synthesis** which convert cholesterol into Pregnenolone.

- Congenital defects in any of the enzymes leads to deficient cortisol secretion and congenital adrenal hyperplasia
- Enzymes → 17 alpha-OH, 21 beta-OH, 11 beta-OH

   17 alpha-OH deficiency:
   Decrease cortisol, decrease androgen
   Increase 11 deoxycorticosterone (weak mineralocorticoid) [responsible for HTN]

   21 beta-OH deficiency:
   Decrease cortisol, Decrease mineralocorticoid
   Increase adrenal androgens [responsible for ambiguous genitalia]

<u>11 beta-OH deficiency:</u>
Decrease cortisol
Increase 11 deoxycorticosterone
Increase adrenal androgens.

- **Other important Actions of Cortisol:**
- It increases blood pressure by increasing the sensitivity of the vasculature to epinephrine and norepinephrine. **In the absence of cortisol, widespread vasodilatation occurs**
- Stimulates gastric acid secretion thus promote **gastric ulcer** formation
- It lowers bone formation thus favoring development of **osteoporosis** in the long term
- Glucagon – increase liver glycogenolysis, but **without cortisol, fasting hypoglycemia rapidly develops**
- **Anti-inflammatory effects** by reducing histamine secretion and stabilizing lysosomal membranes. The stabilization of lysosomal membranes prevents their rupture, thereby preventing damage to healthy tissues
- It causes **hyperkalemia**
- **Actions of Aldosterone:**
  - Increase Na^+ absorption by increasing number of Na^+ channel in luminal membrane
  - Promote activity of Na^+/K^+ ATPase pump
  - Increase excretion of K^+ & H^+
  - For one H^+ secreted, one HCO_3 moves into the ECF
- **Renin-Angiotensin System:**
  - Decrease BP in afferent arteriole – JG cells present in afferent arteriole
  - Decrease Na^+ delivery to macula densa cells – tall columnar cells lined DT near afferent arteriole.
  - * Increase B_1-noradrenergic input to JG cells
  - * Above three factors lead to release of Renin from JG cells which convert Angiotensinogen into Angiotensin-1 which is converted into **Angiotensin-II** by ACE (Angiotensin converting enzyme) **in the lung**.
  - * **Angiotensin-II** [Vasoconstriction & Increase aldosterone secretion]
  - Alveolar capillary contains **ACE**, <u>not</u> Pneumocytes.

- Elevated plasma K^+ (Hyperkalemia) directly stimulate zona glomerulosa to secrete Aldosterone

- **Weightlessness** (<u>Example</u>: standing on the ground, sitting in a chair on the ground, flying in a plane, during an orbital maneuver in a spacecraft etc): b/c blood no longer pools in the extremities, a large portion of the redistributed blood ends up in the atria & large veins the chest & abdomen which stimulate baroreceptors → decrease aldosterone & decrease ADH → lose Na^+ & ECF vol^m.

- 1^0 Hyperaldosteronism (**Conn's syndrome**) – HTN + Hypokalamia
- 1^0 Adrenal insufficiency (**Addison's disease**) – increase ACTH, hyperpigmentation

- **ADH (vasopressin):**
  Maintain osmolarity [Increase Osm → increase secretion of ADH from Post pituitary]
  MA: increase permeability of renal collecting duct for water by placing water channels in the membrane.

- **Atrial Natriuretic Peptide (ANP):**
  - Increase GFR by dilation of afferent arterioles & constriction of efferent arterioles
  - Increase Na+ loss & water loss by inhibition of reabsorption of sodium & water in CD (collecting duct)
  - **Increase secretion in weightlessness**

- **The endocrine Pancreas:**
  - **α cells** : (20% of islet cells) at the periphery, secrete <u>Glucagon</u>
  - **β-cells** : (60-75 % of islet cells) near the center, secrete <u>Insulin + C peptide</u>
  - **Delta cells** : (5% of is let cells) b/w α & B cells, secrete <u>Somatostatin</u>

- Tissues that **require insulin for** effective **glucose uptake** are: adipose tissues, **resting** skeletal muscles. Glucose uptake occur by insertion of glucose transporters in the membrane of above tissues [see biochemistry notes]
- Tissues in which glucose uptake is **not** affected by insulin are: nervous tissue, RBCs, kidney tubules, intestinal mucosa, and beta-cells of pancreas.

- **Insulin decreases formation of ketone bodies by liver.**
- Insulin **pumps K^+ into cells**. Therefore it is used to treat life threatening hyperkalemia (e.g hyperkalemia of renal failure) Simultaneous administration of glucose is required to prevent severe hypoglycemia.

- **Actions of Glucagon:** Mediated by increase cAMP
  1^0 Target tissue → liver hepatocytes
  Skeletal muscles are **not** target tissue for Glucagon

- All hormones which increase degradation of AA increases ureagenesis.

- **Growth hormone:**

  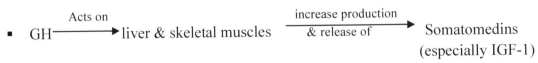
  - GH —Acts on→ liver & skeletal muscles —increase production & release of→ Somatomedins (especially IGF-1)

  - IGF-1 is also called Somatomedin-C

- **IGF-1:** $t_{1/2}$ - very long (20 hrs)
  - Plasma IGF-1 serves as a reflection of 24 hrs GH secretion.
  - GH secreted in pulses & mainly **at night**
  - Increase synthesis of cartilage (chondrogenesis) in the epiphyseal plates of long bones. Increase bone length
  - At puberty, increase in GH secretion is facilitated by the pubertal increase in androgen secretion
  - **Secretion of GH requires the presence of normal plasma levels of thyroid hormones.**

- GH deficiency: Pre-puberty → dwarfism
- Hypersecretion of GH: Pre-puberty → gigantism
  - Post-puberty → Acromegaly

- **Adrenal medulla:**
  - 80% epinephrine & 20% Norepinephrine
  - Plasma **norepinephrine** ($t_{1/2}$ -2 mins only) **levels doubles when one goes from a lying to a standing position.**
  - Secretion of epinephrine by adrenal medulla increase by : exercise, emergency, exposure to cold
- **Actions of epinephrine:**
  Increase metabolic rate (**need presence of thyroid & adrenal cortex hormones**)
  Increase glycogenolysis **in both liver & skeletal muscle** [Glucagon – only liver]
  Increase lactate out put by skeletal muscle
  Lactate → glucose (Cori's cycle in liver)

- Calcium**:**
  - 99% of total calcium – bone (hydroxyapatites)
  - 0.1 % of calcium – interstitial fluid (mostly ca^{+2})
  - 0.5 % of – plasma (50% Ca^{+2} & 50% protein bound)
  - 1 % of – ICF (ca^{+2} & protein bound calcium)
  - Whether calcium & phosphate are laid down in bone <u>or</u> are resorbed from bone depends on the product of their concentration.
  - Increase interstitial fluid conc. of either Ca^{+2} or Phosphate increase bone mineralization
  - Decrease interstitial fluid conc. of either Ca^{+2} or Phosphate promotes bone resorption.
  - **Free Ca^{+2} precisely regulated, <u>not</u> phosphate**

- **Action of PTH:** stimulates Osteoclast & 1-α-hydroxylase [increase production of active form of Vit-D (1-25-(OH)$_2$-D)] – increase Ca^{+2} level by bone resorption (osteoclast) & by absorption of Ca^{+2} from gut and kidney (Vit-D).
- **Action of Vit-D:** increase absorption of **both** Ca^{+2} & Phosphorus (PO4) **from intestine** and increase absorption of Ca^{+2} and **decrease** absorption of **PO4 from kidney**
- Bone resorption leads to increase conc. of **both** phosphate & Ca^{+2}

- **Calcitonin:** [parafollicular cells (c cell) of thyroid gland] decrease plasma ca^{+2} by decrease activity of osteoclast
- **Osteoblast:** deposit bone matrix (collagen), located on surface of bone
- **Osteocyte:** osteoblast when surrounded by mineralize bone, it differentiate into osteocyte.
- **Osteoclast:** resorbed bone, arise from monocytes migrating to bone. Several monocytes fused to form the multinucleated osteoclast.
- **Paget's disease of bone:** increase alkaline Phosphatase, myelophthisic anemia
- **Osteomalacia (rickets in children): increase in osteoid** but **poor mineralization** due to dietary deficiency of Ca^{+2}, Vit-D or sunlight (**also increase osteoblast**)
- **Osteoporosis:** sparse trabaculae
- **Osteoarthritis:** "wear & tear" – enzymatic degradation of type-2 collagen in cartilage

    - Increase alkaline Phosphatase → osteoblastic activity.
    - Increase urinary excretion of hydroxyproline → breakdown product of collagen

* Abnormally high Vit-D promotes bone resorption.
* Receptors for both PTH & Vit-D are on osteoblast. Osteoblast has communication with osteoclast which carries out bone resorption.

* **Thyroid hormones:**
    - Thyroid epithelial cells [follicle cells] [form follicle] synthesize & secrete T4 & T3
    - Thyroid epithelial cells form **thyroglobulin (Tg)** (protein) [Tg was referred to as colloid]
    - Iodine is **stored** as an **iodination of tyrosine residue of thyroglobulin** in follicle lumen.
    - Iodide (I$^-$) **actively** transport in follicle cell.
    - **Thyroperoxidase** is an important enzyme which carry out iodination of tyrosine & coupling of MIT & DIT to form T4 & T3
    - When iodine is abundant → mainly T4 is formed
    - When iodine is scare → mainly T3 is formed
    - T4 - 3,5,3',5'

T3 - 3,5,3' (5'deiodinase) in peripheral tissue; **reverse T3** - 3,5,5'(**inactive**)
- **T4 converts into T3 to exert its effect** in our body [T3 is an active form of thyroid hormone] but **only Free T4 regulates TSH [Free T4 converts into T3 in hypothalamus which inhibits TRH and thus TSH]**
- T4 and T3 are carried into blood by thyroid-binding globulin, transthyretin and albumin. TBG has higher affinity to thyroid hormones but its concentration is lower than other two
- Microsomal Deiodenase removes iodine from **free** DIT & MIT (released by proteolysis of thyroglobulin during secretion of T4 & T3) but **not** from T4 & T3

- **Actions of thyroid hormone:**
  - Permissive <u>or</u> act synergistically with growth hormone (A stippled epiphysis is a sign of hypothyroidism in children)
  - Increase **metabolic rate** by increase Na^+/K^+ - ATPase activity in most tissue.
  - Require for **maturing of nervous tissue.** [Mental retardation if low level in infancy]
  - Require for conversion of carotene – Vit-A (**night blindness & yellow skin in hypothyroid**)
  - Accelerates cholesterol clearance from plasma
  - **Increase number & affinity of beta-adrenergic receptors in heart (causes arrhythmia when in access)**
  - Goiter is an enlarged thyroid gland & **can occur** in hypo-, hyper- & euthyroid.

- **Male reproductive system:**
  LH, FSH, TSH & hCG – all glycoproteins, Alpha subunit is same in all four, only Beta subunit is different in all four
  - **LH** → leyding cells → testosterone
    It acts through cAMP / protein kinase
  - **Testosterone** provides negative feedback to **regulate LH**
  - Androgen binding protein (**ABP**) synthesized by Sertoli cells & secreted into the lumen of the seminiferous tubules, **helps maintain a high local concentration.**
  - FSH + testosterone → increase synthesis of ABP
  - **Testosterone receptors are located on the nuclear chromatin of the Sertoli cell.**
  - **FSH receptors are located on plasma membrane of Sertoli cells**; FSH acts through cAMP / protein kinase
  - **Both** FSH & leyding cell testosterone are **required for normal spermatogenesis.**
  - **Inhibin** provides negative feedback to **regulate FSH**
  - GnRH secreted in **pulsatile** fashion.
  - Methyl testosterone – synthetic androgen – used by athletes.
  - At puberty, if T4 is normal, increase androgen → increase GH → increase IGF-I

- - Near the end of puberty, androgens promote the mineralization (closure) of the epiphysis of long bones. After closure lengthening can **no** longer occur.
  - Androgens stimulate protein synthesis – increase muscle mass

- PANS does <u>not</u> innervate arterioles in systemic tissue (**penis is an exception**)
- **Erection** is caused by dilation of the blood vessels in the erectile tissue of the penis via **parasympathetic response**.
- **Emission** is mediated by **sympathetic transmitters**
- **Ejaculation** → contraction of bulbospongious and ischiocavernosus → (somatic innervation)
  Therefore complete ejaculation requires intact SANS and somatic innervation.

- **<u>The menstrual cycle</u>:**
  Follicular phase → increase estrogen
  Ovulation → LH surge
  Luteal Phase → increase progesterone with estrogen
  Menses → withdrawal of hormones

- **<u>Follicular phase (proliferative phase)</u>:**
  - FSH secretion is slightly elevated which causes proliferation of granulosa cells – increase estrogen (E).
  - E acts locally to increase granulosa cells' sensitivity to FSH, the follicle with best blood supply, secrete more estradiol than others & become dominant follicle.
  - LH (stimulates) → Theca cells → increase androgen (goes to) → granulosa cells → aromatase convert androgen → estrogen.
  - Increase E – stimulate female sex accessory organ & secondary sex characteristics
    Endometrial cell proliferation
    Thinning of cervical mucus
    Inhibits FSH & LH

- **Ovulation:** when **E rises above certain level**, it <u>no</u> longer inhibits FSH & LH. Instead, it stimulates FSH & LH [(-) feedback to (+) feedback loop]
  - Only LH surge is essential for induction of ovulation & formation of corpus lutem therefore if estrogen (E) is still rising, ovulation has <u>not</u> occurred.
  - Follicular rupture occur 24-36 hrs after LH surge
  - LH remove restraint upon meiosis and **first meiotic division is completed** & 1st polar body extruded

- **Luteal phase:** LH surge causes granulosa cells & theca cells to be transformed into Luteal cells.
  - E + FSH → granulosa cells produce LH receptors
  - Luteal cells form progesterone & some E

- Progesterone → Inhibits LH release
  Endometrium become Secretory
  Mucus → thick
  Increase basal temp. (0.5^0 - 1^0 F)

- **Menses:** progesterone inhibits LH which is required for corpus lutem. Decrease LH → demise of the corpus lutem
  - Decrease progesterone due to decrease LH & decrease sensitivity of luteal cells to LH 1 week after ovulation
  - Lower level of progesterone **no** longer support the Endometrium, necrosis of tissue occurs, spiral arterioles break & menses ensues.

- **Decrease P metabolites & rapidly increase E metabolites → follicular phase**
- **Increase P metabolites → luteal phase /pregnancy**

- Length of Luteal phase (last 14 days) doesn't vary

- **Placental hormones:**
  Human chorionic somatomammotropin (hCS) also called human placental lactogen (hPL)
  - hPL → growth stimulating activity, **Anti-insulin activity**
  - hCG requires to maintain pregnancy from implantation to 3rd month.
  - Placenta secrete enough progesterone & estrogen which maintain pregnancy from 3rd month to term
  - Plasma oxytocin is **not** elevated until the baby enters the birth canal
  - Oxytocin → stimulate uterine synthesis of PGs
  - Progesterone & E → stimulate growth of mammary tissue.
  - E → stimulate Prolactin secretion
  - E → inhibits milk synthesis

- At parturition, plasma E drops, withdrawing block on milk synthesis, as a result the number of Prolactin receptors in mammary tissue increase several fold and milk synthesis begins.
- Oxytocin contract myoepithelial cells → milk ejection.
- Suckling of the baby → stimulate oxytocin & Prolactin release (sucking inhibits PIF in hypothalamus)
- Suckling of the baby → inhibits GnRH (FSH & LH) therefore inhibits ovulation & menstruation cease.
- **Aromatase:** convert Testosterone to Estrogen
  Male – Sertoli cells, Adipose tissue
  Female – Granulosa cells, Adipose tissue
- Estradiol (Ovarian follicle) > Estrone (Peripheral tissues) > Estriol (Placenta)

GI Physiology

- **Digestion of food:**

- Phases of gastric secretion:
- **Cephalic phase** – occurs before food enters the stomach – taste and smell send signals to the cerebral cortex which send signal through vagus nerve and release acetylcholine. ACh stimulate gastric secretion. Acidity in the stomach is **not** buffered by food **at this point** and thus acts to inhibit parietal (secretes acid) and G cell (secretes gastrin).
- **Gastric phase** – This phase takes 3 to 4 hours. It is **stimulated by distention of the stomach, presence of food in stomach and increase in pH**. Distention activates long and myentric reflexes which release ACh which release more acid into the stomach. As protein enters the stomach, it binds to hydrogen ion, which raises the pH of the stomach around 6. This leads to increase release of gastrin which in turn releases more HCl.
- **Intestinal phase** – This phase has 2 parts, the excitatory and the inhibitory. When partially-digested food enters the duodenum, it triggers intestinal gastrin to be released. Enterogastric reflex inhibits vagal nuclei, activating sympathetic fibers causing pyloric sphincter to tighten to prevent more food from entering and inhibits local reflexes.
- **Oral Cavity:** Digestion begins in the oral cavity. Saliva is secreted in large amounts (1-1.5 liters/day) by three pairs of exocrine salivary glands (parotid, submandibular, and sublingual) in the oral cavity, and is mixed with the chewed food by the tongue. There are two types of saliva. One is a thin, watery secretion, and its purpose is to wet the food. The other is a thick, mucous secretion, and it acts as a lubricant and causes food particles to stick together and form a bolus. It contains digestive enzymes such as **salivary amylase** [break polysaccharides such as starch into disachharides such as maltose] It also contains **mucin**, a glycoprotein which helps soften the food into a bolus.
- **Swallowing** transports the chewed food into the esophagus, passing through the oropharynx and hypopharynx. The mechanism for swallowing is coordinated by the swallowing center in the medulla and pons. The reflex is initiated in the pharynx as the bolus of food is pushed to the back of the mouth.
- **Esophagus:** The wall of the esophagus is made up of two layers of smooth muscles, which contract slowly, over long periods of time. The inner layer of muscles is arranged circularly, while the outer layer is arranged longitudinally. The epiglottis, a flap of tissue at the top of the esophagus, which closes during swallowing to prevent food from entering the trachea. The chewed food is pushed down the esophagus to the stomach through peristaltic contraction of these muscles. It takes only about seven seconds for food to pass through the esophagus and no digestion takes place in the esophagus.
- **Stomach:** Food enters the stomach through the cardiac orifice where it is further broken apart and thoroughly mixed with gastric acid, pepsin and other digestive enzymes to break down proteins. The acid itself doesn't break down food molecules; rather it provides an optimum pH for the reaction of the enzyme pepsin and kills many microorganisms that are ingested with the food. The parietal cells of the stomach also secrete **intrinsic factor (IF)** which is required for an absorption of Vit-B12. Food in the stomach is in semi-liquid form, which upon completion is known as chyme. It secretes **mucous** which protect stomach mucosa from acid exposure. Pepsinogen is also secreted from the stomach and it **requires H^+ to convert into pepsin** (active form)

S.S.Patel , M.D.

- **Small intestine:** After being processed in the stomach, food is passed to the small intestine via the pyloric sphincter. The majority of digestion and absorption occurs here after the milky chyme enters the duodenum. Here it is further mixed with three different liquids:

- **Bile**, which emulsifies fat to allow absorption, neutralizes the chyme and is used to excrete waste products such as bilin and bile acids.
- **Pancreatic juice** made by the pancrease.
- **Intestinal enzymes** of the alkaline mucosal membranes. The enzymes include maltase, lactase and sucrase (all three of which process only sugars), trypsin and chymotrypsin.
- The pH becomes more basic in small intestine which activate pancreatic and small intestinal enzymes that break down various nutrients into smaller molecules to allow absorption into the circulatory or lymphatic systems. Blood containing the absorbed nutrients is carried away from the small intestine via the hepatic portal vein and goes to the liver for filtering, removal of toxins, and nutrient processing.
- The small intestine and remainder of the digestive tract undergoes peristalsis to transport food from the stomach to the rectum and allow food to be mixed with the digestive juices and absorbed.
- Peristalsis: The circular muscles and longitudinal muscles are antagonistic muscles, with one contracting as the other relaxes. When the circular muscles contract, the lumen becomes narrower and longer and the food is squeezed and pushed forward. When the longitudinal muscles contract, the circular muscles relax and the gut dilates to become wider and shorter to allow food to enter.
- **Large intestine:** After the food has been passed through the small intestine, the food enters the large intestine. The large intestine absorbs water from the bolus and stores feces until it can be egested. Food products that cannot go through the villi, such as cellulose (dietary fiber), are mixed with other waste products from the body and become hard and concentrated feces. The feces is stored in the rectum for a certain period and then the stored feces is egested due to the contraction and relaxation through the anus. The exit of this waste material is regulated by the anal sphincter.

- **Fat digestion:** It requires lipase and bile. The lipase (activated by acid) breaks down the fat into monoglycerides and fatty acids (FA). The bile emulsifies the fatty acids so they may be easily absorbed. **Short and some medium chain FA are absorbed directly into the blood** via intestine capillaries and travel through the portal vein just as other absorbed nutrients do. However, long chain FA and some medium chain fatty acids are too large to be directly released into the intestinal capillaries. They are absorbed into the walls of the intestine villi and reassembled again into triglycerides (TGs). The triglycerides are coated with cholesterol and protein (protein coat) into a compound called a chylomicron. Within the villi, the chylomicron enters a lymphatic capillary called a lacteal, which merges into larger lymphatic vessels. It is transported via the lymphatic system and the thoracic duct. The thoracic duct empties the chylomicrons into the bloodstream via the left subclavian vein. At this point the chylomicrons can transport the triglycerides to liver.

- ❖ **Digestive hormones:**
- **Gastrin:** secreted from G cells of the stomach – stimulates the gastric glands to secrete **pepsinogen** (an inactive form of the enzyme pepsin) and **HCl** – it **stimulates stomach motility and secretion** – Secretion of gastrin is **stimulated by** distension, ACh (parasympathetic stimulation) – The secretion is **inhibited by** low pH (acidity)
- **Secretin:** secreted from the duodenum – stimulates **sodium bicarbonate** secretion from the pancrease and **bile** secretion from the liver & gallbladder – it **inhibits stomach motility and secretion** – The hormone **secreted in response to the acidic chyme**.
- **Cholecystokinin (CCK):** secreted from the duodenum – **stimulates the release of pancreatic enzymes and emptying of bile from the gall bladder** – it inhibits stomach motility and secretion – The hormone is **secreted in response to fat in chyme**.
- **Gastric inhibitory peptide (GIP):** secreted from the duodenum – it **inhibits stomach motility and secretion** – **stimulate insulin secretion** – secreted in response to AA, fat & carbohydrate

- All 4 hormones describe above stimulate insulin release therefore oral glucose will increase insulin secretion more than IV glucose
- **Gastrin & CCK** have **same chemical structure**

* **Salivary secretion:**
    - **Hypotonic** (all secretion in GIT are isotonic. This is an **exception**)
    - Low Na^+ and Cl^- b/c reabsorption of these ions
    - **High K^+ & $HCO3^-$ b/c secretion of these ions**

* **Gastric secretions:**
    - Gastric secretion contains high H^+, K^+, Cl^- but low Na^+

* **Pancreatic secretion:**

Enzymes secreted in **Active** form
    - Pancreatic amylase
    - Pancreatic lipase (needs colipase to be effective)
    - Cholesterol esterase (sterol lipase)
    - Phospholipase A2
    - High $HCO3^-$ & low Cl^-

Enzymes secreted in **inactive** form
    - **Proteases** – Trypsinogen
                    Chymotrypsinogen
                    Procarboxypeptidase
    - **Trypsinogen enterokinase converts trypsinogen into trypsin which then convert all proteases in their active form**
    - **Trypsin inhibitor** is also **secreted by pancreas** with proenzymes

- **Bile salts & micelles:**
  1^0 bile acid (by liver) – Cholic acid
  Chenodeoxycholic acid
  1^0 bile acid – lipid soluble
- Conjugate with glycine → become water soluble but still contain lipid soluble segment
- Because they are ionized at neutral P^H, conjugated bile acids exist as salts of (Na^+) cations & therefore called **bile salts**

  2^0 bile acid (by intestinal bacteria) – Deoxycholic acid (cholic acid) and Lithocholic acid (Chenodeoxycholic acid) **Lithocholic** acid is hepatotoxic → **excreted**

- **Micelle formation:** When bile salts become concentrated, they form micelles. These are water soluble spheres with a lipid soluble interior
- In the **distal ileum** & only in the distal ileum, bile salts are **actively reabsorbed**.

- **Celiac disease:** sensitive to gluten – autoimmune disease – **flattening of villi** & generalized malabsorption – normal function returns if gluten is avoided by removal of wheat or rye flour from the diet – strong association with dermatitis herpetiformis

Renal Physiology

- 7/8 of all nephrons are Cortical nephrons
- 1/8 of all nephrons are Juxtamedullary nephrons

- Juxtamedullary nephrons consist of the long loop of Henle & the terminal region of the collecting ducts.

- Individual nephrons that make up both kidneys are connected in parallel but **flow through single nephron** represents two arterioles & two capillary beds connected **in series**

- **Constrict efferent / dilate afferent** $\rightarrow \uparrow$ glomerular cap pressure $\rightarrow \uparrow$ **filtration**
- **FF = GFR / RPF** [RPF = renal plasma flow, FF = filtration fraction]

- **Filtered load = GFR x Px**   [Px = concentration in plasma]
  (amt / time) = (vol / time) x (amt / vol)
- **Excretion = Ux X V**
  (amt / time) = (vol / time) x (amt / vol)
- Reabsorption = Filtration > Excretion = Filtration – Excretion
- Secretion = Excretion > Filtration = Excretion – Filtration
- Net transport load = Filtered load – Excretion rate = (GFR x Px) – (Ux X V)

	Filtration	Reabsorption	Secretion
Plasma protein	No	—	—
Inulin, Mannitol	Yes	No	No
Glucose, Amino Acid, Urea, Na	Yes	Yes	No
PAH	Yes	No	Yes
Creatinine	Yes	No	Small amount

- Clearance$_a$ = U$_a$ x V / P$_a$
- C$_{INULIN}$ = GFR [b/c no reabsorption and secretion of inulin so it is equal to GFR]
- C$_{PAH}$ = RPF (ERPF) [EPRF – effective renal plasma flow]
- Renal blood flow = ERPF / 1-Hct
- PAH clearance is only 90% as 10% flow perfuse renal capsule and is not cleared.
- PAH – **carrier mediated secretion** – increase PAH leads to increase in secretion initially but later as saturation of carriers occur, clearance decrease and become stable [see protein mediated diffusion]

- ■ **Proximal Tubule (PT):**
  - About 2/3 (66%) of filtered Na$^+$ is reabsorbed in PT
  - About 2/3 of filtered H_2O, K$^+$ & Cl$^-$ follow Na
  - 80-90% of filtered HCO$_3^-$ is reabsorbed & **H$^+$ is secreted**
  - **Osm** at the end of PT is 300 mOsm (**isotonic**)

S.S.Patel , M.D.   62

- The most energy demanding process of nephron
- Normally all CHO, AA, proteins, peptides & ketone bodies are reabsorbed in PT via secondary active transport

■ The loop of Henle:
- Counter current multiplier
- Descending limb is permeable to water
- Ascending loop is permeable to NaCl
- Anything that ↑ flow through loop of Henle or vasa recta will ↓ the ability of the system to maintain a high medullary Osm and reduce the ability of the kidney to form a concentrated urine
- Normally, medullary interstitial fluid is **Hyperosmolar**

■ Collecting Duct (CD):
- **Without ADH**, the CD is **impermeable** to water

■ Distal tubule (DT) & CD:
- ADH – controls the final water & urea reabsorption
- **Aldosterone** – controls the final NaCl reabsorption & K^+ **secretion**
- Regulates pH by absorbing bicarbonate and secreting H^+ into the filtrate
- Arginine vasopressin receptor 2 is also expressed in the DCT

- In Acidosis, H^+ moves inside the cell to buffer & K^+ moves out from the cell therefore **Hyperkalemia occurs in Acidosis & Hypokalemia occurs in Alkalosis except** Diarrhea & carbonic anhydrase inhibitors (Acetazolamide, etc) in which Acidosis & Hypokalemia occur [**Remember Acidosis – Hyperkalemia – Hypercalcemia (↑ free Ca^{+2})**]

- pH = 7.4, Pco_2 = 40 mmHg, HCO_3^- = 22-28 mmol/L [see pathology notes]

- Anion gap – Normal (5-11 mEq/L) = [Na – (Cl + HCO_3^-)]

- **Respiratory compensation:** occurs in Metabolic disturbance
- Metabolic acidosis – hyperventilation
- Metabolic alkalosis – Hypoventilation

- **Renal compensation:** occurs in respiratory &/or metabolic disturbance
- Acidosis (acidic urine) – ↑ loss of H+ in urine, ↑ production of HCO3- & reabsorption
- Alkalosis (alkaline urine) - ↑ loss of HCO3- in urine

Respiratory Physiology

- Total ventilation $V = V_T \times f$ [V_T = tidal volume, f = RR]
- Alveolar ventilation $V_A = (V_T - V_D) \times f$ [V_D = Dead space (150 ml)]
- Dead space does <u>not</u> contain CO_2 at the end of inspiration
- Dead space does contain CO_2 at the end of expiration
- FRC is the volume of gas at the end of passive expiration. FRC is the neutral / equilibrium point for the RS (respiratory system) (2700 ml)
- RV (residual volume) (1200 ml)
- VC (vital capacity) (5500 ml) = TLC – RV
- TLC (total lung capacity) (6700 ml)
- **Positive End Expiratory Pressure (PEEP)** – by not allowing intra-alveolar pressure to return to zero at the end of expiration, the lung will be kept at a larger volume. This will decrease the tendency to develop regional atelectasis

- **Lung compliance (C)** = $\Delta V / \Delta P$ [the ability of the lungs to stretch during a change in volume relative to an applied change in pressure] – Fibrosis is associated with a *decrease* in pulmonary compliance – Emphysema/COPD are associated with an *increase* in pulmonary compliance due to the loss of alveolar and elastic tissue
- ↑ recoil → ↓ compliance → more negative intra-pleural pressure require to inflate the lung
- ↑ negative intra-pleural pressure → ↑ capillary filtration → Pulmonary edema
- Surfactant – ↑ compliance, ↓ recoil, ↓ capillary filtration
- **Pulmonary surfactant** – increases compliance by decreasing the surface tension of water – The main lipid component of surfactant, dipalmitoylphosphatidylcholine – The internal surface of the alveolus is covered with a thin coat of fluid. The water in this fluid has a high surface tension, and provides a force that could collapse the alveolus. The presence of surfactant in this fluid breaks up the surface tension of water, making it less likely that the alveolus can collapse inward

- Airway resistance (R) α 1 / radius^4 [same as vessels – see CVS]
- Increase lung volume α ↓ R
- Increase negative intra-pleural pressure α ↓ R

- Normal people can exhale only 80% of their VC in one second because during forced expiration, intra-pleural pressure become more positive and the airway are closed.

* **Obstructive Pulmonary Disease:**
  - ↑ airway resistance
  - ↓ expiratory flow rate
  - ↑ TLC
* **Restrictive Pulmonary Disease:**
  - ↑ in lung recoil
  - ↓ in all lung volume
  - FEV_1 / FVC - ↑ <u>or</u> N

- $PIo_2 = Fo_2 (Patm - PH_2O) = 0.21 (760 - 47) = 150$ mmHg
- In the Alveoli $PAo_2 = PIo_2 - (PAco_2 / R) = 150 - 40 = 110$ mmHg
- Remember these values – $PAo_2 = 100$ & $PAco_2 = 40$
- R (respiratory exchange ratio)= CO_2 produced (ml/min) / CO_2 consumed (ml/min)

- $\downarrow PAco_2 \rightarrow \uparrow PAo_2$ **by same amount** [Example: $\downarrow PAco_2 = 20$ then $\uparrow PAo_2 = 20$ so $PAco_2 = 20$ & $PAo_2 = 130$]

- Vgas = (A / T) x D x (P1 – P2) [A / T = structural features]
  A = surface area for exchange gases [$\downarrow$ in emphysema, $\uparrow$ in exercise]
  T = Thickness of membrane [$\uparrow$ in fibrosis]
  Above formula suggest that in structural problem more pressure gradient require for gas diffusion therefore **patient with structural problem responds to O_2 supplement**
- Arterial content of O_2 increase, if Hb increase, <u>not</u> if PO_2 increase
- Hemoglobin (Hb) – **four sites**
- Site 4 – Systemic Artery blood (97% of saturation)
- Site 3 – Systemic venous blood (75% of saturation)
- Site 3 – P_{50} for arterial blood [P_{50} is the PO_2 required for 50% of saturation which is 26 mmHg [PO_2 = partial pressure of oxygen

- **<u>Oxygen Dissociation Curve:</u>**

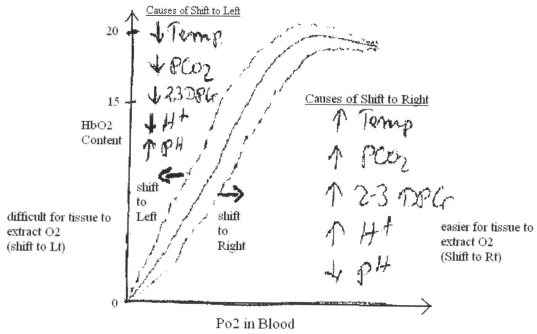

- Stored blood loses 2-3 DPG, causing a shift to left
- Fetal Hb is also shift curve to the left
- **Shifting of curve is due to change in the affinity** of Hb molecule for O2. Oxygen carrying capacity is <u>not</u> changed therefore in Anemia & Polycythemia, there is no shifting of curve as affinity doesn't change. Shifting may occur if hypoxemia occur & 2-3 DPG is produced

* **CO$_2$ Transport:**
  - 5% dissolved
  - 5% carbamino compound
  - 90% plasma bicarbonate
  - Plasma contain no carbonic anhydrase (CA) therefore conversion of $CO_2 \rightarrow HCO_3^-$ occurs in RBC
  - HCO_3^- moves out RBC in **systemic capillaries** and therefore Cl^- moves in RBC in systemic capillaries whereas HCO_3^- moves in RBC in **pulmonary capillaries** and therefore Cl^- moves out RBC in pulmonary capillaries

* **Central Chemoreceptors:**
  - On the surface of Medulla
  - The main **drive for ventilation is CO$_2$ on the central chemoreceptors**
  - $\uparrow CO_2 \rightarrow \uparrow$ Ventilation
  - $\uparrow H^+$ in CSF $\rightarrow \uparrow$ Ventilation but it takes time to increase H^+ in CSF so its response is slower compare to CO_2

* **Peripheral Chemoreceptors:**
  - **Carotid bodies** (send afferent to CNS in CN-9; **most important**) & Aortic bodies (send afferent to CNS in CN-10)
  - H+ & CO_2 receptors (less sensitive in periphery)
  - PO_2 receptors (**more sensitive**) – monitor dissolved O_2 (**not** O_2 content which is oxygen bound to Hb) – they do not begin to fire significantly until the PaO_2 falls to 50-60 mmHg therefore it has **no role in normal ventilation**. Normal ventilation drive is mainly CO_2
  - Sensitivity hypoxia increase in central chemoreceptors with CO_2 retention therefore **in chronic hypoventilation, low PO$_2$ is the only drive for ventilation through peripheral receptors** therefore giving supplemental oxygen in patient with CO_2 retention [eg: COPD] may eliminate drive for ventilation

  - **Medullary Centers** – The DRG (dorsal respiratory group) is involved in the generation of respiratory rhythm, and is primarily responsible for the generation of inspiration – The VRG contains both inspiratory and expiratory neurons. The VRG (ventral respiratory group) is secondarily responsible for initiation of inspiratory activity, after the dorsal respiratory group. The VRG is responsible for motor control of inspiratory and expiratory muscles during exercise

  - **Apneustic center** – located in the lower Pons – it promotes inspiration by stimulation of the inspiratory neurons in the medulla oblongata providing a **constant stimulus [prolong inspiration (Apneustic breathing)]** – It controls the **intensity** of breathing. The apneustic centre is inhibited by pulmonary stretch receptors

  - **Pneumotaxic center [Pontine respiratory group (PRG)]** – The PRG antagonizes the apneustic center (cyclically inhibits inspiration). – The PRG limits the burst of action potentials in the phrenic nerve, effectively decreasing the tidal volume and regulating the respiratory rate – Absence of the PRG results in an increase in depth of respiration and a decrease in respiratory rate

- **Hering-Breuer inflation reflex:** prevent overinflation of the lungs – Pulmonary stretch receptors present in the smooth muscle of the airways respond to excessive stretching of the lung during large inspirations

- <u>High Altitude:</u> Partial pressure of O_2 is decrease at high altitude so **PA_{O_2} & Pa_{O_2} decreased** acutely and remain decrease in person who is living at high altitude for long time. Same way **PA_{CO_2} & Pa_{CO_2} remain decrease.** Hb % saturation remains decrease because partial pressure is decrease at high altitude. P^H is increase (respiratory alkalosis) initially due to hyperventilation but it returns back to normal level in a person who is living at high altitude for long time. **Erythropoietin** secretion **increase** in response to hypoxia which leads to increase RBC in blood after 3-4 wks in a person who is living at high altitude for long time. Increase in RBC brings systemic O_2 content back to normal in a person who is living on high altitude for long time.

- ### <u>Ventilation (V_A) & Perfusion (Q):</u>
- Towards the Apex – lower perfusing pressure & high resistance therefore **less blood flow to the Apex**
- Towards the Base – no loss in perfusing pressure & lower resistance therefore **more blood flow to the Base**
- The ventilation/perfusion ratio is higher in the apex of lung when a person is standing than it is in the base of lung
- **V_A / Q = 0.8 –** in Normal individual
- **V_A / Q > 0.8 –** $\downarrow PA_{CO_2}$, $\uparrow PA_{O_2}$, $\uparrow$ pH (>7.4)
- **V_A / Q < 0.8 –** $\uparrow PA_{CO_2}$, $\downarrow PA_{O_2}$, $\downarrow$ pH (<7.4)

* <u>**Hypoxic vasoconstriction**</u> – **unique to pulmonary circuit** – a physiological phenomenon in which pulmonary arteries constrict in the presence of hypoxia without hypercapnia (high carbon dioxide levels), redirecting blood flow to alveoli with higher oxygen tension

- Alveoli → pulmonary vein (pulmonary end capillary) → LV → systemic arteries
- PA_{O_2} = 100 mmHg [A = Alveolar]
- Pulmonary end capillary PO_2 = 100 mmHg
- Pa_{O_2} = 95 mmHg [a = systemic arteries]

	PA_{O_2}	End capillary PO_2	Pa_{O_2}	
Hypoventilation	$\downarrow$	$\downarrow$	$\downarrow$	
Diffusion Impairment (Structural problem)	$\uparrow$	$\downarrow$	$\downarrow$	Improve A-a gradient with supplemental oxygen
Pulmonary Shunt	$\uparrow$	$\uparrow$	$\downarrow$	A-a gradient does <u>not</u> improve with supplemental oxygen

- Hypoxia <u>never</u> develop in Left to Right shunt

- **Atrial Septal Defect:** PO_2 increase first appears in the Right Atrium

- **Ventricular Septal Defect:** PO_2 increase first appears in the Right Ventricle

- **Patent Ductus Arteriosus:** PO_2 increase first appears in the Pulmonary artery

BIOCHEMISTRY

Basic Concepts

In most of the biochemical reactions, usually the end product of the reaction is the main stimulator / inhibitor of the rate limiting enzyme of that reaction. If end product goes up, it inhibits the rate limiting enzyme and thus inhibits the reaction. If end product level goes down, it stimulates the rate limiting enzyme and thus the reaction. Action of hormones is important too.

Example: Purpose of TCA cycle is to produce ATP. Main end products of TCA cycle are NADH & FADH2 which enter in ETC and give ATP. The rate limiting enzyme of TCA cycle is Isocitrate Dehydrogenase. When **NADH level goes up** [when ETC doesn't use NADH in conditions causing hypoxia], it inhibits Isocitrate dehydrogenase and thus inhibits TCA cycle. When more ATP are used means **increase in ADP** [Because ATP produce energy by giving its phosphate], it stimulate Isocitrate dehydrogenase to meet the need of ATP.

First remember all rate limiting enzymes of all important reaction. In exam, most of the time they ask factors that stimulate / inhibit those reactions by correlating reactions with clinical conditions. Know how our body uses those end products of all important reactions so you can correlate them better with clinical conditions they present on your test.

■ RATE LIMITING ENZYMES OF IMPORTANT REACTIONS:

- Glycolysis – PFK-1
- Glycogenesis – Glycogen Synthase
- Glycogenolysis – Glycogen Phosphorylase
- Gluconeogenesis – Fructose-1,6-Biphosphate (F-1,6-BP)
- HMP Shunt – G6PD
- TCA Cycle – Isocitrate Dehydrogenase
- FA Synthesis – Acetyl co-A Carboxylase
- Beta-Oxidation – Carnitine Acyltransferase-1
- Heme Synthesis – δ ALA Synthase (ALA - aminolavulinate)
- Purine Synthesis – PRPP amidotransferase
- Cholesterol Synthesis – HMG co-A reductase

-	ENZYMES	Stimulated By	Inhibited By
1	Hexokinase (low Km) (in most tissue) Glucose → glucose-6-P		Glucose-6-P
2	Glucokinase (high Km) (in Liver) Glucose → glucose-6-P (irreversible)	Insulin High Glucose	Fasting
3	**PFK-1** (Phosphofructokinase-1) Fructose-6-P → F-1,6 BP (irreversible) [Insulin (+) PFK-2 →F6P→ F-2,6 BP]	AMP F-2,6 BP Insulin	ATP **Citrate** Glucagon
4	**Glycogen Synthase** [form α-1,4 glycosidic bond]	Insulin Glucose	Epinephrine (Epi) Glucagon

5	**Glycogen Phosphorylase** [break α-1,4 glycosidic bond and release glucose-1-P]	Epi, Glucagon AMP Ca^{+2}	Insulin ATP
6	**F-1,6 BP [opposite to PFK-1]**	ATP	AMP
7	Pyruvate Carboxylase [in mitochondria] Pyruvate → Oxaloacetate	Acetyl co-A	
8	Pyruvate Dehydrogenase Pyruvate → Acetyl co-A (irreversible)	Insulin, PEP, AMP	Acetyl co-A, ATP, NADH
9	PEPCK [cytoplasm] [require GTP] [Oxaloacetate → PEP] (PEP = phosphoenolepyruvate)	Glucagon Cortisol	
10	**G6PD** [G6P → 6-Phosphogluconate → Ribulose-5-P → Ribose-5-P] [form **2 NADPH**]	Insulin **NADP**	**NADPH**
11	**Isocitrate Dehydrogenase** [Isocitrate → α-Ketoglutarate]	ADP	**NADH**
12	**Acetyl co-A Carboxylase** [Acetyl co-A → Malonyl co-A]	Insulin Citrate	
13	**Carnitine acyltransferase-1**	Glucagon	Malonyl co-A Insulin
14	**δ ALA Synthase** [glycine + succinyl co-A → δ ALA]	Require Vit-B6	Heme
15	**PRPP amidotransferase** [↑ activity leads to Hyperuricemia]		IMP AMP GMP Allopurinol 6-MP
16	**HMG co-A Reductase** [cholesterol synthesis]	Insulin	Glucagon

- Our body needs energy in the form of ATP and we get ATP from glucose. Period! Substrates to produce glucose are carbohydrate, fat and protein. [from food and from our body storage]

- Carbohydrate from food: Glycolysis [to produce ATP], Glycogenesis [to store in body as a glycogen] Disaccharides like lactose & sucrose are broken to glucose + galactose [by lactase] and glucose + fructose [by sucrase] respectively. These monosaccharide forms are then absorbed into blood and transported to liver and other tissues for Glycogenesis and glycolysis. Once body's need of glucose has fulfilled, remaining glucose is then converted into glycogen in liver and some used in HMP shunt and some in AA synthesis. After glycogen storage, if glucose still remains, is then converted into triglycerides (TGs) in adipose tissues.

- Fat from food: The lipase (activated by acid) breaks down the fat (TGs) into monoglycerides (glycerol) and fatty acids. The bile emulsifies the fatty acids so they may be easily absorbed. **Short- and some medium chain fatty acids are absorbed directly** into the blood via intestine capillaries and travel through the portal vein just as other absorbed nutrients do. However, **long chain fatty acids and some medium chain fatty acids are** absorbed into the fatty walls of the intestine villi and **reassembled again into triglycerides. Chylomicrons carry dietary TGs.** Within the villi, the chylomicron enters a lymphatic capillary called a lacteal, which merges into larger lymphatic vessels. It is transported via the lymphatic system and the thoracic duct which empties the chylomicrons into the bloodstream via the left subclavian vein. At this point the chylomicrons can transport the triglycerides to where they are needed (liver).

- Proteins from food: Pancreatic enzymes clave peptide bonds and releases AA. AA absorbed into intestinal epithelial cells by secondary active transport and from epithelial cells, AA diffuses directly into blood

- During fasting: Glycogenolysis occurs until stored glycogen deprived. After that gluconeogenesis begins to provide glucose to the brain.
- After prolong fasting (>1-wk), brain use ketone bodies (2/3) **&** glucose (1/3)
- In all conditions, RBCs use only glucose because they lack mitochondria.

- Essential AA and Fatty Acid (FA): Essential means **our body can't synthesize them so we have to ingest them in the form of food**.

- Essential AA: PM AT TV HILL: Phenylalanine, Methionine, Arginine, Threonine, Tryptophan, Valine, Histidine, Isoleucine, Leucine, Lysine
- Essential FA: α-Linolenic acid (ALA) (18:3) [ω-3 fatty acids], Linoleic acid (LA) (18:2) [ω-6 fatty acids]

- How do we get energy from food? Glucose is oxidized and released energy. This energy is transferred to NAD^+ by reduction to NADH as part of glycolysis and the TCA cycle. NADH is then enter in ETC to produce ATP.

- **Glycolysis:** Glucose → G-6-P → F-6-P → F-1,6-BP → PEP → Pyruvate
- End product of glycolysis is **Pyruvate.**
- **When oxygen is available / less ATP require**, Pyruvate is converted to acetyl co-A to enter in TCA cycle and produce ATP through ETC
- **When less oxygen available / more ATP required** (Ex: during exercise), Pyruvate is converted to Lactate and produce ATP

PEP $\xrightarrow[\text{ATP} \rightarrow \text{ADP}]{\text{Pyruvate Kinase}}$ Pyruvate (irreversible)

Pyruvate $\xrightarrow[\text{NAD}^+ \rightarrow \text{NADH}]{\text{Pyruvate Dehydrogenase}}$ Acetyl co-A (irreversible)

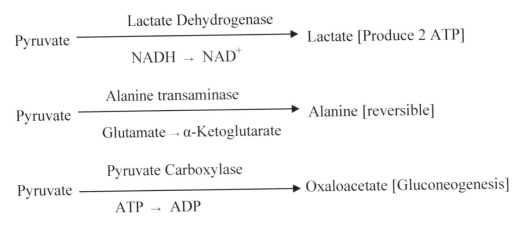

Pyruvate $\xrightarrow[\text{NADH} \rightarrow \text{NAD}^+]{\text{Lactate Dehydrogenase}}$ Lactate [Produce 2 ATP]

Pyruvate $\xrightarrow[\text{Glutamate} \rightarrow \alpha\text{-Ketoglutarate}]{\text{Alanine transaminase}}$ Alanine [reversible]

Pyruvate $\xrightarrow[\text{ATP} \rightarrow \text{ADP}]{\text{Pyruvate Carboxylase}}$ Oxaloacetate [Gluconeogenesis]

- Lactate produced from Pyruvate in anaerobic reaction can be used to synthesis glucose [gluconeogenesis **in Liver** through **Cori's cycle**] [Pyruvate to Lactate produce only 2 ATP **to use** by our body whereas Lactate to Glucose conversion **consumes** 6 ATP of our body so there is a loss of 4 ATP which explains why this cycle can't continue without external energy (food) and we can't survive without eating!] This process also produce NAD^+ which is required to continue glycolysis

- **Glycolysis:** It produces 2 ATP (substrate level phosphorylation), 2 NADH and 2 Pyruvate molecules (Aerobic)
  2 ATP per glucose molecule [Anaerobic]
  6 or 8 ATP (depends upon which shuttle is used to carry NADH) [Aerobic]
  NADH – carried by <u>malate shuttle</u> (**3ATP**) **or** <u>glycerol-3-P shuttle</u> [converts in FADH2 and give **2 ATP**]

- **TCA cycle:** <u>Three</u> important shuttles
  Citrate $\longrightarrow$ FA synthesis
  Succinyl co-A $\longrightarrow$ Heme (to activate ketone bodies)
  Malate $\longrightarrow$ Gluconeogenesis
  Fumarate $\longleftarrow$ Urea Cycle
  Acetyl co A is the entry point in TCA-cycle

- As already mentioned above, end products of TCA cycle are NADH & FADH2 which enter in ETC and produce ATP.

- NADH – carried by <u>malate shuttle</u> (give **3ATP**) **or** <u>glycerol-3-P shuttle</u> (convert in FADH2 and give **2 ATP**)

- **FADH2** [produced by glycerol-3-P shuttle & Succinate dehydrogenase (complex-2)] **directly transfer electron to Coenzyme-Q in ETC.**

Important Concept

- **In Pyruvate Dehydrogenase deficiency**, Pyruvate doesn't convert into acetyl co-A. Increased Pyruvate will then convert into lactate and Alanine so in Pyruvate Dehydrogenase deficiency → ↑ **Lactate & Alanine**
- **Pyruvate Kinase Deficiency** → Anaerobic glycolysis → ↑ **2,3 BPG** → O2 dissociation curve shift to the **Right**

- **Electron in ETC pass in following order:**
  Complex-1 (NADH dehydrogenase)
  Coenzyme-Q
  Complex-3 (cytochrome b/c1)
  Cytochrome C [Inhibited by cyanide]
  Complex-4 (cytochrome a/a3)⟶ transfer electron to O2

- **Uncouplers:** ↓ proton gradient in ETC leads to ↓ ATP synthesis, ↑ O2 consumption, ↑ oxidation of NADH and therefore energy is released as heat. Ex: 2,4 dinitrophenol (2,4-DNP), Aspirin, brown adipose tissue in newborn

- **Gluconeogenesis:** Synthesis of *glucose* from other substrate during *fasting*; Occurs in liver (major) and in the cortex of kidney (small part)
- *Substrate*: Pyruvate, Lactate, Oxaloacetate, Glycerol and Glucogenic AA (except Lysine & Leucine)
- FA cannot be converted directly into glucose in animals, the exception being **odd-chain FA** which yields propionyl CoA, a precursor for succinyl CoA.
- Before **glycerol** can enter the pathway of gluconeogenesis, it **must be converted to their intermediate glyceraldehyde 3-phosphate**
- **Alanine** is converted in Pyruvate which is then used to synthesize glucose

- Gluconeogenesis: Lactate → Pyruvate → **Oxaloacetate** → Malate (in mitochondria) → **Oxaloacetate** (in cytoplasm) → PEP → F-1,6-BP → F-6-P → G-6-P → **Glucose**
- Gluconeogenesis: Glyceraldehyde-3-P → F-1,6-P → F-6-P → G-6-P → **Glucose**

- Our body use this Glucose to generate energy (ATP) during fasting
- Glycolysis: Glucose → G-6-P → F-6-P → F-1,6-BP → PEP → Pyruvate

- Important reaction of glycolysis *intermediate* when excess of glucose is available: F-1,6-BP ↔ Glyceraldehyde-3-P + Dihydroxyacetone Phosphate (DHAP) [fructose bisphosphate Aldolase] (↔ means reversible process) (Enzyme has written in bracket [] with each end product)

- **In Liver** (after eating), Glycerol (**came from food**) ↔ Glycerol-3-P [glycerol kinase] [*used for TGs synthesis in adipose tissue for storage*]
- **In adipose tissue**, DHAP (produced during glycolysis from F-1,6-BP in liver) ↔ Glycerol-3-P [glycerol-3-P dehydrogenase] [*used in synthesis of TGs for storage*]

- **During fasting**, *in adipose tissue*, TGs ↔ free FA + Glycerol [Glucagon stimulate Hormone sensitive Lipase] **Glycerol from adipose tissue** now goes to liver.
- **In Liver**, Glycerol (*came from adipose tissue*) ↔ Glycerol-3-P [glycerol kinase] ↔ DHAP [glycerol-3-P dehydrogenase] ↔ Glyceraldehyde-3-P [Triosephosphate isomerase] → F-1,6-P → F-6-P → G-6-P → *Glucose*
- Glucose-6-P & Glycerol kinase enzymes – present only in Liver that's why gluconeogenesis (major) occurs in Liver. Glucokinase (glycolysis) is also present in liver only.

- **Beta Oxidation:** When glycogen store depleted, TGs from adipose tissue break into free FA & glycerol via hormone-sensitive lipase. Free FA is then converted into acetyl co-A which is used in TCA cycle to produce ATP but **when acetyl co-A is exceeded and TCA cycle can't handle the load** (low TCA intermediate especially Oxaloacetate which is also used for gluconeogenesis), **acetyl co-A is then used to form ketone bodies**.
  - Acetoacetate is the first ketone bodies to form.
  - Acetone & β-hydroxybutyrate are formed from acetoacetate
  - Acetone is 3-carbon ketone bodies which are **not** used as energy fuel. Acetone is excreted as a waste product and that's why we get specific **fruity smell** in patient with **Diabetic Ketoacidosis** which is due to acetone.
  - **Free FA** is needed to be **activated** first before they are carried to mitochondria for beta oxidation. It is done **by the enzyme fatty acyl-CoA synthetase**.
    Fatty acid + CoA + ATP ↔ Acyl-CoA + AMP + PP$_i$ [by fatty acyl co-A synthase]
  - **Carnitine shuttle:** Fatty acyl co-A then transfer fatty acyl group to Carnitine via Carnitine acyltransferase-1. Fatty acyl Carnitine is a shuttle across the inner membrane. Carnitine acyltransferase-2 transfer fatty acyl group back to a co-A to formed fatty acyl co-A in the mitochondria.
  - Fatty acyl co-A is *then* degraded to acetyl co-A + acyl co-A. This process continues until it gives acetyl co-A + acetyl co-A for FA with **even number of carbons**. For FA with **odd number of carbons**, it continues until it gives acetyl co-A + **propionyl co-A**.
  - During each step, it gives one FADH2, one NADH. Acetyl co-A enters in TCA cycle and gives ATP. That's how beta oxidation provides energy.

  - **Propionyl co-A:** Propionyl co-A is a product of **odd chain fatty acid oxidation**, a product of metabolism of Isoleucine & Valine and a product of alpha-ketobutyric acid [which is a product of Threonine and Methionine], Propionyl co-A → Methylmalonyl co-A → Succinyl co-A [First reaction is conducted by **Propionyl co-A Carboxylase** which requires **biotin** as a cofactor. Second reaction is catalyzed by **Methylmalonyl-CoA mutase** which requires **Vit-B12** as a cofactor.] Succinyl co-A is then enter in TCA cycle

  - **FA synthesis,** *from glucose which is still there after body's demand has over, through glycolysis:* Oxaloacetate + Acetyl CoA ↔ Citrate (Citrate synthase)
  - **Citrate is transported to the cytoplasm** where it again converts to acetyl co-A. Acetyl co-A is converted into Malonyl Co-A by acetyl Co-A Carboxylase enzyme
  - Fatty acids are formed by the action of **Fatty acid synthase** from acetyl-CoA and malonyl-CoA precursors.

  - **Glycogen synthesis,** *from glucose which is still there after body's demand has over, through glycolysis:* Glucose → Glucose-6-P → Glucose-1-P → **UDP glucose → UDP and (1,4-α-D-glucosyl)$_{n+1}$** → Branches are made by Branching enzyme
  - *Only* those Glucose molecules *which are bound to UDP nucleotide* used in glycogen synthesis.
  - Enzymes responsible for above reactions respectively are: Glucokinase / Hexokinase → Phosphoglucomutase → Uridyl Transferase (also called UDP-glucose pyrophosphorylase) → **glycogen synthase** → Branching enzyme [amylo-α(1:4)-α(1:6) transglycosylase]

- **Glycogen synthase:** catalyses the reaction of UDP-glucose and $(1,4\text{-}\alpha\text{-D-glucosyl})_n$ to yield UDP and $(1,4\text{-}\alpha\text{-D-glucosyl})_{n+1}$. In other words, *this enzyme converts excess glucose residues one by one into a polymeric chain for storage as glycogen.*

- <u>**Glycogenolysis:**</u> Glycogen $\rightarrow$ Glycogen $_{n-1}$ + Glucose-1-P by glycogen Phosphorylase. It breaks down glucose polymer at α-1-4 linkages until 5 linked glucoses are left on the branch. Now debranching enzymes involve that moves the remaining glucose units to another non-reducing end. This results in less glucose units available to glycogen Phosphorylase. The final action of the debranching enzyme leads to the original glucose-1-P connected 1,4 to another branch being released. Glucose-1-P $\rightarrow$ Glucose-6-P by phosphoglucomutase. *Glucose-6-P is then enters in glycolysis to provide ATP.*

- <u>**HMP shunt (Pentose phosphate pathway):**</u> <u>Glucose-6-phosphate</u> does HMP shunt. <u>Fructose-6-phosphate</u> produced in HMP shunt is a re-entry to glycolysis.
- **Important of HMP shunt:** To generate **NADPH** [for reductive biosynthesis reactions within cells] and **ribose-5-phosphate** [for the synthesis of the nucleic acids and nucleotides]
- **Importance of NADPH:** To maintain the reduced state of glutathione (GSH). Reduced Glutathione converts reactive H_2O_2 into H_2O by oxidizing itself (GSSH). In G6PD deficiency, there is very low NADPH so glutathione remains in its oxidizing phase so RBC can't handle oxidative stress leads to hemolysis.

- Pyruvate dehydrogenase, Alfa-Ketoglutarate dehydrogenase, Branched-chain ketoacid dehydrogenase → **require Thiamin (Vit-B1)**, co-A, NAD, FAD, lipoic acid.
- ↑ **Transketolase in RBCs** in thiamin (Vit-B1) deficiency.

- <u>**Amino Acid Synthesis:**</u> There are 20 main amino acids. Out of 20, 8 are essential AA. Our body synthesizes remaining 12 AA.
- Amino acids are synthesized from TCA cycle intermediate [**Glutamate**].
- Alpha-Ketoglutarate + NH_4^+ ↔ Glutamate
- Afterwards, **Alanine** and **Aspartate** are formed by **transamination** of Glutamate. All of the remaining amino acids are then constructed from Glutamate or Aspartate, by transamination of these two amino acids with one α-keto acid.
- NH_4^+ is the source of nitrogen for all the amino acids
- **Alanine** and **Aspartate** are synthesized by the transamination of Pyruvate and Oxaloacetate, respectively. **Glutamine** is synthesized from NH4+ and glutamate, and asparagine is synthesized similarly. **Proline** and **Arginine** are derived from glutamate. **Serine**, formed from 3-phosphoglycerate, is the precursor of **glycine** and **cysteine**. **Tyrosine** is synthesized by the hydroxylation of phenylalanine (an essential amino acid)
- <u>**Importance of AA:**</u> **Nitric oxide**, a short-lived messenger, is formed from Arginine. **Porphyrins** are synthesized from glycine and succinyl CoA, which condense to give δ-aminolevulinate which is a part of Heme synthesis.
- **Aminotransferases** (AST & ALT) – both **require** Vit-B6 (**Pyridoxine**)
  In muscle – transfer amino group to glutamate
  In liver – Alanine to Aspartate

- **Glutamate Dehydrogenase** convert Glutamate to α-Ketoglutarate (**TCA cycle intermediate**)
- **AST & CPS-1** (Carbamoyl Phosphate Synthetase -1) are **direct donor of nitrogen** in urea cycle

- ■ **Urea cycle (Ornithine cycle):** It produces urea from ammonia. Ammonia is toxic to the brain. Urea cycle takes place **only in liver**. Both **mitochondria & cytosol**
- It consumes 4 ATP and release 5 ATP so **we get 1 ATP from urea cycle**
- Reactions: $NH_4^+ + 2ATP + HCO_3^- \rightarrow$ **Carbamoyl Phosphate** [CPS-1] + 2ADP + P [Mitochondria] CPS-1 + Ornithine $\rightarrow$ Citrulline + P [Ornithine Transcarbamoylase] [Mitochondria] Citrulline + aspartate + ATP $\rightarrow$ Argininosuccinate + AMP + PP [Argininosuccinate synthase] [Cytosol] Argininosuccinate $\rightarrow$ Arginine + **Fumarate** [Argininosuccinate lyase] [cytosol] Arginine + $H_2O \rightarrow$ Ornithine + Urea [Arginase] [Cytosol]
- Fumarate $\rightarrow$ Malate [Fumarase] $\rightarrow$ Oxaloacetate [malate dehydrogenase]
- Oxaloacetate $\rightarrow$ Aspartate [transaminase] / Oxaloacetate $\rightarrow$ PEP [*Gluconeogenesis*]

- ■ **Importance of Essential FA:** Used to make **Eicosanoids** [Prostaglandins, Prostacyclins, Thromboxane and Leukotrines]
- ▪ Eicosanoid biosynthesis begins when cell is activated by mechanical trauma, cytokines, growth factors or other stimuli. Phospholipids from cell membrane $\rightarrow$ **Arachidonic Acid** [Phospholipase A_2] $\rightarrow$ **Prostaglandins (PG)** [Cyclooxygenase (COX)] / Arachidonic acid $\rightarrow$ HPETE [Lipoxygenase] [**Leukotrines synthesis**] Arachidonic acid $\rightarrow$ **PGH** [cyclooxygenase] $\rightarrow$ Thromboxane A_2 [thromboxane synthase] Arachidonic acid $\rightarrow$ **PGH** [cyclooxygenase] $\rightarrow$ Prostacyclins [prostacyclin synthase] Arachidonic acid $\rightarrow$ **PGH** [cyclooxygenase] $\rightarrow$ PGE_2 [PGE synthase] $\rightarrow$ PGF_2
- ▪ **Clinical Importance:** Steroids inhibits Phospholipase [inhibit synthesis of both prostaglandins and Leukotrines] NSAIDs inhibits COX [inhibit synthesis of prostaglandins] Ziluton inhibits Lipoxygenase [inhibit synthesis of Leukotrines] Low dose Aspirin inhibits thromboxane synthase [inhibits platelate aggregation]

- ▪ **Glucose Transport:**
  GLUT-1 – Brain, RBCs (do not need insulin for uptake)
  GLUT-3 – most tissue (do not need insulin for uptake)
  GLUT-2 – Liver
  GLUT-4 – Adipose tissue & Skeletal M. (**Insulin stimulated glucose uptake**)

4. **Citrate shuttle** – transport Acetyl co-A group from mitochondria to cytoplasm for FA synthesis.

5. **Carnitine shuttle:** After FA is activated to fatty acyl co-A, Fatty acyl co-A then transfer fatty acyl group to Carnitine via Carnitine acyltransferase-1. Fatty acyl Carnitine is a shuttle across the inner membrane. Carnitine acyltransferase-2 transfer fatty acyl group back to a co-A to formed fatty acyl co-A in the mitochondria.

6. **Farnesyl Phosphate:** an intermediate in cholesterol synthesis pathway, **used for:**
   - Synthesis of Co-Q
   - Synthesis of dolichol phosphate, (required cofactor in N-linked glycosylation in RER)
   - Prenylation of proteins that need to be hold in the cell membrane by lipid tail

- **Enzymes In Inner Mitochondrial Membrane:**
  Succinate Dehydrogenase (complex-2)
  F0-F1-ATP Synthetase
  Carnitine Acyltransferase-2

- **Enzymes In Outer Mitochondrial Membrane:**
  Fatty Acyl co-A Synthetase
  Carnitine Acyltransferase-1

- **Carbamoyl Phosphate Synthase (CPS):**
  Cytoplasm – Pyrimidine Synthesis
  Mitochondria – Urea cycle
  [Both are different enzymes with different locations but similar name]

- <u>Fatty **Acyl** Synthase</u>: activate FA by attaching co-A (first step in both FA synthesis & Beta-Oxidation)
- <u>Fatty **Acid** Synthase</u>: FA synthesis
  [Both are different enzymes so don't confuse]

PROCESSES IN MITOCHONDREA:
- Ketone body synthesis
- FA oxidation
- Production of Acetyl co-A
- TCA cycle
- ETC (electron transport chain)

PROCESSES IN CYTOPLASM:
- Glycolysis
- FA synthesis
- Cholesterol synthesis
- HMP shunt

PROCESSES IN BOTH MITOCHONDREA & CYTOPLASM:
- Gluconeogenesis
- Urea cycle
- Heme synthesis

- **Lipoproteins:** Lipid + Protein
- **Chylomicrons** - carry **triacylglycerol** (fat) **from the intestines to the liver**, skeletal muscle, and to adipose tissue.
- **VLDL** - carry (newly synthesized) **triacylglycerol from the liver to adipose tissue.**

- **IDL** - intermediate between VLDL and LDL, not usually detectable in the blood.
- **LDL** - carry **cholesterol from the liver to cells** of the body. [bad cholesterol]
- **HDL** - carry **cholesterol from the body's tissues to the liver**. [good cholesterol]

■ Chylomicron metabolism:

- After lipids absorb from small intestine, these lipids [triglycerides, phospholipids, and cholesterol] are **assembled with apolipoprotein B-48 into chylomicrons**. These nascent chylomicrons are secreted into the lymphatic circulation bypass the liver circulation and are drained via the thoracic duct into the bloodstream.
- In the circulation, HDL particles donate **apolipoprotein C-II** and **apolipoprotein E** to the nascent chylomicron; the chylomicron is now considered mature. **Apolipoprotein C-II activates lipoprotein lipase** (LPL), an enzyme on endothelial cells lining the blood vessels. LPL catalyzes a hydrolysis reaction that ultimately releases glycerol and fatty acids from the chylomicrons. Glycerol and fatty acids can be absorbed in peripheral tissues, especially adipose and muscle, for energy and storage.
- The hydrolyzed chylomicrons are now considered **chylomicron remnants**. The chylomicron remnants absorb into liver via interaction with apolipoprotein E. This interaction causes the **endocytosis** of the chylomicron remnants, which are subsequently hydrolyzed within lysosomes. Lysosomal hydrolysis releases glycerol and fatty acids into the cell, which can be used for energy or stored for later use.

■ VLDL metabolism:

- The liver is another important source of lipoproteins, principally VLDL. Triacylglycerol and cholesterol are assembled with **apolipoprotein B-100** to form VLDL particles. (nascent VLDL)
- In the circulation, HDL donates its apolipoprotein C-II and apolipoprotein E to VLDL particles. (mature VLDL)

- Now Apolipoprotein C-II activates LPL, causing hydrolysis of the VLDL particle and the release of glycerol and fatty acids. These products can be absorbed from the blood by peripheral tissues, principally adipose and muscle. The hydrolyzed VLDL particles are now called **VLDL remnants or intermediate density lipoproteins (IDL)**. The VLDL remnants absorb into liver via interaction with apolipoprotein E. They can be further hydrolyzed by hepatic lipase.
- Hydrolysis by hepatic lipase releases glycerol and fatty acids, leaving behind IDL remnants, called low density lipoproteins (LDL), which contains relatively high cholesterol content. LDL circulates and is absorbed by the liver and peripheral cells. **Binding of LDL to its target tissue occurs through an interaction between LDL receptor and apolipoprotein B-100 or E on the LDL particle**. Absorption occurs through **endocytosis**, and the internalized LDL particles are hydrolyzed within lysosomes, releasing lipids, chiefly cholesterol.

- LPL (lipoprotein lipase) → induced by Insulin
- HSL (hormone stimulated lipase) → induced by Epinephrine

- **COLLAGEN SYNTHESIS:**
- **Hydroxyproline** is an amino acid unique to collagen
- Glycine (Gly) is found at almost every third residue [Gly – x-y-Gly-x-y- etc.]
- Proline (Pro) makes up about 9% of collagen
- Proline & Lysine – hydroxylated in RER by prolyl and lysyl **Hydroxylase (require Vit-C)**
- Procollagen (triple helical structure) **glycosylated in golgi** & secreted from cell
- Cross-linking involves **Lysyl Oxidase (require O2, Cu+2)**

- **Tetrahydrofolate (THF):** THF is a carrier of activated one-carbon unit, plays an important role in the metabolism of amino acids and nucleotides. This coenzyme carries one-carbon units at three oxidation states, which are interconvertible: most reduced—**methyl**; intermediate—methylene; and most oxidized—formyl, formimino, and methenyl. Methionine → S-adenosylmethionine [methionine adenosyltransferase] → Adenosylhomocystine [Methyltransferase] → Homocystine → **Methionine [Homocystine methyltransferase** transfer methyl group from N^5-Methyl-THF] [This enzyme **requires Vit-B12** as a cofactor therefore in Vit-B12 deficiency, stored folate (N^5-Methyl-THF) can not be used and so secondary folate deficiency is created which produce Megaloblastic anemia] / Homocystine → **Cystathione** [cystathione synthase] [**require Vit-B6**]
- Cystathione → Cystine + α-ketobutyrate [cystathione γ lyase]
- α-ketobutyrate → Propionyl-CoA [α-ketobutyrate dehydrogenase]

- **Vit-B12:** It is used as a cofactor in Propionyl co-A metabolism which is a product of Odd chain FA, Valine, Isoleucine, Methionine & Threonine
- **Methylmalonic Aciduria** (seen in Vit-B12 deficiency) – distinguished Megaloblastic anemia from folate deficiency.

- **Heme Transport And Storage:**
- Feroxidase (also known as Ceruloplasmin, Copper protein) oxidize Fe^{+2} to Fe^{+3} for transport and storage.
- Transferrin carries Fe^{+3} in blood
- Ferritin stores normal amount of Fe^{+3} in tissue
- Hemosiderin binds excess Fe^{+3} to prevent escape of free Fe+3 into blood where it is toxic.

Delta ALA $\xrightarrow{\text{ALA dehydrogenase}}$ Porphobilinogen

Protoporphyrin (9) $\xrightarrow{\text{Ferrochelatase, Fe+2}}$ Heme

- **Lead** inhibits both ALA dehydrogenase & Ferrochelatase.

- **Vit-B$_6$ deficiency:** ↓ Protoporphyrin & ↓ δ ALA
- **Iron deficiency:** ↑ Protoporphyrin & **N** δ ALA
- **Lead poisoning:** ↑ Protoporphyrin & ↑ δ ALA

- **Purine & Pyrimidine Metabolism:**
- Purines are synthesized as **nucleotides** (bases attached to ribose 5-phosphate).
- pyrimidines are **assembled before being attached to** 5-phosphoribosyl-1-pyrophosphate (PRPP)
- Purine Synthesis: Ribose-5-Phosphate [HMP shunt] → PRPP [by ribose-phosphate diphosphokinase] → 5-phosphoribosylamine [**Amidophosphoribosyltransferase**] → **IMP** [*It is a precursor of both adenine & guanine*] [amino acids involved in synthesis of IMP are glycine, glutamine, and aspartic acid] [Also used THF as a cofactor] IMP → XMP → **GMP** / IMP → adenylosuccinate → **AMP**
- Pyrimidine Synthesis: Glutamine → Carbamoyl Phosphate [Carbamoyl Phosphatase II] → Carbamoyl aspartic acid → dihydroorotate → orotate → OMP [used PRPP] → UDP → UTP → CTP [Glutamine & ATP] [*Uracil is a precursor of both C & T*]
- Purine Degradation: Final common product is **Uric acid**. When cell dies (apoptosis), nuclease frees nucleotides. **Guanine:** Nucleotide → Guanosine [nucleotidase] → Guanine [Purine nucleoside Phosphorylase] → Xanthine [Guanase] → **Uric acid** [Xanthine oxidoreductase] **Adenine:** Nucleotide → Adenosine → **Inosine** [Adenosine deaminase, deficiency of which causes Severe Combined Immuno Deficiency (SCID)] / Nucleotide → IMP [AMP deaminase] → **Inosine** [nucleotidase]; Now from **Inosine** → Hypoxanthine [Purine nucleoside Phosphorylase] → Xanthine [Xanthine oxidoreductase] → **Uric acid** [Xanthine oxidoreductase]
- Purine Salvage: Salvage pathways are used to recover bases and nucleosides that are formed during degradation of RNA and DNA. Hypoxanthine → IMP [HGPRT] Guanine → GMP [HGPRT] Adenine → AMP [Adenine phosphoribosyltransferase]
- * **Clinical Biochemistry:**

- **GLYCOGEN STORAGE DISEASES:**

- **von Gierke's Disease:** glucose-6-phosphatase deficiency
  Severe fasting hypoglycemia, lactic acidosis, **Hyperuricemia**, Hepatomegaly, **Ketosis**, hyperlipidemia

- Medium-chain Acyl co A Dehydrogenase **(MCAD) deficiency:** severe fasting hypoglycemia, **No** ketosis, **Dicarboxylic Acidosis**

- Pompe's Disease: (**P**ump - heart) – lysosomal alfa-1,4 glucosidase deficiency
  Cardiomegaly (usually death occur by age of 2 yrs)
  Glycogen like material **in inclusion** bodies

- McArdle's Disease: (**M**uscle) Muscle glycogen Phosphorylase deficiency
  Muscle cramps & weakness on exercise
  Glycogen present **in muscle biopsy**

- **Myopathic Carnitine Deficiency:** Carnitine deficiency in muscle
  Muscle cramps & weakness on exercise
  Triglycerides (TGs) present **in muscle biopsy**

- **Her's Disease:** **H**epatic glycogen Phosphorylase deficient
  Mild fasting hypoglycemia, Hepatomegaly

- **Cori's Disease:** debarnching enzyme deficiency
  Short outer branches, **single glucose residue at outer branch**

- **Anderson's (Amylopectinosis):** branching enzyme deficiency
  Very few branch toward periphery.
  Infantile hypotonia, cirrhosis, usually death occur by age of 2 yrs

- **Lesch – Nyhan Syndrome:**
- Defective purine metabolism
- Deficient HPRT (HGPRT)
- Child tendency to compulsively bite his finger (**self mutilation**)
- Mental retardation
- Hyperuricemia is due to ↓ IMP (Hypoxanthine $\xrightarrow{\text{HPRT}}$ IMP)

- **Tay Sachs Disease :**
- Hexosaminidase A deficient
- Ganglioside accumulate in cells
- **Charry red macula, No** Hepatomegaly and cervical lymphadenopathy

- **Niemann – Pick:**
- Sphingomyelinase deficiency
- Sphingomyelin accumulate in cells
- Characteristic **foamy macrophage,** charry red macula, **Hepatomegaly** & cervical Lymphadenopathy [Hepatomegaly is absent in Tay Sachs]

- **Gaucher's Disease:**
* Gluocerebrosidase deficiency
* glucocerebroside accumulate in cells
* characteristic Macrophage (**crumpled paper inclusion**)

- Ashkenazi Jews (Eastern European) → two diseases → Tay Sachs and Gaucher's disease (type – I)
- **Ceremide** is common substance from all sphingolipid derived. Serine is AA join with fatty acyl co–A to form ceremide.

- **Phenylketonuria:**
- Phenylalanine Hydroxylase Deficiency (Phenylalanine → tyrosine)
- **Musty odor** from child, mental retardation
- Aspartame (**artificial sweeteners**) must be **strictly avoided** by phenyketonurics
- ↑ Phenylalanine level in pregnant woman → mental retardation in Infants

- **Homogentisate Oxidase Deficiency:**
- accumulation of homogentisic acid in blood & excretion in urine
- **Ochronosis** (accumulation of **black/brown pigments** in cartilages)

- **Maple Syrup Urine Disease:**
- Branched chain ketoacid dehydrogenase deficiency
- impaired metabolism of Valine , Leucine , Isoleucine
- **Maple syrup odor in urine**
- Ketosis, coma, & death if not treated

- **Acute Intermittent Porphyria:**
- Uroporphyrinogen – 1 synthase deficient
- Episodic variable expression
- Acute abdomen ("**belly full of scars**") , brief psychosis
- **No** photosensitivity ($\uparrow \delta$ ALA,PBG)
- Never give <u>Barbiturates</u>, Pyrazinamide, Gresiofulvin

- **Porphyria Cutanea Tarda:**
- Uroporphyrinogen decarboxylase deficient
- **Photosensitivity** ($\uparrow$ uroporphyrin 1) [urinary uroporphyrin - **diagnostic test**]
- chronic inflammation to overt blistering and shearing in exposed area of skin – **Tx**: stop alcohol & estrogen use .

- **Homocystinuria:** Arthrosclerosis in childhood, recurrent DVT

$$\text{(Homocystine} \xrightarrow[\text{Vit-B6}]{\text{Cystathione Synthase}} \text{Cystathione)}$$

- **Causes:** Cystathione synthase deficiency, Vit- B_6 deficiency, Homocystine methyltransferase deficiency, Folic acid & Vit- B_{12} deficiency
- * Methionine is degraded via the Homocystine–Cystathione Pathway; so **methionine** is **elevated** in patient with **cystathione synthase deficiency** via activation of Homocystine methyltransferase by excess substrate homocystine.

- **Genetic Deficiency of the Urea cycle:** (Both mitochondrial enzyme)
- Carbamoyl-P-Synthase and Ornithine Transcarbamoylase deficiency
- Both have same sign & symptoms but increase in uracil & orotic acid seen in Ornithine Transcarbamoylase deficiency differentiate both
- Increase in NH_4^+ which is toxic to the brain.
- <u>Tx</u>: Low protein diet [urea is produced from AA degradation]

- **Hartnup Disease** : defect in epithelial transport of neutral AA including Tryptophan
- Sign & Symptoms are **similar to Pellagra**
- Niacin – helpful in controlling symptoms
- Defective transport leads to dietary AA in stool & excess **free AA in urine**

- **Cystinuria**: Most common aminoaciduria characterized by defect in reabsorption of "**COAL**" → Cystine , Ornithine , Arginine , Lysine
- Associated with **Staghorn calculi in kidney**

Galactosemia/Galactosuria	Fructosemia/Fructosuria
▪ **Galactokinase deficiency**	▪ **Fructokinase deficiency**
-↑ galactose in blood	- ↑ fructose in blood
- **cataract** (Aldose reductase)	- **No** cataract
- galactokinase trap galactose in cell by phosphorylation as galactose-1-phosphate	- fructokinase trap fructose in cell by phosphorylation as fructose-1-phosphate
▪ **Gal-1-Uridyltransferase Deficiency**	▪ **Aldolase B Deficiency**
- convert galatose-1-phosphate into glucose-1-phosphate	- convert fructose-1-phosphate into DHAP & Glyceraldehydes
- If it deficient, galactose-1-phosphate accumulate in cells and produce symptoms	-If it deficient, fructose-1-phosphate accumulate in cells and produce symptoms.
- Liver, **Brain** & other tissue.	- Liver , **kidney**
- Symptoms evident while on Breast milk, so **early onset** of symptoms after birth	- Symptoms are **not** evident while on Breast milk, **so late onset** of symptoms after birth
- **cataract**	- **No** cataract
- Hypoglycemia, Lactic acidosis, Jaundice, **Mental retardation**	- Hypoglycemia, Lactic acidosis, Jaundice, **Proximal Renal tubular disorder** resembling Fanconi's syndrome
- Avoid milk & milk product	- Avoid Honey, table sugar which contain sucrose

- **Menkes Disease:** X-linked recessive
  Mutation in the gene encoding a Cu^{+2} efflux protein
  Cu^{+2} accumulate in the cell create Cu^{+2} deficiency.

- **HYPERLIPIDEMIAS:**

- **Type-1** [Familial hyperchylomicronemia]- ↑ Chylomicrons (↑ TGs) – **lipoprotein lipase deficiency – Xanthomas present** but **No** ↑ **risk for atherosclerosis**
- **Type-2a [Familial hypercholesterolemia]** - ↑ LDL only (**LDL receptors deficiency**) - ↑ Cholesterol

- Type-2b [Combined hyperlipidemia] - Decreased LDL receptor and Increased Apo B - ↑ LDL & VLDL (↑ Cholesterol & TGs)

- Type-3 [Familial Dysbetalipoproteinemia] - Defect in Apo E synthesis - ↑ Chylomicrons remnants & IDL (↑ Cholesterol & TGs)

- Type-4 [Familial Hyperlipemia] - Increased VLDL production and Decreased elimination - ↑ VLDL (↑ Cholesterol & TGs)

- **Type-5** [Endogenous Hypertriglyceridemia] – carbohydrate induced (DM, Alcohol) - ↑ VLDL (↑ TGs) but **Normal Cholesterol**

- **Fragile X-Syndrome:**
- **CGG** repeat sequence
- Mental retardation, **enlarge testis**, prominent jaw, large ears

- **Ehlers-Danlos Syndrome :**
- **defect in type-I & type-III collagen synthesis** and structure
- Hypermobile joints, **Aortic dissection** (MCC of death), poor wound healing

- **Osteogenesis Imperfecta :**
- **Blue sclera**, brittle bones
- **Defective synthesis of type-I collagen**

- **Albinism :** deficiencies of **tyrosine hydroxylase** (copper dependent tyrosinase) – <u>blocking production of melanin from aromatic AA tyrosine</u> – white hair, pink irises, very pale skin, and a history of burning easily when exposed to the sun – Patients are at **increase risk of Squamous cell CA and Melanoma**

* **Miscellaneous:**

- Histidine is the only AA with good buffering capacity at physiologic pH.

* Fat free diet – **decrease Prostaglandins** (essential FA products)

- Km = **[S] concentration** at which half Vmax produced. S = substrate
  Km – measure affinity of the enzyme
  Low Km (high affinity) – less substrate require
  High Km (low affinity) – more substrate require
  Competitive inhibitors – Km-↑, **Vmax – no effect**
  Non-competitive inhibitors – **Km – no effect**, Vmax - ↓

CELL BIOLOGY

- Replication: DNA synthesis
- Transcription: RNA synthesis
- Translation: Protein synthesis

- DNA: Deoxyribonucleic acid
- RNA: Ribonucleic acid

Basic Concepts

Nucleic acid = Chain of nucleotides
Nucleotides = Nitrogenous base + Sugar + Phosphate
Nucleosides = Nitrogenous base + Sugar

DNA	RNA
- **2 strands** of chain of nucleotides	- **Single strand** of chain of nucleotides
- **Deoxyribose** sugar [doesn't contain –OH group at 2nd position]	- **Ribose** sugar
- Complementary base to **A is T**	- Complementary base to **A is U**

Nitrogenous Bases: A, C, G, T, U
Purines: 2 rings [A, G] [Short name 2 rings]
Pyrimidines: 1 ring [C, T, U] [Long name 1 ring]
Base pairing: A-T [DNA], A-U [RNA], G-C [Both DNA & RNA]

A-T / A-U – **double** bond, G-C – **triple** bond

A = Adenine
C = Cytosine
G = Guanosine
T = Thymine

A is identified by NH3 group

Uracil (U) is a precursor of both C & T [C contains –NH2 & T contains –CH3]
Amination of U → C [Deamination of C gives U]
Methylation of U → T [Demethylation of T gives U]

Deamination of A & G gives Hypoxanthine & Xanthine respectively

Because of base pairing, **amount of purines & pyrimidines are same in both DNA & RNA** therefore amount of A = amount of T [DNA], amount of A = amount of U [RNA] and amount of G = amount of C

Ribose Sugar – contain –OH group at 2nd position
Deoxyribose Sugar – doesn't contain –OH group at 2nd position

RNA is **anti-parallel & complementary** to DNA **template strand**; RNA is **identical** to DNA **coding strand** (except U substitutes for T in RNA)

Sequences are always specified as 5' → 3'

S.S.Patel , M.D.

- Denaturation occurs by heat & Renaturation occurs by cooling
- Supercoiling – more twisting
  - DNA gyrase (topoisomerase-2) – negative supercoiling (remove positive)
  - Topoisomerase-1 – positive supercoiling (remove negative)
- In nature, DNA remains in a slight negative supercoiling
- Histone Proteins (Lysine & Arginine) – +ve charged, help condensing DNA
- **core histones** – H2A, H2B, H3 and H4
- **linker histones** – **H1** and H5
- Without H1 – (10 nm fibers) sensitive to Endonucleases [10 nm fibers are first fibers to destroyed in apoptosis]
- Basic P^H – decrease Histone activity – fibers susceptible to endonucleases

- **DNA Synthesis**: DNA is double stranded structure. First we need something to start the process and then we need something to separate it then need something to maintain the process and at the end we need something to end the process. During this process we need something which make sure process is going smoothly without mutations.
- **DNA synthesis always occur in 5'→ 3'** direction and newly synthesize strand is anti-parallel & complementary to template strand so **template strand would be 3'→ 5' direction**
- **To start the process** – Protein binds to DnaA box in Prokaryote (Pro)
- **Separation of DNA double strands** – Helicase [DnaB protein]
- **To continue process** – need **SSB protein** (single strand binding protein) which prevent reannealing (rejoining of strands), **DNA gyrase** is needed to relieves the stress by creating negative supercoiling, need **Primase & RNA polymerase** to prime each DNA template to begin synthesis
- **Maintaining the process** – DNA is synthesized in two forms. Continuous [**Leading strand**] & Short fragment forms [**Lagging strand**]; both forms require DNA polymerase 3. Short fragments are called **Okazaki fragments**. After beginning of synthesis, RNA primers are removed by **DNA polymerase 1 (exonuclease)**. Short fragments are joined by **Ligase**.
- **Checking mutations** – In bacteria, **all three DNA polymerases** (I, II, and III) have the ability to proofread, using **3'→ 5' exonuclease activity**.
- **Termination** – Because bacteria have circular chromosomes, termination of replication occurs when the two replication forks meet each other on the opposite end of the parental chromosome.
- **DNA synthesis in Eukaryotes**: Process occurs same way as above with following differences
- DNA replication in eukaryotes occurs only in the S phase of the cell cycle. However, pre-initiation occurs in the G1 phase.
- The G1/S checkpoint (or restriction checkpoint) regulates whether eukaryotic cells enter the process of DNA replication and subsequent division. Cells which do not proceed through this checkpoint are quiescent in the "G0" stage and do not replicate their DNA.
- Synthesis of leading strand occurs by DNA polymerase δ
- Synthesis of lagging strand occurs by DNA polymerase α
- In eukaryotes only the polymerases that deal with the elongation (γ, δ and ε) have proofreading ability (**3'→ 5' exonuclease activity**)

- **Termination** – Because eukaryotes have linear chromosomes, DNA replication often fails to synthesize to the very end of the chromosomes (telomeres), resulting in telomere shortening.
- Within the germ cell line, which passes DNA to the next generation, the enzyme telomerase extends the repetitive sequences of the telomere region to prevent degradation. **Telomerase can become mistakenly active in <u>somatic cells</u>, sometimes <u>leading to cancer formation</u>**.
- **Telomerase** is a **reverse transcriptase enzyme** that carries its own RNA molecule, which is used as a template when it elongates telomeres.

Important Concepts can be asked from replication
Direction of synthesis, Direction of templates, Function of SSB, Function of DNA gyrase, Proof reading enzymes and its direction, Telomeres & its importance

---

- **Ribosomes:** 70s (30s & 50s) in Pro; 80s (40s & 60s) in Eu
- **tRNA:** Acceptor arm – carry AA [amino acid]; Anti-codon arm – anti-codon complementary & anti-parallel to codon in mRNA.
- **mRNA:** carry coded information for protein synthesis
- **rRNA:** central component of the ribosome, provide a mechanism for decoding mRNA into amino acids and to interact with the tRNA during translation by providing peptidyl transferase activity.
- **snRNA (small nuclear RNA):** participate in splicing mRNA (remove introns)
- **RNA:** tRNA – smallest species; mRNA & hnRNA – largest species. On electrophoresis – smallest species migrate farthest.

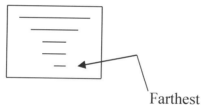

Farthest

- <u>**RNA Synthesis**</u>: **RNA synthesis always occur in 5'→ 3'** direction and newly synthesize strand is anti-parallel & complementary to template strand so **template strand would be 3'→ 5' direction**
- Only one DNA strand is act as template (Both strands used in DNA synthesis)
- RNA synthesis **doesn't require primers**
- It **occurs in cytoplasm in prokaryote** and **in nucleus in eukaryote**
- mRNA is **not modified in prokaryote** but mRNA is **modified** through RNA splicing, 5' end capping, and the addition of a polyA tail **in eukaryotes**
- Transcription is divided into **5 stages**: pre-initiation, initiation, promoter clearance, elongation and termination
- **Pre-initiation**: RNA polymerase with other cofactors simply binds to DNA to initiate process. Proximal (core) Promoters [TATA promoters] are found around -30 bp to the start site of transcription.
- **Initiation**: **In prokaryote**, <u>a sigma factor</u> (number 70) that helps in finding the appropriate -35 and -10 base pairs downstream of promoter sequences to initiate

transcription. **In eukaryotes**, transcription factors mediate the binding of RNA polymerase and the initiation of transcription.

- RNA polymerase in Prokaryotes: a core enzyme consisting of 5 subunits [2 α subunits, 1 β subunit, 1 β' subunit, and 1 ω subunit]
- RNA polymerase in Eukaryotes: **RNA polymerase I** synthesizes a pre-rRNA 45S, which matures into 28S, 18S and 5.8S rRNA which will form the major RNA sections of the ribosome. **RNA polymerase II** synthesizes precursors of mRNA and most snRNA. **RNA polymerase III** synthesizes tRNA, rRNA 5S found in the nucleus and cytosol.
- **Promoter clearance**: RNA polymerase clears promoter. It is an ATP dependent process
- **Elongation**: RNA polymerase traverses the template strand to create an RNA copy. It produces an exact copy of the coding strand (except that thymine is replaced with uracil, and the nucleotides are composed of a ribose sugar)
- **Termination**: In Prokaryotes: **Rho-independent transcription termination**, RNA transcription stops when the newly synthesized RNA molecule forms a G-C rich hairpin loop, followed by a run of U's, which makes it detach from the DNA template. **"Rho-dependent" type of termination**, a protein factor called "Rho" destabilizes the interaction between the template and the mRNA, thus releasing the newly synthesized mRNA from the elongation complex. In Eukaryote: It is **less well understood**. It involves cleavage of the new transcript, followed by template-independent addition of polyA at its new 3' end, in a process called polyadenylation.
- **Modification in Eukaryotes**: RNA splicing [in which introns are removed and exons are joined; splicing is done in a series of reactions which are catalyzed by the spliceosome, a complex of small nuclear ribonucleoproteins (snRNP)], 5' cap (7-methyguanine), 3' cap (poly-A sequence)

Important concepts can be asked from transcription
Sigma & Transcription factor, Different RNA polymerase in eukaryotes, Modification in eukaryote

---

- **Synthesis of Protein**: Occurs in **cytoplasm** where ribosomes are located
- Same as replication and transcription, Translation proceeds in four phases: activation, initiation, elongation and termination

---

Basic Concepts
- The **ribosome** consists of **three sites**: the **A site**, the **P site**, and the **E site**. The A site is the point of entry for the aminoacyl tRNA (except for the first aminoacyl tRNA, fMet-tRNA$_f^{Met}$, which enters at the P site). The P site is where the peptidyl tRNA is formed in the ribosome. The E site which is the exit site for the tRNA after it gives its amino acid to the growing peptide chain.
- **Prokaryotic Initiation Factors (IF)**: IF1 blocks the A site to insure that the fMet-tRNA can bind only to the P site and that no other aminoacyl-tRNA can bind in the A site during initiation, while IF3 blocks the E site and prevents the two subunits from associating. IF2 is binds fmet-tRNA$_f^{Met}$ and helps its binding with the small ribosomal subunit.

- **Eukaryotic Initiation Factors (eIF):** There are many different eIF but eIF2 is the most important one. The eIF2 is a GTP-binding protein responsible for bringing the initiator tRNA to the P-site of the pre-initiation complex. It has **specificity for** the methionine-charged **initiator tRNA**, which is distinct from other methionine-charged tRNAs specific for elongation of the polypeptide chain. Once it has placed the initiator tRNA on the AUG start codon in the P-site, it hydrolyzes GTP into GDP, and dissociates. This signals the beginning of elongation.
- **Start codon:** AUG [Methionine]
- **Stop codon:** UAG, UGA, UAA
- **Shine-Dalgarno sequence (AGGAGG):** It exists in **Prokaryotic only**. It is **a ribosomal binding site** generally located 6-7 nucleotides upstream of the start codon AUG **on mRNA**. The complementary sequence (**CCUCCU**), is called the **anti-Shine-Dalgarno sequence** and is **located at the 3' end of the 16S rRNA** of small 30s ribosomal subunit. When the Shine-Dalgarno sequence and the anti-Shine-Dalgarno sequence pair, **initiation begins**.
- In Eukaryotic, when 40s subunit of ribosome binds to 5' cap on mRNA through initiation factors, **initiation begins**.
- **Elongation in both prokaryote & eukaryote (eEF2):** Once initiator tRNA with methionine (formyl-methionine in prokaryote) is inserted at P-site and large ribosomal subunit join the complex, A-site open and elongation begins. So when new amino acid (AA) attached with tRNA is inserted to A-site, tRNA attached to AA in P-site released tRNA and form peptide bond with newly added AA in A-site. This process is catalyzed by Peptidyltrasferase enzyme, an activity intrinsic to the 23S ribosomal RNA in the 50S ribosomal subunit. A-site AA still has its tRNA and new peptide bond. When new AA is come to join A-site amino acid, tRNA of A-site amino acid release and peptide bond form b/w A-site AA and newly came AA. This process is going on until it reaches to stop codon. **Translocation** is the process in which tRNA is moved to E-site for exit. This requires **GTP**
- **Termination in Both:** Once stop codon comes in way of elongation process, termination of translation occurs and releasing factors release newly formed peptide chain.
- **Post-translational modification:** It occurs **only in Eukaryote**. This may include the formation of disulfide bridges or **attachment** of any of a number of biochemical functional groups, such as acetate, phosphate, various lipids (**Dolichol phosphate**) **and** carbohydrates (**Phosphorylation of mannose in Golgi apparatus**).
- When AA is attached to tRNA, it is called "charged" tRNA. It consumes 2 ATP. When AA is inserted to A or P sites, it consumes 2 GTP. So **it requires 4 high energy phosphate bonds to insert one AA**
- Puromycin (similar to the tyrosinyl aminoacyl-tRNA) binds to the ribosomal A site and participates in peptide bond formation, producing peptidyl-puromycin. However, it does not engage in translocation and quickly dissociates from the ribosome causing a premature termination of polypeptide synthesis.
- Streptomycin causes misreading of the genetic code in bacteria and inhibits initiation by binding to the 30s ribosomal subunit
- Tetracyclines block the A site on the ribosome, preventing the binding of aminoacyl tRNA

- Chloramphenicol blocks the peptidyl transfer step of elongation on the 50s ribosomal subunit
- Macrolides and Lincosamides bind to the 50s ribosomal subunits inhibiting the Peptidyltrasferase reaction or translocation or both
- **Important concepts from translation can be asked in exam:** When do initiations occur in both? How many phosphate bonds require in the process of inserting one AA? Mechanism of action of different antibiotics on translation? Which factor is inhibited by pseudomonas & diphtheria? [Ans: eEF2]

- **DNA repair:**
- **Thymine Dimers:** due to UV radiation; Excision endonucleases recognize & excise it. (This enzyme is deficient in Xeroderma Pigmentosa) DNA Polymerase & Ligase are repair enzymes.
- **Mismatched Bases:** deficiency in the ability to repair mismatched base pairs in DNA leads to Hereditary Non-Polyposis Colorectal Cancer (HNPCC)

- **Regulation of Gene Expression:**

- **Prokaryote:** Lactose Operon; Attenuation

- **Lactose Operon:**
- Lactose: induce gene expression for lactose metabolism by preventing the repressor protein binding to operator sequence
- Glucose: repress gene expression for lactose metabolism by decreasing cAMP in the cell and thus preventing cAMP dependent activator binding to CAP site (cAMP dependent Activator Protein site).
- In the absence of lactose, repression protein binds to operator protein & prevents gene expression.

- **Attenuation**: Premature termination of transcription (not possible in Eukaryote b/c in eukaryote, transcription and translation not occur simultaneously. Both transcription & translation are independent events in Eu)
- High Histidine: rho-independent terminator to form; RNAP stops transcription.
- Low Histidine: prevent terminator formation; RNAP continues transcription & transcription of message produce all enzymes require for Histidine biosynthesis.

- **Eukaryote:** (regulation of gene expression)
  - Upstream Promoter Elements:
    - TATA box – (-25) general transcription factor (TFIID) binds here
    - GC rich – SP-1 binds here
    - CCAAT box – (-75) NF-1 binds here
  - Enhancers: (response elements) – activator proteins bind here.
  - Silencers: repressor proteins bind here.
  - Transcription factors:
    - DNA binding domain:
      Zinc fingers (steroid hormone receptors)

Leucine Zippers (cAMP dependent transcription factors)
Helix-turn-helix (Homeodomain protein)
- ▪ Activation Domain:
    1. Binds to other transcription factors
    2. Recruit chromatin modifying proteins such as histone acetylase (favor gene expression) <u>or</u> deacetylase (favor inactivate chromatin)
- ▪ <u>Homeodomain Proteins</u>**:** control embryonic gene expression & are regulated by Homeobox (HOX) / homeotic gene & paired box (PAX) gene.

- ▪ **<u>Waardenburg - Klein Syndrome:</u>**
- • Mutation in PAX3 gene
- • Dystonia Canthorum (Lat displacement of inner corner of eye)
- • Pigmentary abnormality
- • Congenital Deafness, defects in structures arising from the neural crest

- ❖ **Neucleolus:** rRNA synthesis & then transport them to Ribosome in cytoplasm

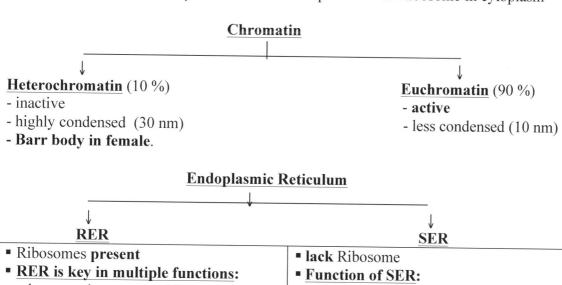

Chromatin

Heterochromatin (10 %)
- inactive
- highly condensed (30 nm)
- **Barr body in female**.

Euchromatin (90 %)
- **active**
- less condensed (10 nm)

Endoplasmic Reticulum

RER	**SER**

▪ Ribosomes **present**
▪ **RER is key in multiple functions:**
  – lysosomal enzymes with a mannose-6-phosphate marker added in the *cis*-Golgi network
  – Secreted proteins
  – integral membrane proteins
  – N-linked glycosylation
▪ **Abundant RER in neuron cell body** stains intensely with basic dyes is referred to as **Nissl substance**
	▪ **lack** Ribosome
	▪ **Function of SER:**
	  – lipid & steroid synthesis
	  – Gluconeogenesis via G-6-Phosphatase
	  – **Detoxification**
	  – regulation of calcium concentration

- ▪ **<u>Golgi Apparatus:</u>**
- - Cis face – RER
- - Trans face – Plasma membrane
- - **Post-translational modification**

- **Peroxisome:** contain enzyme which produce H_2O_2 which is degraded by enzyme catalase – detoxification & long chain FA (fatty acid) metabolism – degradation of ethanol to acetaldehyde occurs in peroxisome & SER

- **Mitochondria:**
  - Outer membrane – highly permeable
  - Inner membrane – impermeable
    - Inner membrane compartmentalized into numerous **cristae**, which expand the surface area of the inner mitochondrial membrane – enhance its ability to produce ATP
  - Matrix – the space enclosed by inner membrane – contains a highly-concentrated mixture of hundreds of enzymes

* **Cytoskeleton:** Microtubule, Intermediate filaments & Microfilaments
- Microtubule: polymers of α- and β-tubulin dimers
  - involved in many cellular processes including mitosis, cytokinesis, and vesicular transport (anterograde & retrograde)
- Intermediate filaments:
  - **V**imentins – being the common structural support of many cells (endothelial cells, **V**ascular smooth muscle, fibroblast, chondroblast)
  - Keratin – found in skin cells, hair and nails
  - Neurofilaments of neural cells
  - Lamin – giving structural support to the nuclear envelope
- Microfilaments:
  - Composed of Actin filaments (thinnest filaments of the cytoskeleton)
  - responsible for resisting tension and maintaining cellular shape
  - participation in some cell-to-cell or cell-to-matrix junctions
  - essential to transduction
  - along with myosin in muscle contraction

- **Gap junction:** area of communication b/w adjacent cells
  - directly connects the cytoplasm of two cells, which allows various molecules and ions to pass freely between cells
  - One gap junction is composed of two connexons (or hemichannels) which connect across the intercellular space

- **Cilia:** two types of cilia: motile cilia [constantly beat in a single direction] and non-motile or primary cilia, which typically serve as sensory organelles
  - two central microtubule surrounded by nine microtubule
  - Nine microtubule connect each other with **Nexin link**
  - **Dynein arm** is attached to each **A** sub-tubule
  - Dynein arm binds to ATP

- **Hemidesmosomes** anchor epithelial cell to basement membranes.
- **Hydrophobic interactions** are responsible for retaining integral membrane proteins within cell membranes (lipid bilayer)

- **Receptors in cAMP & PIP2 pathways,** All have characteristic 7-helix membrane spanning domains.
- **Trimeric G protein** include Gi, Gs, Gq & Gt, all have 7-helix membrane spanning structure.
- **Zinc finger receptors** – Steroids, Thyroxine, Vit-A, Vit-D.

- **I-cell Disease (Mucoliposis):** A **deficiency in N- acetylglucosamine Phosphotransferase** results in I- cell disease in which whole family of enzyme is sent to the wrong destination.
  - **Lysosomes missing** the **hydrolase enzyme** which normally degrade glycoconjugates
  - This enzyme is <u>present in other body fluid & plasma in I-cell disease.</u>
  - The **absence of the mannose-6-phosphate on the hydrolase** results in their secretion into other body fluids rather than their incorporation in lysosomes.
  - Phosphorylation of mannose done by N- acetylglucosamine Phosphotransferase.
  - I- cell disease is characterized by **huge inclusion bodies in cells**
  - <u>Symptoms of I-cell disease</u> : skeletal abnormality , coarse features , mental retardation, restricted joint movement

- **Fabry's Disease:** Sphingolipidosis in which ceremidetrihexoside accumulate in cells leading to renal failure, Telangiectasia and skin rashes. Alfa-galactoside A (lysosomal enzyme) is deficient. **X-linked**

- **Hunter's Disease:** (mucopolysaccharidosis type-2) – Iduronate sulfate sulfatase deficiency – dermatan & heparin sulfate accumulate in cells. **X-linked**

- **Hurler Disease, Scheie Disease, Hurler/Scheie Disease:** (mucopolysaccharidosis type-1) – Alfa-L-iduronidase deficiency
  Severe symptoms – <u>Hurler's Disease</u>
  Normal intelligence & who live into Adult life – <u>Scheie Disease</u>
  Normal intelligence but severe symptoms – <u>Hurler/Scheie Disease</u>
  Characterized by accumulation of **Dermatan & heparin sulfate in cells**
  Autosomal Recessive

- **Chediak-Higashi Syndrome: defect in microtubule polymerization** – Delayed fusion of phagosomes with lysosomes in leucocytes thus preventing phagocytosis of bacteria

- **Cilium Diseases:** a defect of the primary cilium in the renal tube cells can lead to polycystic kidney disease (PKD) – Lack of functional cilia in Fallopian tubes can cause ectopic pregnancy – **Kartagener's syndrome** (Primary Ciliary Dyskinesia, Immotile cilia syndrome)**:** genetic defect in dynein arm – situs inversus, recurrent sinusitis

GENETIC DISEASES

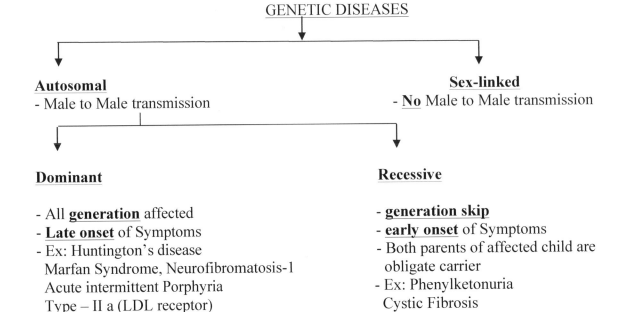

Autosomal
- Male to Male transmission

Sex-linked
- **No** Male to Male transmission

Dominant

- All **generation** affected
- **Late onset** of Symptoms
- Ex: Huntington's disease
  Marfan Syndrome, Neurofibromatosis-1
  Acute intermittent Porphyria
  Type – II a (LDL receptor)

Recessive

- **generation skip**
- **early onset** of Symptoms
- Both parents of affected child are
  obligate carrier
- Ex: Phenylketonuria
  Cystic Fibrosis
  Tay Sachs
  Pyruvate Kinase deficiency

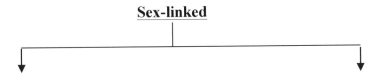

Sex-linked

X – linked Dominant

- Either sex can be affected
- Fragile X Syndrome

X – linked Recessive

- **Only males** affected
- G-6-PD
- Lesch Nyhan
- Duchenne Mussculodystrophy
- Hemophilia A & B
- Fabry's Disease

- • **Mitochondrial Inheritance:** Sperm lost its tail during fertilization which contain
  mitochondria that's why mitochondrial disease inherited **only maternally**
- - **All offspring of an affected females** are affected
- - Mitochondrial genes code for – components of ETC & oxidative phosphorylation, some
  mitochondrial t-RNA molecules.
- - Present as myopathies & neuropathies (**Laber's optic neuropathies**)

- In the exam, we get <u>pedigree chart</u> **or** <u>description of disease</u> with male or female or both are affected and we have to identify Autosomal / sex-linked recessive or dominant diseases. They give a list of diseases and we have to pick only 1 correct answer. *First* look at the chart <u>or</u> description of question that *who is transmitting disease?* Male (black square) / Female (black circle) / Carrier (half black & half white); **If Affected male is transmit disease to his son then we are dealing with Autosomal diseases**; If Affected male is **not** transmitting disease to his son then we are dealing with Sex-linked diseases. **If affected mother is transmitted disease to <u>all</u> of her offspring then we are dealing with Mitochondrial Inheritance.** *Now look at generation;* **if all generation affected** then Dominant Disease; **if generation skips** then Recessive Disease. Now you just need to remember name of disease according to their transmission (Autosomal / Sex-linked recessive or dominant). So now we know how to pick disease from the given list. Try to memorize diseases name I have written in the chart above because those are the most commonly asked diseases on the exam.

- **<u>Hardy-Weinberg Rule</u>:** $P^2 + 2pq + q^2 = 1$

  - p^2 = Frequency of Homozygote Dominant in population
  - q^2 = Frequency of Homozygote recessive in population
  - $2pq$ = Frequency of Homozygote individual
  - p = gene frequency
  - q = frequency of disease allele

■ MUTATIONS:

- **Point Mutation:** Point mutations that **occur within the protein coding region** of a gene **by change in base** may be **classified into three kinds**, depending upon what the new codon codes for
  - **Silent mutations:** in which new codon code for the same amino acid
  - **Mis-sense mutations:** in which new codon code for a different amino acid. <u>Example</u>: Sickle cell disease
  - **Non-sense mutations:** in which new codon code for a stop leads to premature termination of the protein
- **Insertions:** add one or more extra nucleotides into the DNA. Insertions in the coding region of a gene may **alter splicing of the mRNA** (splice site mutation), or cause **a shift in the reading frame** (frame shift), both of which can significantly alter the gene product. <u>Examples</u> of splice site mutation are beta thalasemia, Gaucher's disease, Tay Sachs
- **Deletions:** remove one or more nucleotides from the DNA. Like insertions, these mutations can alter the reading frame of the gene.

- **Large Segment Deletion:** unequal crossover in meiosis (**Sex-link** disorders) – Cri-du–chat, $\propto$ - thalasemia

- **Triplet Repeat Expansion:** expansion in coding regions cause protein product to be longer than normal and unstable

- Huntington's disease, Fragile X Syndrome
- Disease often **shows anticipation** in pedigree

---

* **Southern Blot Test:** Analyzed DNA
- It uses a <u>hybridization probe</u> – a single DNA fragment with a specific sequence whose presence in the target DNA is to be determined
- Analyses are based on RELP (Restriction Fragment length Polymorphism)
- **Mechanism:** Mutation in restriction site (the recognition sites for restriction endonucleases) leads to increase in fragment size
- **Steps:** Restriction endonucleases are used to cut high-molecular-weight DNA strands into smaller fragments. In normal DNA, it cuts normal size fragments but in mutated DNA it cuts larger fragments. These fragments are then placed on electrophoresis gel. These fragments are then identified by hybridization probe.
- By detecting abnormal fragments using hybridization probe, we can tell which family member is normal and which is carrier. Presence of two normal fragments mean normal person, presence of one normal and one large fragment means carrier.

* **Western Blot Test:** Analyzed **protein**
- ^{125}I (or) Enzyme linked antibody is used as probe
- Eg: Confirmation of HIV

* **Northern Blot Test:** Analyzed **RNA** extracted from tissue
- use to determine which gene is expressed
- ^{32}p DNA probe is used
- Eg: expression of enzyme in different tissues

* **PCR:** It is a technique by which DNA polymerase is used to amplify a piece of DNA
- Heat-Stable DNA Polymerase (Taq Polymerase) & Deoxynucleoside triphosphates (dNTPs) from which the DNA polymerases synthesizes a new DNA strand
- Detection of DNA by expected size (gel electrophoresis) or by sequence (probing a dot blot)
- Flanking primers (**on either sides**) complementary to the either $5'$ or $3'$ regions

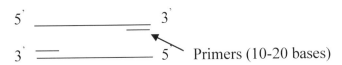

- **When mutation is large** (repeat sequences as in Huntington, myotonic Dystrophies) use **southern blot** to detect sequences by probe.

- **Gene Deletion:** detected by two methods.
  - Southern blot → use probe from cDNA / genomic library
  - PCR → using primers specific for genes

S.S.Patel , M.D.

- **Fluorescence Activated cell sorting (FACS):** useful for determining the stage of development (or) activation of cell but **not** tell anything about DNA

- **Cystic Fibrosis**: Mutation affects post-translational modification (folding of AA chain into a stable structure)

- **Palindromes: DNA sequences** recognized by restrictive endonucleases
- palindrome is a base sequence in which the sequence of one strand read in 5´→3´ is the same as the opposite strand read in 5´→3'

- **Genomic Libraries:** made from nuclear DNA, cleaved by restriction endonucleases
- It contains all types of sequence found in genome (Exon, intron, promoter, enhancer, spacer DNA, etc)
- **cDNA Libraries:** derived by isolating mRNA from a tissue expressing the gene
- **Reverse transcriptase** is used to prepare complementory DNA (cDNA) using the mRNA as a template
- Contain **only exons** (coding sequence) [**No** introns]

* **Vectors for recombinant DNA & Cloning:**

- **Plasmid pBR 322:** Restriction site, Replication origin, **Resistance to antibiotics**
- **Expression Vectors:** to produce protein; also require promoter & shine-Dalgarno sequence
- cDNA is usually cloned into expression vector b/c **no** introns in cDNA

- **Multi factorial inheritance** is non-mendelian inheritance pattern. Characteristics that exhibit broad range of values like height, eye color, etc. inherited in this manner

- **Skewed X inactivation:** It means nonrandom x inactivation. In women, normally one x chromosome is inactivate randomly. When x inactivation is nonrandom and towards normal chromosome means normal chromosome becomes inactive, the mutant chromosome express and show symptoms. *In recessive disease*, normally women are carrier and do not express symptoms but in skewed inactivation, sometimes normal x chromosome inactivates and mutant remain active and show symptoms.

Microbiology

* **Viruses:**

1. Give name of RNA & DNA viruses

(−) RNA viruses	**(+) RNA viruses**	**DNA viruses**
- Paramyxovirus	- Calcivirus	- Herpes virus
- Orthomyxovirus	- Picornavirus	- Hep B virus
- Rhabdovirus	- Flavivirus	- Papova virus
- Filovirus	- Togavirus	- Parvovirus
- Bunyavirus	- Coronavirus	- Poxvirus
- Arenavirus	- Retrovirus (HIV)	- Adénovirus
- Reovirus		
- Delta virus		

2. How to identify different viruses

- Viruses are identified by <u>Shape</u>, <u>envelope/non-envelope</u>, <u>ds/ss nucleic acid (DNA/RNA)</u>, <u>nucleic acid shape (circular/linear)</u>

- <u>Shape</u>: Only 2 shape to remember: Icosahedral & Helical. **(+) RNA virus:** All (+) sense RNA viruses are **Icosahedral shaped <u>except</u>** corona virus which is Helical shaped. **(−) RNA viruses:** All (−) sense RNA viruses are **Helical shaped <u>except</u>** Reovirus which is icosahedral shaped. **DNA viruses:** All DNA viruses are Icosahedral **<u>except</u>** Pox virus which is brick shaped "complex"

- <u>Envelop / Non-envelop</u>: **RNA viruses:** All RNA viruses are enveloped except Reovirus [(−) RNA], Picorna & Calcivirus [(+) RNA]; **DNA viruses:** Herpes family, Hep B, and Poxvirus are enveloped (all other are non-enveloped)

- <u>ds / ss nucleic acid</u>: **RNA viruses:** All RNA viruses are **single stranded <u>except</u>** Reovirus. **DNA viruses:** All DNA viruses have ds DNA **<u>except</u>** Parvovirus which has ss DNA

- <u>Nucleic acid shape</u>: **RNA viruses:** All RNA viruses have LINEAR nucleic acid **<u>except</u>** Bunyavirus & Arenavirus. These two have CIRCULAR nucleic acid. **DNA viruses:** All DNA viruses have LINEAR nucleic acid **<u>except</u>** Hepatitis B & Papova (HPV). These two have CIRCULAR nucleic acid.

- In exam, first we need to recognize virus from symptoms, then we need to screen all answer and apply all of above factors (one by one) to avoid "trap" in answers!

Q-1   A mother brought her 1 yr old child with c/o diarrhea and dehydration. Which of the following is the most likely structure of the causative virus?
a) **single strand (+) RNA virus**
b) double strand (+) RNA virus
c) single strand DNA virus
d) double strand DNA virus
e) single strand (-) RNA virus

Q-2   A child was sent home from day care center because of development of flu like symptoms. After few days, he developed bright red facial rash which looks like "slapped cheek" appearance. Which of the following is the most likely structure of the causative virus?

---

a) single strand (+) RNA virus
b) double strand (+) RNA virus
c) **single strand DNA virus**
d) double strand DNA virus
e) single strand (-) RNA virus

Q-3 A 40 yo IV drug abuser presented to the hospital with c/o fever, malaise and jaundice. Blood work showed elevated LFT consistent with viral hepatitis. Which of the following is the most likely structure of the causative virus?
a) single strand (+) RNA virus with circular nucleic acid
b) double strand (-) RNA virus with linear nucleic acid
c) **double strand DNA virus with circular nucleic acid**
d) single strand DNA virus with circular nucleic acid

Q-4 A mother bring her 6 yo child to your office for several lesions on his body. On examination, lesions appear to be flash colored papules with central umbilication. Which of the following is the most likely structure of the causative virus?
a) single strand enveloped (+) RNA virus
b) double strand non-enveloped (-) RNA virus
c) **double stranded enveloped DNA virus**
d) double stranded non-enveloped DNA virus

Q-5 A 35 yo male came in with c/o painful swallowing. His social history is significant for multiple sexual partners. Lab showed low CD4 counts. Which of the following is the most likely structure of the causative virus?
a) **single strand icosahedral shaped (+) RNA virus**
b) double strand helical shaped (+) RNA virus
c) single stranded icosahedral shaped DNA virus
d) double stranded helical shaped DNA virus

- In all five questions, we first identify the causative virus by sign and symptoms. Then we need to screen all options to see what they have asked. Then apply all 4 factors: Shape, Envelope/Non-envelope, Nucleic acid and Nucleic acid shape. I have tried to include all 4 factors in different ways these 5 questions. Viruses are as follow: Reovirus, Parvovirus, Hep B, Pox virus and HIV
- This is how they present the question and ask about following points by giving 4/5 different but very similar options: difference b/w replication of DNA&RNA viruses, positive & negative sense RNA virus replication, replication site

3. What is the difference b/w positive sense and negative sense RNA viruses?
- Positive sense RNA: **Can use their genome directly as if it were mRNA**
- Negative sense RNA: **Needs to convert their genome into positive sense by RNA-dependent RNA polymerase**
- Replication: Positive sense mRNA – Protein synthesis – forms new virion
- Retrovirus (HIV): Use DNA intermediates to replicate. **Reverse transcriptase** converts the viral RNA into a complementary strand of DNA, which is copied to produce a double stranded molecule of viral DNA. After this DNA is integrated, expression of the encoded genes may lead the formation of new virions

4. Which is the site of viral replication?
- **DNA viruses:** All replicate in nucleus **except** Pox virus which replicate in cytoplasm
- **RNA viruses:** All replicate in cytoplasm **except** HIV & Influenza which replicate in nucleus

5. How replications in DNA viruses occur?
- Most DNA viruses use the host cell's enzymes to synthesize their DNA and other proteins
- **Hep B virus** has its own DNA polymerase with **reverse transcriptase activity** which synthesizes RNA intermediate that is then used to make the genomic DNA
- **Replication:** DNA – mRNA – Protein synthesis – forms new virion

---

Q: A 35 yo M came in with c/o shortness of breath, chest pain started 2 days ago. The pain relieved on leaning forward. The patient was feeling fine before that. His past medical history is not significant. On further inquiry you found that the patient had cold two weeks ago. Which of following is true about replication of causative virus?
a) use RNA-dependent RNA polymerase to convert their genome into (+) sense RNA
b) **use their genome directly as mRNA and then use host cell enzymes**
c) use reverse transcriptase to convert viral RNA to DNA and then use host cell enzymes
d) use host cell enzyme to synthesize their DNA and other protein
e) use reverse transcriptase to convert DNA to RNA and then use host cell enzymes

In this example, I have included all 5 possible options for viral replication according to + & - sense RNA virus replication, HIV replication, Hep B replication and DNA virus replication. The virus in this example is coxsackie A virus, (+) sense RNA virus.

Life cycle of virus: Attachment → Penetration (endocytosis/fusion) → Replication, Protein synthesis and assembly of viral proteins & viral genome replication → released from cell (lysis)

---

6. What is an importance of segmented viruses?
- Segmented viruses are responsible for **pandemics**. Genetic shift (Reassortment) is responsible for pandemics which only seen in segmented viruses
- Reovirus (Rotavirus), Orthomyxovirus (**influenza virus**), Bunyavirus, Arenavirus

---

Q: A 60 yo M presented to your clinic during winter season with high grade fever, muscle ache, sore throat, cough, headache and malaise for 2 days. You told the patient that it is flu and you asked the patient to take Tylenol as needed. The patient got better in 3 days. Which of the following factor make this virus responsible for pandemics?
a) **genetic shift**
b) genetic drift
c) lack of immunity
d) fomite transmission

The same way they can present clinical scenario for rotavirus, bunyavirus or arenavirus

---

7. Which DNA virus has **self coded envelope**?
- Only Pox virus

8. Give name of an important **viruses in Calcivirus family**
- Hep E, Norwalk

9. Give name of an important **viruses in Flavivirus family**
- Hep C, Dengue virus, Yellow fever virus

10. Give name of an important **viruses in Paramyxovirus family**
- Measles, Mumps, Respiratory syncytial virus and Parainfluenza

11. Give name of an important viruses in Picornavirus family
- **Hep A**, Enterovirus (Polio virus, **Coxsackie A** & Echo), Rhinovirus

12. Give name of an **important viruses in Herpes family**
- HSV, VZ, EBV, CMV, HHV-8

13. "Clue words" to diagnose important viruses from <u>inclusion bodies</u>
* **Intracytoplasmic**
  - Rabies (Negri bodies)
  - Poxvirus (Guarnieri – acidophilic)
  - **HPV (<u>Perinuclear</u> – <u>koilocytic cells on pap smear</u>)**
  - **Chlamydia (<u>elementary body</u> – <u>infective form</u>, <u>Iodine stain</u>)**

* **<u>Intranuclear</u>**
- **Herpes (Cowdry's body)**

* **<u>Both Intracytoplasmic & Intranuclear inclusion bodies:</u>**
- **CMV (<u>Owl's eye inclusions</u>)**

Q: A 30 yo M with h/o HIV presented with several lesions on his body. On examination, lesions appear to be flash colored papules with **central umbilication**. Which of the following inclusion bodies will you see?
a) Negri body
b) **Guarnieri body**
c) cowdry's body
d) owl's eye inclusion body

Q: A 21 yo F came to your office for physical examination. She is sexually active. On pap smear you saw **perinuclear inclusion body**. Which of the following is the most likely causative agent?
a) Chlamydia
b) **Human papilloma virus**
c) Gonorrhea
d) Herpes virus

Q: A 21 yo F came to your office for physical examination. She is sexually active. She was c/o vaginal discharge. On pelvic exam, cervix was tender on slight movement. You sent smear for

---

examination. Gram stain was negative, **iodine stain** showed **intracytoplasmic inclusion body**. Which of the following is the most likely causative agent?

a) **Chlamydia**
b) Human papilloma virus
c) Gonorrhea
d) Herpes virus

Q: A 35 yo F present with c/o blurred vision and black spots in her visual field. PMH is significant for HIV diagnosed ten years ago. On fundoscopic exam, it shows characteristic white perivascular infiltrate with hemorrhage. Which of the following inclusion body will you see in this patient?

a) Negri body
b) Guarnieri body
c) cowdry's body
d) **owl's eye inclusion body**

14. Important points to know about Rabies virus (Rhabdovirus family)
    - Bullet shaped – carrier (**dogs, bat, skunk**) – fever, headache, malaise, uncontrolled excitement, <u>hydrophobia</u> – **fatal once developed** – **Dx:** Negri bodies (Intracytoplasmic inclusion in brain tissue) – Post-exposure prophylaxis with human rabies immunoglobulin & 4 doses of vaccine (1,3,7,14th day)

15. Influenza virus: (A, B & C)
    - <u>Two important glycoproteins</u>: Hemagglutinin (HA) & Neuraminidase (NA). HA mediates binding of virus to the target cells and NA involved in releasing of progeny virus from infected cells. During replication, after HA binds the virus to the target cells, it is cleaved by protease and then cells import the virus by endocytosis. That's why these proteins are target for anti-viral drugs.
    - Influenza A: more common in human, more severe than B&C, the virus can be subdivided into differet serotypes based on the Ab (antibody) response to these viruses. There are 16 H and 9 N subtypes known, but only H 1, 2 and 3, and N 1 and 2 are commonly found in humans. Eg: H1N1 (Spanish flu), H2N2, H3N2, H5N1 (current threat)
    - Influenza B: almost exclusively infect human, only one species, lower mutation rate, these all factor make it less favorable for pandemics
    - Influenza C: has one species, less common

16. Most common cause of <u>Aseptic meningitis</u> [Sign & Symptoms of meningitis (headache, fever, stiff neck, phtophobia) but <u>patient appears less toxic</u>]
    - ECHO virus (belongs to Enterovirus – Picornavirus family)

17. Most common cause of viral encephalitis [headache, altered consciousness, receptive aphasia, problem with memory (s&s related to temporal lobe)]
    - HSV-1 (Herpes simplex virus) [**temporal lobe** most common site]

18. Most common cause of viral pink eye
- Adenovirus

19. Most common cause of common cold
- Rhinovirus, Coronavirus
- Runny nose, nasal congestion, cough, sore throat; symptoms are less severe than influenza; sometimes associated with pink eye

20. Causes of diarrhea due to virus
- Rotavirus – diarrhea in **Infants (<2 yrs)**
- Norwalk virus – diarrhea in **kids & adults**

21. Cause of Hand Foot Mouth disease
- Coxsackie A virus [papulovesicular Erythematous lesions]

22. Most common cause of acute Pericarditis
- Coxsackie A virus [Chest pain relieved by leaning forward]

23. Give the name of virus family of Measles (Rubeola) & Rubella (German Measles)
- Measles (Rubeola): Paramyxovirus
- Rubella (German Measles): Togavirus

24. "Clues" to diagnose Measles (Rubeola)
- Coryza, cough, conjunctivitis, **koplik spots** (grayish white dots on the buccal mucosa)
- **Vit-A** should be **given in pt with measles**

25. "Clues" to diagnose Mumps
- **Swelling of the parotid gland**, orchitis
- **Elevation of serum amylase**
- [Contagious 1 day before and 3 days after the swelling appear]

26. "Clues" to diagnose Rubella (German Measles)
- Retroauricular, **Posterior cervical & Post-occipital lymphadenopathy**
- [Contagious 2 days before the rash begin and 5 days after the rash appear]

27. "Clues" to diagnose Roseola (Exanthema Subitum)
- High grade fever → resolve by 3-4 day → maculopapular rash appears after fever resolve
- Caused by HHV 6 (Human herpes Virus-6)

28. "Clues" to diagnose Varicella (chicken pox)
- Pruritic rash consisting of papules, vesicles, pustules and crusted lesions in **crops in various stages**
- Caused by Varicella Zoster virus [VZV]
- [contagious 2 days before the rash begin and until all the lesions are crusted]

29. "Clues" to diagnose Molluscum Contagiosum
- Papules with **central umbilication**
- Caused by Poxvirus, immunocompromised person (HIV/AIDS)

30. TORCH infections
- **Toxoplasmosis** – more serious in first trimester → **intracranial calcifications**, IUGR , microcephaly, **blindness**

- **Other (Syphilis)** – can be transmitted to fetus at any stage of pregnancy → fever, anemia, failure to thrive, maculopapular rash, hepatosplenomegaly (<2yrs) → Hutchinson teeth, saber skin, saddle nose, clutton joints (late manifestation).

- **Rubella** – IUGR, **Cataract**, **PDA** (Patent Ductus Arteriosus), **Deafness**, blueberry muffin lesions.

- **CMV** – IUGR, **Chorioretinitis**, **Periventricular calcification**.

- **Herpes** – infection occur due to passage through an infected birth canal → first time infection in mother has high rate of transmission – fever, jaundice, poor feeding, lethargy, **small fluid filled blisters** on the body, seizure, irritability

---

Q: A premature newborn baby develops jaundice, fever and rash on the body. On examination, spleen and liver were enlarged. CT scan of head showed **periventricular calcification**. Which of the following is the most likely causative agent?
a) Toxoplasmosis
b) Syphilis
c) **Cytomegalovirus**
d) Herpes virus

Q: A premature newborn baby develops jaundice, fever and rash on the body. On examination, baby has enlarged spleen and liver, bulging fontanelle. The patient also developed seizure. CT scan of head showed **intracranial calcification**. Which of the following is the most likely causative agent?
a) **Toxoplasmosis**
b) Syphilis
c) Cytomegalovirus
d) Herpes virus

CMV & Toxoplasmosis presents very similarly but periventricular calcification on CT scan gives a clue towards diagnosis of CMV. Toxoplasmosis causes multiple brain lesions so it shows multifocal intracranial calcification on CT scan.

Q: A newborn developed fever, jaundice, poor feeding and lethargy. You also noticed few small **fluid filled blisters** on skin. On reviewing patient's file, you noticed that mother had similar skin lesions around genital area during delivery of the baby. Which of the following is the most likely diagnosis?

---

a) Toxoplasmosis
b) Syphilis
c) Cytomegalovirus infection
d) **Herpes virus infection**
e) Rubella

Q: A mother brings her newborn baby because baby was developing white spots in eyes. On examination, baby's both pupils were white, has continuous machinery murmur, microcephaly and characteristic blueberry muffin rash on skin. Which of the following is the most likely diagnosis?
a) Toxoplasmosis
b) Syphilis
c) Cytomegalovirus infection
d) Herpes virus infection
e) **Rubella**

Q: A mother brings her newborn baby for fever, irritability, failure to thrive. On examination, patient has no bridge to nose, small blisters on palm and sole. Which of the following is the most likely diagnosis?
a) Toxoplasmosis
b) **Syphilis**
c) Cytomegalovirus infection
d) Herpes virus infection
e) Rubella

Q: A mother brings her newborn baby because baby was developing white spots in eyes. On examination, baby's both pupils were white, has continuous machinery murmur, microcephaly and characteristic blueberry muffin rash on skin. Which of the following is the most likely diagnosis?
a) **patent ductus arteriosus**
b) ASD
c) VSD
d) Tetralogy of fallot

The reason I include question with patent ductus arteriosus is because this is how they present different clinical scenario for particular organism and ask question related to it so if you don't recognize the organism or condition, you will most likely get it wrong on the exam.

31. Clinical importance of **Papova virus (HPV)**
  ▪ It is responsible for **cervical CA (HPV type: 16, 18, 31, 33, 35)** – **cauliflower like growth / varrucous lesions**
  ▪ **HPV 1&4** – **planter warts** – **fomite spread** – **varrucous lesions**

32. Herpes Viruses**:**
  ▪ **Human Herpes Virus-6:** causes exanthema subitum (high grade fever followed by maculopapular rash)

- **Cytomegalovirus:** <u>CMV Mononucleosis</u>: fever, sever malaise; compare to EBV, it is associated with less pharyngitis & spleenomegaly; <u>CMV infection in immunocompromised</u>: pneumonitis, GI disease & retinitis; <u>CMV Pneumonitis</u>: very severe, usually in immunocompromised (**HIV, transplant patient**) start with fever, dry cough, rapidly progress to dyspnea and hypoxemia; CXR shows diffuse bilateral interstitial infiltrates; <u>CMV GI disease</u>: gastroenteritis, hepatitis, pancreatitis, colitis; sign & symptoms: nausea, vomiting, **diarrhea**, jaundice; <u>CMV retinitis</u>: most common cause of blindness in AIDS, less common in transplant patient; blurred vision, black spots in visual field, fundoscopic exam shows white perivascular infiltrate with hemorrhage (pizza pie appearance)
- **Epstein-Barr Virus:** <u>Infectious Mononucleosis</u>: high grade fever, sore throat (exudative tonsillar enlargement), lymphadenopathy & hepatosplenomegaly; development of maculapapular rash in patient treated with amoxicillin/ampicillin (80% of patient); spleenomegaly is more common and very prone to rupture even with minor trauma so always advise to avoid sports for 3-4 weeks; atypical lymphoytosis is also seen in infectious mono; <u>Burkitt's lymphoma</u>: tumor of B-lymphocyte; the most common tumor of childhood in Africa (endemic variant) is associated with Epstein-Barr virus and malaria, most commonly involve jaw or other facial bone; Sporadic variant (non-African) most commonly involve ileo-cecal region; Immunodeficiency-associated Burkitt's lymphoma is most commonly associated with HIV/AIDS, mainly CNS lymphoma
- **Herpes Simplex Virus:** HSV-1 typically affect above the waist area & HSV-2 genital area, CNS infection in neonates; the patient usually present with constitutional symptoms like fever, malaise, develop localize **pain**, tingling, **burning** or itching followed by vesicular lesions; <u>HSV encephalitis</u>: headache, **altered mental status**, receptive aphasia, problem with memory (last two are s&s of temporal lobe which is the most common site)
- **Varicella Zoster Virus:** causes chicken pox in childhood & shingles in elderly – Pruritic rash consisting of papules, vesicles, pustules and crusted lesions in **crops in various stages** in chicken pox – burning, painful, itchy rash followed by vesicles on skin, usually localized to dermatomes, in shingles

33. Which virus is a **causative agent for Kaposi sarcoma**?
- HHV-8 [Human Herpes Virus 8] [Microscopically looks like angiosarcoma]
- Kaposi's sarcoma lesions are nodules that may be red, purple, brown, or black, and it is not a true sarcoma (not arising from mesenchymal tissue). It is a tumor of lymphatic endothelium and forms vascular channels that fill with blood cells, giving the tumor its characteristic bruise-like appearance. Highly vascular. Most common in AIDS. It is one of the <u>AIDS defining condition</u>.

34. For which virus we do Tzank test? What are we looking for in Tzank test?
- For Herpes virus
- Swab is stained by Giemsa staining and look under microscope for the presence of characteristic **multinucleated giant cells**

35. What does Monospot test check? Is it specific?
- Heterophile antibodies (react with animal RBCs)
- It is **non-specific**

36. What is **an important of different Hep-B markers**? [HBsAg, Anti-HBcAb, HBeAg, Anti-HBeAb, Anti-HBsAb] [Ag=antigen; Ab=antibody]
- HBsAg: active disease / persistent (chronic) disease
- Anti-HBc IgM Ab: **1st Ab to appear** in Hep B, suggest current infection
- Anti-HBc IgG Ab: suggest **remote** or **current** infection
- HBeAg: higher rates of viral replication and enhanced **infectivity**
- Anti-HBeAb: a dramatic decline in viral replication
- Anti-HBsAb: protective Ab, Immunization
- Sequence of marker: HBsAg, anti-HBcAb, HBeAg, anti-HBeAb, anti-HBsAb

37. What is **a window period**? How do we diagnose Hep-B and HIV infection when patient is in window period?
- equivalence zone of Ab production so screening test become negative during that time frame
- Hep-B: **Anti-HBcAb, Anti-HBeAb [Both present in window period]**
- HIV: **Anti-p24 Ab present in window period**

38. Diagnosis of acute infection (current infection) due to important Hepatitis viruses
- Hep-B: HBsAg, IgM to HBcAg
- Hep-A: IgM to HAV
- Hep-C: PCR HCV RNA

39. What does Anti-HCV Ab indicate?
- It indicates exposure to Hepatitis C Virus (screening test) but it doesn't tell if infection is current. To diagnose current HCV infection, order PCR of HCV RNA

40. Most common virus causes hepatocellular CA
- Hep B virus [Hep C also cause cirrhosis and hepatocellular carcinoma]. Pt with Hep C has high chance of developing hepatic CA than Hep B, but Hep B is more prevalent than Hep C

41. Transmission of different Hepatitis viruses
- Hep-A: fecal-oral transmission
- Hep-B: blood products, body fluids
- Hep-C: blood products
- Hep-D: blood
- Hep-E: fecal-oral

42. Important points to know about Hep-D virus
- Delta virus, **incomplete virus, co-infection with Hep B required / super infection in previously infected with Hep B**, In combination with Hep B, it has **highest mortality** rate of all the hepatitis infections

43. Important points to know about Hep-E virus
- **high mortality in pregnant women**

44. Common feature of all hemorrhagic fever [Ebola, Dengue, Yellow fever]
- Fever + bleeding diathesis [Low platelet counts, DIC, shock]
- Yellow fever is distinguished from others by severe proteinuria
- Viral families: Arenavirus, Filovirus, Bunyavirus, Flavivirus

45. Diagnosis of HIV
- **ELISA** – screening test (screen for **antibody** against HIV in patient's serum)
- **Western blot test** – confirmatory test (check antibody against p24, p17, gp120 and gp41), should demonstrate **presence of antibody to atleast 2 out of 3 antigens** [p24, gp41 and gp120]; if antibody to only one antigen present, then consider it negative and order **HIV PCR** to confirm the diagnosis

46. Which is the capsid protein in HIV? Importance of it
- It is p24 [Gag structural gene]
- Anti-p24 Ab is present during window period

47. Give name of envelope proteins. Which envelope protein binds to CD4+ cells?
- gp 120, gp 41
- **gp 120 binds to CD4+ cells**
- gp 41 helps in cell fusion

48. Which HIV gene down regulates host cell's immunity (MHC-1, MHC-2)?
- **Nef gene**

49. Which gene is responsible for production of important viral enzymes? Function of these enzymes
- Pol gene [Reverse transcriptase, Protease & Integrase]
- Reverse transcriptase: converts the viral RNA into a complementary strand of DNA, which is copied to produce a double stranded molecule of viral DNA
- Integrase: integration of the viral DNA into the host cell's genome
- Protease: The Env polyprotein (gp160) is cleaved by protease in Golgi complex and processed into the two HIV envelope glycoproteins gp41 and gp120

50. Clinical presentation of Hantavirus (Bunyavirus family)
- Myalgia, fever & **ARDS,** carrier – rats & **mice**, transmits through urine, droppings or saliva

51. Viral encephalitis
- Arboviruses [viruses transmitted through arthropod vectors]
- Flavivirus [West Nile, St. Louise, Japanese, Powassan], Togavirus [Eastern, western, Venezuelan]; all transmitted through mosquito except powassan which is transmitted through tick (ixodes); Herpes Simplex virus
- Headache, fever, myalgia, **altered mental status**, s&s related to temporal lobes in herpes simplex encephalitis
- Headache & fever seen in both meningitis & encephalitis but altered mental status leads toward encephalitis

52. Clinical presentation of Lassfever (Arenavirus family)

- Non-specific symptoms like fever, retro-sternal pain, mucosal bleeding, proteinuria, etc, 15-20% mortality; reservoir – rodents; spread through inhalation of tiny particle of rodents excretion, person-person transmission; <u>Dx</u>: ELISA, <u>Tx</u>: Ribavirin; <u>Complications</u>: deafness, spontaneous abortion

53. What are eclipse period and latent period?

- Eclipse period – No internal (nor external) virus
- Latent period – No external virus

54. Immunization

- **<u>Live Attenuated Vaccine</u> :**
- <u>Viral</u>: MMR, Yellow fever, Varicella
- <u>Bacterial</u>: BCG, oral typhoid

- **<u>Inactivated Vaccine</u> :**
- <u>Viral</u>: Polio, Rabies, Hepatitis **A** (whole)
- <u>Fractional</u>
  <u>Protein based</u> – Subunit → Hep B, Influenza, acellular Pertussis
  Toxoid → Diphtheria, Tetanus
  <u>Polysaccharide based</u> – Pure → Pneumococcal, Hib, meningococcal
  Conjugate → Hib, Pneumococcal

- **Influenza & Yellow fever** vaccines are **contraindicated** in persons with hypersensitivity to egg.
- **IPV & MMR** are **contraindicated** in persons with hypersensitivity to neomycin/ streptomycin.

- **<u>Contraindications to vaccines</u> :**
- severe allergic reaction to prior doses of vaccine (or) to a component
- Encephalopathy following Pertussis vaccine
- **Immunocompromised state & pregnancy**
- Only **MMR** is contraindicated in HIV infected patient **<u>with severe immunocompression</u> & <u>Symptomatic</u>**. All other vaccine can be given in HIV positive symptomatic person.
- Previous febrile illness is **<u>not</u>** a contraindication (C/I) for giving MMR
- **C/I to MMR are:** pregnancy, **<u>severe</u>** immunodeficiency (asymptomatic HIV is **<u>not</u>** a C/I), recent immunoglobulin administration, allergy to neomycin

- **Immunization:** Usually vaccines [DTaP, Hib, PCV, IPV] and Hep B (if **<u>not</u>** given at birth) are given at 2, 4, 6 months and then boosters if appropriate.
- All **pre-term infants** should receive vaccines according to their <u>chronological age</u>, **not** their gestational age. Hep B vaccine should be administer at birth (Wt should be >2 kg)

- <u>Hep-B vaccine</u> → **at birth**.
- <u>DTaP, Hib, PCV, IPV</u> → Started at 2 months of age.
- <u>MMR, Varicella</u> → started at 12 months of age.

- Influenza → started at 6 months of age.
- DTaP → 2nd & 3rd dose 4-6 weeks apart, 4th dose 6 months after 3rd dose.
- Hib → All doses 4-6 weeks apart, **if first dose is given after 15 months of age** then **no** need for other doses, booster b/w 12-15 months of age
- PCV → All doses 4-6 weeks apart, **no doses for healthy child of ≥ 24 months of age**, booster b/w 12-15 months of age
- MMR → 2nd doses→ 4-6 weeks after 1st dose/at 4-6 yrs f age.
- Meningococcal Vaccine (serotypes A, C, Y, W - 135) → **not** protective for those **< 2 yrs of age**. That means give vaccine after 2 yrs of age
- If mother is HBsAg positive → HBIG + HB Vaccine at birth.
- OPV (oral polio vaccine) is **not** used in USA

- **Immunization in internationally adopted child without written documentation** – Give all necessary immunization according to recommendation for unimmunized child + screen for Hep B, Hep C, HIV, Syphilis and TB

* **Parasites:**
1. What is the difference b/w intermediate host and definitive host?
- **Intermediate host** in which larval stage develop
- **Definitive host** in which adult parasite reach sexual maturity

2. What happen when men as an intermediate host
- Serious diseases occur in men [cystodes – tapeworms]

3. Give an example of conditions in which men as an intermediate host
- Cysticercosis – T.solium (pork) – eat **eggs** of T.solium
- Hydatid liver cyst – E.granulosus – eat **eggs** of E.granulosus
- Alveolar Hydatid cyst – E.multilocularis – eat **eggs** of E.multilocularis

4. Parasite causing Sparganosis; Clinical importance of it
- Diphyllobothrium Latum [D.latum]
- **causes Vit-B12 deficiency**

5. **Carrier of Toxoplasmosis** (T. gondii)
- Cat

6. Which form of Toxoplasma can cross placenta
- **Tachyzoite** – a rapidly dividing for of Toxoplasma

7. Which form of maternal toxoplasmosis can infect fetus?
- **Primary infection in mother during pregnancy**
- If mother had previous infection with Toxoplasma, antibodies from mother prevent infection in fetus

8. Presence of IgM against Toxoplasma in newborn indicates what? Clinical importance of it
    - It indicates **recent (transmission from mother)** infection in newborn
    - If it is not treated, <u>progressive blindness</u> occurs
    - Primary infection (transmission from cat) **after** birth is usually asymptomatic

9. Parasite causing Chagas disease. [common in Brazil]
    - T. cruzi [transmitted through Reduviidae family bug]

10. Important sign specific to Chagas disease
    - Unilateral swelling of eye [Romana's sign] [bug bites near eye]
    - Affect heart (myocarditis, cardiomyopathy), Dysphagia

11. Parasite causing African sleeping sickness
    - T. bruzi [tsetse fly] [<u>Winterbottom's sign</u>: swelling in posterior triangle lymphnodes]

12. Parasite causing Kala-azar
    - Leishmania Donovani [sand fly]

13. Which form of L. Donovani is present in liver & spleen?
    - Amastigotes [**tissue protozoa**]

14. Parasite causing Babesiosis [Similar to malaria; it causes <u>hemolysis</u>]
    - Babesia microti [**Ixodes tick** – same tick causes **Lyme disease**] [**blood protozoa**]

15. Parasite causing Giardiasis
    - Giardia Lamblia [cyst – fecal-oral route; <u>camping</u>]

16. Parasite causing amoebiasis
    - Entamoeba Hystolytica [cyst with four nuclei – fecal-oral; <u>trip to Mexico</u>]

17. Parasite causing vaginosis
    - Trichomonas vaginalis [<u>Sexually transmitted</u>]

18. Which <u>free living amoeba present in contact lens</u> solution causes keratitis & granulomatous Amoebic Meningitis?
    - **Acanthamoeba**

19. Which <u>free living amoeba present in fresh warm water</u> causes Amoebic Meningitis?
    - **Naegleria** [diving in fresh warm water]

20. Mosquitoes inject which form of plasmodia in human blood?
    - **Sporozoites**

21. Which form of plasmodia causes relapse?
    - **Hypnozoites** [remains dormant in liver] (P.vivax and P.ovale)

22. Which form of plasmodia is responsible for malarial paroxysm?
- **Merozoites** release by lysis of infected RBC causes malarial paroxysm

23. Which form is picked up by mosquitoes from patient infected with malaria?
- **Sexual form**

24. Name of liver and bladder flukes. How do they transmit?
- **Schistosoma mansoni** [contact with water, skin penetration – mature in mesenteric veins] [**Cholangiocarcinoma**]
- **Schistosoma haematobium** [contact with water, skin penetration – mature in bladder veins] [**Bladder carcinoma**]

25. "Buzz word" for pinworm infection [Enterobius Vermicularis]
- **Perianal itching**

26. How do you diagnose pinworm infestation?
- Swab of Perianal area [show ova with flattened side]

27. Which worm causing rectal prolapse?
- **Trichuris trichura (whipworm)** [Dx: stool (barrel-shaped eggs with bipolar plug)]

28. Life cycle of round worm [Ascaris lumbricoides]
- Ingestion of eggs – larva invade intestinal wall – enter in blood – migrate to other tissues (liver, lung, heart, etc.) – migrate back to GI

29. How does hookworm [Necator Americans] transmit?
- Filari form larva penetrate intact skin of bare feet
- Blood sucker causes anemia

30. "Clues" to diagnose **Cryptosporidium** [Causing diarrhea in patient with **AIDS**]
- **Acid fast oocyst in stool**

31. "Clues" to diagnose Trichinella spiralis
- **Muscles pain & Eosinophilia**
- Transmission occur via ingestion of viable encysted larvae in meat

* **Fungi:**
1. Which fungus is found in reticular endothelial system cells like macrophage?
- **Histoplasmosis** [soil enriched with bird/bat feces]

2. "Clues" to diagnose Coccidioidomycosis [California, Arizona]
- **spherules with endospores**

3. "Clues" to diagnose Blastomycosis
- **Broad base bud**, rooting woods, [**no capsule** but **double refractile walls**]

4. "Clues" to diagnose Cryptococcosis
- **India ink preparation, Urease positive yeast**

5. "Clues" to diagnose Pneumocystis Carinii Pneumonia (PCP)
- **Silver stain cyst** on bronchoalveolar lavage

6. "Clues" to diagnose Aspergillosis
- **45°branching hyphea** when mount in 10% KOH preparation, positive allergic skin test, neutropenic patient, fungus ball on CXR

7. "Clues" to diagnose Candida
- **germ tube formation at 37°C, Pseudohyphae**, whitish lesions, bleed when scrape

8. "Clues" to diagnose Sporothrix schenkii
- **rose gardener, throne injury**

9. "Clues" to diagnose Paracoccidioides
- **"pilot's wheel" appearance** due to multiple yeast sprouting out of a single parent cell

10. "Clues" to diagnose tinea infections
- **Annular lesions expand peripherally and clear centrally**

11. "Clues" to diagnose tinea versicolor
- White, scaling lesions that tend to coalesce, **"spaghetti and meatball"** appearance on KOH preparation

12. Causative agent for tinea versicolor
- Malassezia furfur (Pityrosporum orbiculare)

13. When should we start prophylaxis for PCP and Cryptococcosis in HIV patient
- PCP: Start TMP + SMX when CD4+ count fall below 200
- Cryptococcosis: Start Fluconazole when CD4+ count fall below 100

14. Difference b/w bacteria, virus, fungi and parasites
- Bacteria: **No** nuclear membrane, **No** histone, **No** introns, **No** mitochondria (membrane bound organelles) but **have** ribosomes and cell wall (peptidoglycans)
- Virus: Acellular, **No** cell wall, **No** ribosomes, **No** mitochondria
- Fungi: Ergosterol in cell wall
- Parasites: **No** cell wall

* **Bacteria:**
1. What is unique to gram (+) bacteria only?
- **Teichoic acid**

2. What is unique to gram (−) bacteria only?
- **Outer membrane & Periplasmic space**

3. What forms **capsule in bacteria**?
- Polysaccharide gel **except** Bacillus Anthrax which contain polypeptide of poly D-glutamate
- It **protects bacteria from host immune system**

4. Where do **metabolic process / electron transport take place in bacteria**?
- Cytoplasmic membrane (lipoprotein)

5. What is the **purpose of Porins**?
- Passive transport of material

6. What is **responsible for shock in gram (−) bacterial infection**?
- Outer membrane (lipopolysaccharides – lipid A)

7. Which **factor in streptococci is responsible for rheumatic fever**?
- M protein

8. Give name of important bacteria
- **Gram positive bacteria:** Staphylococci, Streptococci, Bacillus, Listeria, Corynebacterium, Nocardia, Actinomyces, Clostridium
- **Miscellaneous:** Rickettsia, Mycoplasma, Chlamydia
- **Gram negative bacteria:** Neisseria, Moraxella, Enterobacteraceae, H.Pylori, C.Jejunii, Pseudomonas, Legionella, Haemophilus, Vibrio

9. Color of gram (+) & gram (−) bacteria
- Gram (+) – Purple/Blue [same color as Non-Acid Fast bacteria]
- Gram (−) – Pink/Red [same color as Acid Fast bacilli]

10. Important characteristics of **all Staph**? How is it **differing from Strep**?
- Arrange in clusters, **catalase positive**
- **Streptococci are catalase negative**, arrange in chain

11. How would I **differentiate Staph aureus from other staph**?
- Staph aureus is **Coagulase positive**

12. How would I **differentiate Staph Epidermidis from Staph Saprophytics**?
- Staph Epidermidis is **Novabiocin sensitive**

13. Important characteristics of Staph Aureus
- **Catalase positive**
- Coagulase positive (**β hemolytic**)
- **Ferment mennitol**
- Evades phagocytosis by **protein A**

14. How would I differentiate Strep Pyogens from Strep Agalactiae?
- Strep Pyogens is **Bacitracin sensitive**
- Strep Agalactiae give **cAMP test positive** [Cl. Perfringens also has this property]

15. How would I differentiate Viridans group (Strep mutans) from strep pneumonia?
- Strep Viridans is **optochin resistant,** and is **NOT** lysed by bile

16. How would I differentiate Enterococcus fecalis from Strep Bovis?
- Enterococcus fecalis **grows in high salt solution (6.5% NaCl)**

17. What are alpha, beta & gamma hemolysis?
- Alpha hemolysis – reduction of iron in hemoglobin giving green color on blood agar; Examples: Strep Viridans group and Strep Pneumonia
- Beta hemolysis – complete rupture of red blood cells, giving distinct, wide, clear areas around bacterial colonies on blood agar; Examples: Strep Pyogens and Strep Agalactiae
- Gamma hemolysis: no hemolysis take place; Examples: Enterococcus fecalis and Strep bovis

18. On what basis we classify strep in class A, B, D, etc?
- According to the specific carbohydrate in the Cell wall
- Group A: Strep Pyogens
- Group B: Strep Agalactiae
- Group D: Enterococcus fecalis and Strep bovis
- Non-grouped: Strep Viridans group and Strep Pneumonia

19. Clinical importance of all of above streptococci
- Strep Pyogens: Sore throat, responsible for Rheumatic fever, Glomerular nephritis
- Strep Agalactiae: Septicemia, meningits in neonates [No. 1 cause] [E.coli is 2nd]
- Strep Viridans: Bacterial endocarditis [affect **mitral** valve]
- Strep Pneumonia: pneumonia, meningitis [> 18 yrs old] [produce **IgA protease which lyses IgA in respiratory tract and facilitate infection**]
- Enterococcus fecalis: UTI [Dipstick test – **positive leukocyte esterase & negative** nitrite test. (Nitrite test is positive in E.coli)]
- Strep Bovis: affect **tricuspid** valve in **colon cancer patient**

20. Characteristics of Bacillus
- Obligate Aerobes, rod-shaped, beta-hemolytic, Catalase positive, substantial portion usually contain an oval endospores at one end, making it bulge [spore forming bacteria]

21. Clinical importance of Bacillus Anthrax
- Cutaneous anthrax [necrotic skin lesion – **black eschar**]
- Inhalational anthrax [**woolsorters' disease** – mortality is nearly 100% - can be used in **biological war**]
- Ingestion [vomiting of blood, severe diarrhea – 25-60% mortality rate] – produced both **toxin** (consisting of **three proteins**: the protective antigen, the edema factor and the

lethal factor) and a **capsule** (consisting of a polymer of glutamic acid – protects from phagocytosis by host cells)

22. "Clues" to diagnose B. cereus
   ▪ **Diarrhea within 2-6 hrs of eating fried rice**

23. "Clues" to diagnose Listeria monocytogen
   ▪ Spontaneous abortion in <u>Pregnant</u> women; septicemia, meningits / wide spread granulomas in <u>newborns</u> (3rd MCC of meningitis in newborn)

24. Characteristic of Listeria and Tx of its infection
   ▪ **Beta hemolytic**, tumbling motility, **gram (+) rods**; <u>Tx</u>: **Ampicillin**

25. Source of Listeria infection in humans
   ▪ **Unpasturized milk products** (pregnant mothers should avoid soft cheese like feta, brei, camembert, queso blanco)

26. "Clue" to diagnose diphtheria
   ▪ **Gray white pseudomembrane in throat**, Volutin granules

27. How does diphtheria toxin work? Which toxin is similar to diphtheria toxin?
   ▪ It works by <u>inhibiting protein synthesis</u> by catalyzing the ADP-ribosylation of the elongation factor eEF-2 (<u>inactivates eEF-2</u>) (ADP-ribosylation can be reversed by administration of high Nicotinamide)
   ▪ It is **similar to Pseudomonas toxin**

28. Which important organ is affected in diphtheria?
   ▪ Heart [Cardiomyopathy]

29. Give name of selective and differential cultural media for diphtheria
   ▪ Loffler's medium (selective)
   ▪ Tellurite agar (differential)

30. "Clue" to diagnose Actinomycosis. Treatment of it
   ▪ **Yellow sulfur granules** from sinus tract
   ▪ <u>Tx</u>: Penicillins

31. "Clue" to diagnose Nocardia. Treatment for it
   ▪ **Partially acid fast**, gram (+) rods
   ▪ **Tx:** Sulfonamides

32. "Clue" to diagnose Cl. Botulinum
   ▪ **honey has given to the infant (<1 yr old), droopy head**

33. "Clue" to diagnose Pseudomembranous colitis [caused by Cl. Difficile]
   ▪ **Greenish watery diarrhea**, recent use of Clindamycin [<u>Tx</u>: Metronidazole]

34. Clinical importance of Cl. Perfringens
   - Food poisoning [**unheated frozen meat**]
   - **Gas gangrene** [Produce Lecithinase (alpha toxin) which damage cell membrane]

35. How does **tetanus toxin** work?
   - It blocks release of glycine & GABA

36. Which two factors are we looking for when we give Tetanus Toxoid (TT)?
   - **Vaccination history & Wound (clean or dirty)**
   - Last TT dose (< 10 yrs) & clean wound – No need to give tetanus prophylaxis
   - Last TT dose (> 5 yrs) & dirty wound – Give TT prophylaxis
   - No previous vaccination & clean wound – Give TT prophylaxis
   - No previous vaccination & dirty wound – Give TT + **tetanus immunoglobulins**

37. "Clue" to diagnose Mycoplasma
   - **Positive cold agglutinin test**, Atypical Pneumonia in school children

38. Characteristics of Mycoplasma. Treatment of its infection
   - Require **cholesterol**, purines, pyrimidines for **to culture**
   - **No cell wall**
   - Fried egg colonies on Eaton's media
   - Tx: Macrolides [Erythromycin]

39. "Clue" to diagnose Acute Epiglottitis
   - **Stridor**, difficulty swallowing, **thumbprint sign** on lateral view of neck x-ray

40. Characteristics of H. Influenzae
   - Require factor X (protoporphyrin) & factor V (NAD) to culture / **Co-culture with Staph. Aureus**
   - **Encapsulated** causes Acute Epiglottitis, Meningitis
   - **Unencapsulated** causes Conjunctivitis, Otitis media, Sinusitis
   - **Tx:** Ceftriaxone [3rd generation cephalosporin]

41. Characteristic of Neisseria
   - Both **Catalase & Oxidase positive**
   - Diplococci, kidney bean shaped

42. Clinical importance of Neisseria
   - N. Meningitides: causes meningitis in age group 1-18 years
   - N. gonococcus: causes gonorrhea, Septic arthritis

43. Important characteristics of N. gonococcus
   - Facultative **intracellular** [Seen in neutrophils in gonorrhea]
   - Its **pili undergo antigenic and phase variation** causing recurrent infection and resistance to antibiotics

44. Clinical importance of Moraxella Catarrhalis. Treatment of infection causing by it
   - It causes Sinusitis, Bronchitis, Otitis Media
   - <u>Tx</u>: Amoxicillin, Amoxicillin + Clavulanate

45. How would you differentiate Enterobacteriaceae from other gram (−) bacteria?
   - Enterobacteriaceae is **<u>oxidase negative</u>.** It also **reduces nitrates to nitrites**

46. Give name of bacteria in enterobacteriaceae
   - Citrobacter, Escherichia, Enterobacter, Klebsiella, Shigella, Yersinia, Proteus, Salmonella

47. Which enterobacteriaceae bacteria doesn't have flageller antigen (H)?
   - Shigella & Yersinia [That's why they are **not motile**]

48. "Clue" for diagnosis of Proteus infection
   - **Big staghorn calculi, Urease positive organism** [<u>produce alkaline urine</u>]

49. Which is the only bacterium from enterobacteriaceae catalase negative?
   - Shigella [All other are catalase positive]

50. Give name of important non-lactose fermenting enterobacteriaceae bacteria
   - Salmonella, Shigella, Proteus

51. Give name of important **lactose fermenting** enterobacteriaceae bacteria
   - E.coli, Enterobacter, Klebsiella

52. Clinical importance of Yersinia
   - <u>Causes</u>: Mesenteric adenitis (**pseudoappendicitis**), **Plague** [Bubonic, Septicemia and Pneumonic], **Reactive arthritis** [Association with **HLA-B27**]

53. Patients with **Hemochromatosis** are susceptible to which organisms?
   - **Vibrio vulnificus**, Listeria monocytogenes, **Yersinia enterocolica**, Salmonella, Klebsiella pneumoniae and Escherichia coli [**Iron loving bacteria**]

54. Diarrhea producing different E.coli
   - Enterotoxigenic E.coli [ETEC]: Produce toxin which is responsible for diarrhea. **LT enterotoxin** [similar to Cholera toxin] and ST enterotoxin cause **increase in cAMP** in cells and subsequent secretion of fluid and electrolytes in intestinal lumen; **Traveler's Diarrhea**
   - Enteropathogenic E. coli (EPEC): Adherence to the intestinal mucosa causes a rearrangement of actin in the host cell, changes in intestinal cell ultra structure due to "attachment and effacement" is likely the prime cause of diarrhea in those afflicted with EPEC. **It lacks fimbriae**
   - Enteroinvasive E.coli [EIEC]: EIEC are **highly invasive**, and they utilize adhesin proteins to bind to and enter intestinal cells. They produce **<u>no</u> toxins**, but severely damage the intestinal wall through mechanical cell destruction.

- Enterohemorrhagic E.coli [EHEC]: moderately-invasive and possesses a phage-encoded **Shiga toxin** that can elicit an intense inflammatory response. **O157:H7 strain produce HUS [hemolytic uremic syndrome]**

55. **Important points to remember** about all of the above E coli
- ETEC: LT toxin = Cholera toxin; traveler's diarrhea
- EPEC: lacks fimbriae; rearrangement of actin causes diarrhea
- EIEC: no toxin; diarrhea occurs due to intestinal wall destruction
- EHEC: toxin = Shigella toxin; O157:H7 strain causes HUS

56. Which capsular antigen do E coli possess?
- K capsular antigen

57. Which capsular antigen do salmonella possess?
- Vi capsular antigen

58. **Reservoir / Transmission of important bacteria**
- S typhi: **Fecal-oral** transmission [Human]
- S enterica: Raw chicken and **egg yolk [Poultry]**
- Campylobacter jejunii: **Poultry**, colonizes the GI tract of many bird species
- H pylori: **Fecal-oral** transmission [Human]
- Legionella: **air-conditions** (cooling towers)
- Francisella (tularemia): **rabbit hunting**, deer fly and tick bite
- Chlamydia psittaci: **birds**, turkey
- Coxiella Burnetti: **Domestic live stock** [cattle, sheep, goats, cats and dogs]; Infection results from **inhalation of contaminated particles in the air**
- Borrelia burgdorferi: **Ixodes tick** [tick should be attached for more than 24-hrs]
- R rickettsii: **Hard tick** (dermacentor)
- R prowazakii: **human louse**
- R typhi: **flea bite**
- Bartonella Henselae: **cat**
- Brucella: Milk product

59. "Clue" to diagnose Klebsiella
- **Pneumonia in chronic alcoholics**, big capsule, **Mucoid colonies**, red-current jelly sputum

60. Clinical importance of H pylori
- **Gastric ulcer, Gastric lymphoma**

61. Clinical importance of C jejunii
- Bloody diarrhea followed by **Guillian Barre Syndrome [Ascending paralysis]**

62. "Clue" to diagnose Legionella
- **BCYE agar** (Buffered Charcoal Yeast Extract), **Air-conditions, cooling towers**, chronic smoker, Atypical pneumonia, **hyponatremia** & elevated **LFT**

63. "Clue" to diagnose Pseudomonas
- **Green pus, grape like order**

64. Clinical importance of Pseudomonas
- Burn patient: Septicemia, **produce elastase causing necrotic skin lesions**
- Otitis externa: **Necrotic / granulation tissue** in the ear canal in **DM patient**
- Ecthyma gangrenosum: ulcer on foot with **black necrotic center** in **DM patient**
- Cystic Fibrosis: recurrent lung infection
- Hot tub Folliculitis: occurs after sitting in a hot tub that was not properly cleaned
- Hospital acquired infection: appear 48 hours or more after hospital admission

65. What is an Alpha toxin? Give name of bacteria that produce it
- Alpha Toxin: Damage cell membrane
- Examples: Staph Aureus, Cl Perfringens, Pseudomonas, Diphtheria
- **Alpha toxin of Pseudomonas and Diphtheria is similar to each other**

66. Important points to remember about **Mycobacterium Tuberculosis**
- Produce **Niacin; waxy envelope** (responsible for **Caseous necrosis**)
- **Cord factor (trehalose dimycolate): Interferes with phagocytosis** by macrophages by preventing the fusion of the phagosome with the lysosome [It also present in Nocardia]
- **Tuberculin + mycolic acid**: delayed HS, damage is done by immune system. **No** endotoxin / exotoxin

67. When will you consider PPD test positive?
- It should be considered positive if induration after 48-hrs is
- ≥ 5 mm in HIV (+) / recent TB exposure
- ≥ 10 mm in high risk population [health workers]
- ≥ 15 mm in low risk population

68. "Clue" to diagnose Francisella (tularemia). Treatment of it.
- **rabbit hunting**, ulceroglandular disease. **Tx:** Tetracycline

69. "Clue" to diagnose Chlamydia
- Intracytoplasmic **inclusion body on iodine stain**

70. Which inclusion body form of Chlamydia is infectious?
- **Elementary body**

71. Characteristics of Chlamydia
- **Can't make ATP, Lack muramic acid**

72. "Clue" to diagnose **Lyme disease** (Borrelia burgdorferi)
- **Erythema (chronicum) migrans** [circular, outwardly expanding rash - "bull's-eye" rash]

73. Organism present in **Human bite** / animal bite. **Treatment** of it.
- Pasturella multocida. **Tx:** Amoxicillin + Clavulanate

74. How would you identify different Rickettsia infection easily?
- **R**ocky mountain spotted fever - **R. Rickettsii**
- E**p**idemic typhus – R. **P**rowazakii
- Endemic typhus – R. typhi

75. "Clue" to diagnose Bartonella Henselae
- Cat **scratch** fever, Bacillary Angiomatosis in patient with AIDS

76. "Clue" to diagnose Bordetella Pertusis
- Severe hacking cough followed by intake of breath that sounds like "whoop", **Lymphocytosis**

77. Which stage in Pertusis is infectious?
- Catarrhal stage

78. How does Pertusis toxin work?
- Catalyze ADP ribosylation of **Gi** protein and **increase cAMP**

79. Which other toxin work by increasing cAMP?
- ETEC, Cholera [Both catalyze ADP ribosylation of **Gs** protein]

80. "Clue" to diagnose Vibrio cholera. Which cultural media do we use to grow cholera?
- **"rice water" stool**, coma shaped organism
- TCBS medium (selective), Alkaline bile salt agar [very sensitive to acid so grow in Alkaline pH]

81. Give name of Urease positive organism
- **Proteus, Ureaplasma, H.pylori & Cryptococcus**

82. Importance of Lysogenic phage conversion. Give name of bacteria that undergoes Lysogenic phage conversion
- Lysogeny is characterized by integration of the bacteriophage nucleic acid into the host bacterium's genome.
- Importance: increase the pathogenic capability of the bacteria for a host
- Examples: C. diphtheria, S. Pyogens, Cholera, Shiga toxin, Cl. Botulinum

83. Organism causing Scarlet fever. "Clue" to diagnose it. Treatment for the same.
- Group A **β**-hemolytic Streptococci
- **Maculopapular/Sandpaper rash**, "Strawberry" tongue, circumoral pallor
- **Tx:** Penicillins, Erythromycin

84. Important points to remember about Mycobacterium Avium intracellularae
- Present in soil and water
- Infection occur in patient with AIDS usually when CD4+ counts go **below 50**
- Sx: fever, diarrhea, malabsorption, anorexia
- Azithromycin is given as a prophylaxis when CD4+ counts go below 50

85. Important points to remember about **Primary Syphilis (Chancre)**
   - <u>Painless</u> ulcer with **rolled edge & punch out base**

86. How would you differentiate Chancroid (Haemophilus Ducreyi) from Primary syphilis, Lymphogranuloma venerum and Granuloma Inguinale?
   - **In Chancroid**, ulcer is **painful**, gray base & foul smelling

87. Important points to remember about granuloma Inguinale (Donovanosis)
   - Papule rapidly evolves into <u>painless</u> ulcer characterized by irregular border and brief red granular base

88. Important points to remember about Lymphogranuloma venerum (L1, L2 or L3 of Chlamydia trachomatis)
   - <u>Painless</u> shallow ulcer and associated with nonspecific symptoms. **Inguinal adenopathy** is inflammatory & **does not appear at the same time as** the ulcer

89. Which important infectious agents are not killed by Autoclave?
   - Endotoxin & Prion [Bacterial spores (contain dipicolinic acid) can be destroyed by autoclave]

90. Clinical **importance of Prion**
   - Responsible for Creutzfeldt-Jacob Disease

91. "Clue" to diagnose Creutzfeldt-Jacob disease
   - **Presence of Myoclonus** in patient with Dementia

92. What are conjugation, transformation and transduction?
   - **Conjugation** – direct DNA transfer b/w bacteria via sex pili
   - **Transformation** – uptake of naked DNA from environment
   - **Transduction** – DNA transferred via a bacteriophage vector
     - <u>General</u> – non-specific DNA transfer
     - <u>Site-specific</u> – specific genomic information is transferred
   - **Examples of Bacteria which are able to Transform** – Haemophilus species, Strep. Species, H.pylori, N. gonorrhea

93. What is the difference b/w direct and indirect fluorescence antibody (Ab) test?
   - **Tissue** sample from patient (Ex. Sputum) – **Direct** Fluorescent Ab test (**detect Antibody**)
   - **Serum** from patient – **Indirect** Fluorescent Ab test (**detect Antigen**)

94. Organism responsible for **rat bite fever in US**
   - Streptobacillus moniliformis

122

95. Important Clinical Presentation

Clinical Presentation	Organisms
A mother brought her **1 yrs** old child with diarrhea, dehydration	Rotavirus
A mother brought her **4 yrs** old child with c/o abd pain, vomiting, diarrhea. Many child at day care center develop this symptoms	Norwalvirus (Norovirus)
A mother brought her 4 yrs old child to the hospital with high grade fever & cough. It was **started as mild cold like symptoms** and progress to present symptoms. On exam, pt has **barky cough** and intermittent inspiratory <u>stridors</u>. X-ray of neck showed **narrow subglottic space.**	Parainfluenza virus (Croup)
A mother brought her 3 yrs old child with **sudden onset** of high grade fever, inspiratory <u>stridors</u>. On exam, pt was **drooling saliva**. Child was sitting in tripod position with neck hyperextended. Neck X-ray showed thumb print sign.	H. Influenza type B (bacteria) (Acute epiglottitis)
A mother brought her **6 months** old child with lethargy, difficulty feeding. It was **started as fever, rhinorrhea, sneezing**. On exam, pt is very tachypnic, respiratory rates in 60's. CXR showed hyperinflated lungs.	RSV (Bronchiolitis)
A child was sent home from day care center because of development of facial rash & fever. On exam, rash was bright red looks like "**slapped cheek**". Pt also has joint pain	Erythema Infectiosum (Fifth Disease) (Parvo)
A mother brought her 6 yrs old child with rash on the body. Pt had fever, runny nose and diarrhea. As per mother, pt had fever for 3 days and **rash appeared after fever resolved**. On exam, pt looks in no acute distress. Exam was within normal range except rash	Roseola (HHV-6)
A 6 yrs old child was brought in by her mother for development of rash. Pt had **fever, runny nose, cough, red eyes**. Pt developed rash after 3 days of initial symptoms. Rash first appeared on face and then spread towards body. It was maculopapular. On exam, in mouth pt has **grayish white spots on buccal mucosa.**	Measles
A 6 yrs old child was brought in by her mother for fever, headache, sore throat and swelling around jaw area. On exam, pt has **enlarged parotid gland.**	Mumps
A 6 yrs old child was brought in by her mother for development of fever & rash. Rash was first appeared on face and spread downward. As rash was spreading downwards, it was clearing from face. On exam, pt has **postauricular, cervical & postoccipital lymphadenopathy.**	Rubella
A 21 yrs old girl came in with fever, **burning and painful blisters on lips**. On exam, she had cervical lymphadenopathy.	Herpes Simplex (HSV-1)
The dentist comes to your office for c/o fever, malaise and development of **burning pain** on right hand fingers. On exam, there were few **vesicles** of 1.5 mm.	Herpetic whitlow
A 23 yrs old sexually active female comes to your office for fever & malaise. On exam, she has low grade fever, inguinal lymphadenopathy and **painful blister on labia & around clitoris.**	HSV-2

She uses oral contraception pills.	
A 21 yrs old girl came in with fever, headache, stiff neck and **change in mental status**. Her past medical history includes **recurrent cold sores**. On exam, she has receptive aphasia & hard time remembering stuff.	HSV encephalitis
A **65 yrs old** male comes to your office for development of **painful rash** on abdominal area (<u>or</u> on the face). On exam, rash was distributed in area of one dermatome (or sensory area of one branch of trigeminal nerve). You also noticed few ulcers with crusts.	Herpes Zoster (Varicella Zoster Virus - VZV)
A mother brought her 6 yrs old boy for fever, malaise and development of painful & pruritic rash. Rash was started on face and spread downwards. On exam, **rash was consisting of papules, pustule, vesicles and crusted lesions**.	Chicken Pox (VZV)
A 30 yo M with h/o **HIV** presented with several lesions on his body. On examination, lesions appear to be flash colored papules with **central umbilication**.	Molluscum Contagiosum (Pox virus)
A mother brought her 6 yrs old boy for fever, malaise and development of rash. On exam, pt has **vesicular rash on face, hands & fee**t.	Hand, Foot & Mouth disease (Coxsackie A)
A 30 yrs old male came in with c/o **chest pain**, 7/10 in severity, worse with deep inspiration and **better when leans forward**. Pt had cold like symptoms one week ago. On exam, pt has **friction rubs** over precordium.	Pericarditis (Coxsackie A Virus)
A 21 yrs old came in with c/o crusting of <u>**both**</u> eyes in the morning. Pt also has fever, runny nose and joint pain. On exam, both eyes are red and have **clear** secretion and **postauricular lymphadenopathy**	Viral Conjunctivitis (adenovirus)
A **65 yrs old** man comes with c/o right eye **redness**. On exam, pt also has **vesicular lesion** on forehead.	Herpes zoster ophthalmicus
A 23 yrs old college student came in with c/o right eye redness & **pain**. On exam, pt has **corneal vesicles & dendritic ulcers**. Pt also has a history of recurrent similar episodes in past.	HSV keratitis / conjunctivitis
A 21 yos old came in with c/o crusting of <u>**right**</u> eye. On exam, right eye is red and has **purulent** discharge. Both right eyelids are swollen and there is no lymphadenopathy	Bacterial Conjunctivitis (Pneumococcus, Haemophilus)
A newborn baby develops purulent eye discharge on **5th day** after delivery. On exam, eye looks red and **copious purulent discharge** is present. Cornea is edematous and ulcerated. Both eye lids swollen	Gonorrheal conjunctivitis
A newborn baby develops **mucoid** discharge **few days** after birth. Pt also has fever and dry cough. CXR is suggestive of **pneumonia**.	Chlamydia conjunctivitis
A child with **chronic** red eye present with blurred vision. On exam, Pt has **mucoid** discharge, **eye lids have white lumps**, linear scars, and eyelashes are turned inward. Cornea is cloudy.	Trachoma (Chlamydia trachomatis)
A 21 yo F came to your office for physical examination. She is sexually active. On pap smear you saw **perinuclear inclusion body**. (or **koilocytosis** on pap smear)	HPV
A 21 yo F came to your office for physical examination. She is	Chlamydia

sexually active. She was c/o vaginal discharge. On pelvic exam, cervix was tender on slight movement. You sent smear for examination. Gram stain was negative, **iodine stain** showed **intracytoplasmic inclusion body**.	
A 21 yo F came to your office for physical examination. She is sexually active. She was c/o **vaginal discharge**. On pelvic exam, **cervix was tender** on slight movement. You sent smear for examination. Gram stain showed gram negative **intracellular diplococci**.	Gonorrhea
A 18 yrs old boy comes to your office with lesion on his finger. On exam, it looks like a **verrucous lesion** on finger.	Wart (HPV 1&4)
A 28 yrs old man comes to your office for physical exam. He is sexually active with multiple male and female partners. On exam, he has **cauliflower like mass** around anus.	Genital warts (HPV)
A 35 yrs old man comes to the hospital via EMS for confusion, agitation and paranoia. As per family member, he was return from his **trip in jungle** where he was **exposed to** wild animal including **bats**. Initially it was started as fever, malaise and headache. While in the hospital pt was **unable to drink water or any liquid**. Any liquid will provoke spasm of his body. Pt **died** in 3 days.	Rabies
A 60 yo M presented to your clinic during **winter season** with **high grade fever, muscle ache**, sore throat, cough, headache and malaise for 2 days. Pt looks more ill. Pt's symptoms resolved in 3 days.	Flu
A 25 yrs old presents to your clinic in **spring** season with mild fever, sore throat, cough and nasal congestion. Pt doesn't look that ill.	Common cold
A 23 yrs old female came with fever and headache. On exam, pt has mild **neck stiffness**. Analysis of cerebrospinal fluid show increase in WBC with lymphocyte predominant and normal glucose	Aseptic (Viral) Meningitis (ECHO virus)
A 33 yrs old male came with fever, headache, stiff neck and **altered mental status**. Analysis of cerebrospinal fluid show increase in WBC with lymphocyte predominant and normal glucose. Pt was admitted in ICU and recovered slowly.	Viral encephalitis
A 23 yrs old female came with fever, headache and photophobia. On exam, pt has **neck stiffness** and upon **bending of her head, she lift her legs**. Analysis of cerebrospinal fluid show increase in WBC with **neutrophils** predominant and **low** glucose	Bacterial Meningitis
A 38 yrs old HIV positive person comes to the hospital with fever, headache and photophobia. On exam, pt has **neck stiffness** and upon **bending of her head, she lift her legs**. Analysis of cerebrospinal fluid shows only 40 WBC with **lymphocyte** predominant and **low** glucose	Cryptococcal meningitis
A premature newborn baby develops jaundice, fever and rash on the body. On examination, spleen and liver were enlarged. CT scan of head showed **periventricular calcification**.	CMV
A premature newborn baby develops jaundice, fever and rash on the	Toxoplasmosis

body. On examination, baby has enlarged spleen and liver, bulging fontanelle. The patient also developed seizure. CT scan of head showed **intracranial calcification**.	
A newborn developed fever, jaundice, poor feeding and lethargy. You also noticed few **small fluid filled blisters on skin**. On reviewing patient's file, you noticed that mother had similar skin lesions around genital area during delivery of the baby	Herpes
A mother brings her newborn baby for fever, irritability, failure to thrive. On examination, patient has **no bridge to nose, small blisters on palm and sole.**	Syphilis
A mother brings her newborn baby because baby was developing white spots in eyes. On examination, baby's **both pupils were white**, has **continuous machinery murmur**, microcephaly and characteristic **blueberry muffin rash on skin.**	Rubella
A 15 yrs old boy comes to your clinic with high grade fever & sore throat. On exam, **tonsils are covered with exudates**. Cervical lymphadenopathy is present. Pt also has **hepatospleenomegaly**. You prescribed **amoxicillin**. Pt comes again with **maculapapular rash**.	Epstein Barr Virus [infectious mononucleosis]
A 10 yrs old African boy comes to the clinic with jaw swelling. On exam, it is a hard mass. Biopsy of mass consistent with B cell lymphoma	EBV (Burkitt's lymphoma)
A 45 yrs old male comes with blurred vision & black spots in visual field. PMH is significant for **AIDS**. On fundoscopic exam, there are white perivascular infiltrate with hemorrhage looks like **pizza pie appearance**	CMV retinitis
A 45 yrs old kidney transplant patient on immunosupression therapy came in with fever, **diarrhea** and dry cough which rapidly progress to dyspnea. Pt's oxygen saturation was low. CXR shows diffuse bilateral interstitial infiltrates.	CMV pneumonitis
A 38 yrs old male came with red, purple and brown **nodular lesions** on body. Pt's PMH is significant for **HIV**. Lesions look like angiosarcoma microscopically.	Kaposi sarcoma (HHV-8)
A 9 yrs old boy comes to the clinic for **fever**, malaise, **loss of appetite**, abd pain, diarrhea & vomiting. On exam, pt has **jaundice** and right upper quadrant tenderness. Blood test was **positive** for **IgM** against **HAV**, negative for HBV and HCV	Acute Hep A
A 38 yrs old female comes to your office with **loss of appetite**, wt loss, malaise, **fever and jaundice**. A blood test is significant for markedly elevated transaminases. Hepatitis serology showed **positive** results for the presence of **HBsAg, HBc IgM antibody** and negative result for the presence of HBsAb.	Acute Hep B
A 32 yrs old **IV drug abuser** comes to your office for physical exam. Exam was only significant for mild jaundice so after complete physical exam, you ordered liver function test with routine blood test which showed elevated transaminases. You ordered	Chronic Active Hep B

hepatitis panel which showed **positive** results for the presence of **HBsAg, HBeAg, HBc IgG Ab**.	
A 32 yrs old **IV drug abuser** comes to your office for physical exam. After complete physical exam, you ordered hepatitis panel which showed **positive** results for the presence of **HBsAg, HBc Ab**.	Asymptomatic Hep B carrier
A 32 yrs old male come to your office for follow up after having acute hepatitis b virus infection. You order follow up hepatitis panel which showed **positive** result for **HBsAb, HBc IgG Ab**, negative for HBsAg	Recovered from acute self-limited HBV
A 23 yrs old college student comes to your office for routine physical exam. He born in foreign country and has no record of vaccination but he told you that he received all of his vaccines. You ordered some blood test which showed **positive HBsAb** and **negative** for **HBsAg, Anti-HBcAB**	Vaccinated against HBV
A 32 yrs old **IV drug abuser** comes to your office for physical exam. Exam was only significant for mild jaundice so after complete physical exam, you ordered liver function test with routine blood test which showed elevated transaminases. You ordered hepatitis panel which showed **positive result for HCV antibody**, negative result for HBV and HAV	Chronic Hep C
A 32 yrs old male comes to your office with **loss of appetite**, wt loss, malaise, **fever and jaundice**. He is an IV drug user. A blood test is significant for markedly elevated transaminases. Hepatitis panel showed **positive** result for **HBsAg, HBc IgM Ab, Anti-HDV IgM Ab** and negative for HBsAB, HAV & HCV	Hep B & Hep D co-infection
A 32 yrs old male IV drug abuser comes to your office with **loss of appetite**, wt loss, malaise, **fever and jaundice**. A blood test is significant for markedly elevated transaminases. Hepatitis panel showed **positive** result for **HBsAg, HBc IgG Ab, Anti-HDV IgM Ab** and negative for HBsAB, HAV & HCV	Hep D superinfection in pt with chronic Hep B infection
A recent epidemic of severe hepatitis occurred in India which was found to be transmitted through **fecal-oral route**. It was reported that there was a **high mortality** rate in **pregnant women**.	Hepatitis E
A 30 yrs old recently migrated from Iran comes to the emergency room via EMS after having grand mal seizure. Pt is afebrile. No recent illness. Neurological exam unremarkable. CT scan of head showed multiple calcifications with **multiple enhanced "cystic" lesions** with surrounding edema.	Neurocysticercosis
A 32 yrs old with **AIDS** brought to the emergency room via EMS after having grand mal seizure. Pt is afebrile. No recent illness. Neurological exam unremarkable. CT scan of head showed multiple calcifications with **multiple "ring" enhancing lesions** with surrounding edema. (Toxo lesions are "**solid**" enhancing lesions)	Toxoplasmosis
A 35 yrs old recently migrated from Europe comes to your office with c/o RUQ pain and jaundice. Physical exam was unremarkable except jaundice. Blood work was normal. Hepatitis panel was	Hydatid Cyst (Echinococcus Granulosus)

negative. US ABD showed large fluid filled cyst in liver with **multiple daughter cyst inside the cyst**. (<u>or</u> honeycomb appearance of cyst)	
A 35 yrs old recently migrated from Europe comes to your office with c/o chronic cough, chest pain and dyspnea. Physical exam was unremarkable except decrease breath sounds. Blood work was normal. US Chest showed large fluid filled cyst in alveoli with **multiple daughter cyst inside the cyst**. (<u>or</u> honeycomb appearance of cyst)	Alveolar hydatid cyst (Echinococcus Multilocularis)
A 15 yrs old migrated from third world country comes to your office with chronic abd pain, wt loss, constipation and discomfort. Stool sample showed **multiple proglottid segments**.	Diphyllobothrium latum (D. Latum)
A 18 yrs old boy comes to your office with c/o weakness of legs and arm, tingling and numbness now getting progressively worse. Pt is recently migrated from India. His history is significant for **tape worm infection in past for which he didn't complete the treatment**. On exam, pt has bilateral spastic paresis and diminished pressure, vibration and touch sensation. Lab study is significant for anemia and **MCV of 106**. Stool sample showed **multiple proglottid segments**.	Subacute combined degeneration of spinal cord from Vit-B12 deficiency (related with D. Latum)
A 20 yrs old boy recently migrated from **Brazil** comes to your clinic with c/o chronic shortness of breath. Chest x-ray showed **pulmonary edema**. Echocardiography reveals **biventricular dilatation with massive cardiac enlargement**. An endomyocardial biopsy shows diffuse interstitial fibrosis, myocyte necrosis, chronic inflammation, and the presence of **intracellular protozoan parasites**.	Chagas disease (Trypanosoma Cruzi) (T. Cruzi)
A 20 yrs old boy recently migrated from Brazil comes to your office with c/o **difficulty swallowing**, wt loss. Pt has difficulty with **both solid and liquid**. Barium swallow revealed **"bird's beak" appearance** of esophagus. (<u>or</u> "rat's tail" appearance of esophagus). Biopsy showed diffuse interstitial fibrosis, chronic inflammation and the presence of **intracellular protozoan parasites**.	Chagas disease (Achalasia)
A 30 yrs old recently migrated from **Africa** comes to the hospital with c/o fever, headache, fatigue, joint pain and **somnolence**. On exam, pt has swollen **lymphnodes in posterior triangle of neck**. Examination of lymphnode aspirate showed motile **parasites**.	African sleeping sickness (T. bruzi)
A 35 yrs old comes to your office with c/o **persistent diarrhea**. He **went to Mexico** couple of days ago. You sent stool for ova and parasites which showed numerous thin-walled cysts measuring 10-20 μm in diameter. Detail exam showed **four nuclei in most of the cysts**.	Entamoeba histolytica (E. Histolytica)
A 35 yrs old man comes to your office with c/o fever, chills, headache and fatigue. He has recently visited eastern seaboard beach. On exam, he has an icterus. On blood smear you saw **protozoa within erythrocyte**.	Babesia microti (transmitted by ixodes tick)

A 21 yo college student comes to your office with c/o frothy greenish vaginal discharge. Pap smear show flagellated **protozoa**	Trichomonas vaginalis
A 21 yo college student comes to your office with c/o thin, grayish white discharge with **fishy order**. Microscopic exam of discharge show epithelial cells with smudge border (**"clue" cells**)	Bacterial vaginosis
A 45 yo female with h/o diabetes present to you with c/o curdy white vaginal discharge. Microscopic exam of discharge show pseudohyphae.	Candida vaginitis
A 30 yo returning from camping develop severe headache, fever, nausea and vomiting. Pt went for **diving into lake** during camping. Despite of aggressive medical therapy, he died.	Naegleria fowleri
A 24 yo presents to you with c/o red eye and pain after removing lens. Other symptoms include tearing and sensitivity to light. On slit lamp exam, pt has **"ring-like" corneal ulcer**. He **doesn't wash his contact lens** each time before and after wearing.	Acanthamoeba keratitis
A 5 yo child brought to the physician office for c/o parianal itching which interrupts pt's sleep. You asked the parents to put transparent tape to child's perianal area at night. Next day, under microscope it shows oval eggs that are flattened on one side.	Enterobius vermicularis
A 4 yo boy was brought in by his mother for fever, nonproductive cough and **wheezing**. Blood work was significant for **eosinophilia**. His mother reported that he **passed worms in his feces**.	Ascaris lumbricoides (roundworm)
A 8 yo boy was brought in by his mother for epigastric pain, nausea and vomiting. His blood work was significant for **anemia** and **eosinophilia**. Examination of stool shows oval shaped eggs, measuring 60 μm by 40 μm, colourless, not bile stained and with a thin transparent hyaline shell membrane.	Necator americanus (Hookworm)
A 15 yo presents to your office with **rectal prolapse**. Review of exam was positive for chronic bloody diarrhea. Exam of stool showed **barrel shaped eggs** with bipolar plugs	Trichuris trichura (Whipworm)
A 35 yo presents to your office with nausea, vomiting and diarrhea started 12 hrs after ingestion of food. Pt was sent home and treated as food poisoning. Pt comes back in one week with c/o severe **muscles pain** and breathing difficulty. Blood work was significant for **eosinophilia**.	Trichinella spiralis
A 45 yo male presents to you with chronic diarrhea and weight loss. Exam of stool showed **acid fast oocyst**.	Cryptosporidium
A 60 yo chronic smoker comes to you with c/o cough for 2 months. His CXR showed **mass** with hilar lymphadenopathy. Biopsy of mass showed **multiple yeasts within macrophage**.	Histoplasmosis
A 60 yo chronic smoker who recently moved from **California** comes to you with c/o cough for 2 months. His CXR showed **mass** with hilar lymphadenopathy. Biopsy of mass showed **spherules with endospores**.	Coccidioidomycosis
A 30 yo immigrant has CXR which showed **mass** with hilar lymphadenopathy. Biopsy of mass showed fungal organisms with a	Paracoccidioidomycosis

few very distinctive **"pilot's wheel" yeast forms**.	
A 45 yo male comes to your office with fever, dry cough. His past medical history is significant for **HIV**. His last **CD4** count was **138**. Pt's vitals were significant for low oxygen saturation. CXR showed **bilateral infiltrates**. Bronchoalveolar lavage showed **silver stain cyst**.	PCP (Pneumocystis Pneumonia)
A 28 yo male came in with c/o **pain on swallowing**. On exam, pt's mouth has **white plaques** on tongue and buccal mucosa. You scrape the lesion and sent to lab. It was growing large, round, white colonies with **pseudohyphae** on agar plate.	Candida albicans
A 28 yo male came in with c/o **pain on swallowing**. On exam, pt's mouth has **white plaques** on tongue and buccal mucosa. You scrape the lesion and sent to lab. It was incubated at **37° c**. It started making **filamentous (germ) tubes**.	Candida albicans
A 45 yo female receiving **chemotherapy** for breast cancer came in with high grade fever and cough. She was coughing up dark **blackish material** in her sputum. CXR showed **air crescent sign** (radio opaque mass surrounded by radio lucent)	Aspergillosis (Aspergillus fumigates)
A 45 yo female receiving **chemotherapy** for breast cancer came in with high grade fever and cough. She was coughing up dark **blackish material** in her sputum. When incubated, it was growing **septate hyphae** which was **branching at 45°**.	Aspergillus fumigates
A 45 yo female with **diabetes** came in with high grade fever, left eye swelling, facial pain and **black discharge from nose**. It was rapidly growing **broad hyphae without septa**. Despite of aggressive treatment patient died.	Mucormycosis
A 24 yo male came in with **white scaly lesions** on his body. All lesions **tend to coalesce**. After staining with KOH, it has typical appearance so called "**spaghetti and meat ball**"	Tinea versicolor (Malassezia furfur)
A 40 yo male came in fever, rash and joint pain. He recently went to hiking in mountain and remembers having a **tick bite**. On exam, **red macular rash** was present on abdomen and both extremities. The patient mentioned that it was **started on ankles and wrists first and then spread upwards**.	Ricketssia ricketssiae (Rocky Mountain Spotted Fever - RMSF)
A 48 yo homeless came to ER with fever, joint pain and **rash** that **started on chest and spread to his extremities**. He remembered having multiple **flea bites**. The patient's condition improved on antibiotics.	R. typhi (endemic Murine typhus)
A 35 yo male came in with abrupt onset of high grade fever, severe headache and prostration. He also developed **rash** which **started on trunk and then become generalized, involving entire body except palm, soles & face**.	R. prowazekii (epidemic typhus)
A 27 yo female came in with fever, headache, cough and malaise. She remembered getting **bite by mite**. At the biting site, she has **black eschar**. On exam, she has regional lymphadenopathy.	Scrub typhus (O. Tsutsugamushi)
A 37 yo **veterinarian** came in with c/o fever, malaise and non-productive	Q-fever (Coxiella

cough. CXR showed right lower lobe opacity consistent with **pneumonia**. Serological test is positive for ricketssial group disease.	Burnetii)
A 50 yo male came in with fever with chills, headache and myalgia. The patient went for **hiking** with his family one month ago. Lab study showed **low WBC, low platelets and elevated liver function test**. Blood smear showed **morulae within neutrophils**.	Ehrlichioses (E. Chaffeensis)

IMMUNOLOGY

1. What happen when organism enter to the body?

Organisms enter in the body
↓
Chemotaxis [IL-8, LTB4, C5a, Organisms] (**Phagocytic cells** - macrophage, neutrophil, etc.)
↓
Opsonization (**IgG** via Fc receptor & **C3b** via CR3 receptor)

↓	↓
Macrophage & other antigen presenting cells	Neutrophils, Eosinophils, Basophils
↓	↓
Engulfment of organisms and <u>process antigens to T-cells</u>	Engulfment & <u>Killing of organisms</u>
↓	↓

Extracellular organisms	Intracellular organisms	Oxygen dependent	Oxygen independent
↓	↓	↓	↓
<u>CD 4 T-cell</u> IL-4 (activate B-cell) γ interferon (activate macro-phage) ↓	<u>CD 8 T-cell</u> Kill organism by Perforin, granzymes, **γ interferon,** Fas & Fas ligand (induce apoptosis)	H_2O_2, superoxide anion, Hydroxyl radicals, HOCl	lysozymes, defensins, lactoferins, hydrolytic enzymes

Macrophage (secrete IL-1, IL-6, TNF-α)
B-cell (secrete Immunoglobulins)

- When organism enter in the body, IL-8, LTB4, C5a and Organisms itself act as a chemotactic agents to attract phagocytic cells (macrophage, neutrophil, etc.) Meanwhile IgG via Fc receptor and C3b via CR3 receptor attach to organism and mark them for engulfing by phagocytic cells. Now depends upon phagocytic cell, organisms are either presented to T-cells or killed directly. Macrophage and other antigen presenting cells present organisms to T-cells whereas neutrophils, eosinophil kill them directly.
- **Macrophage** present <u>extracellular</u> organisms to <u>CD 4</u> cells while <u>intracellular</u> organisms to <u>CD 8</u>.
- <u>When organisms are presented to CD4 cells</u>, they secrete IL-4 (which activate B-cells) & gamma interferon (which activate macrophage, now to kill organisms). Macrophage secrete IL-1, IL-6 and TNF-α (acute phase reactants) and B-cells (transform into plasma cells) secrete immunoglobulins to kill organisms [**B-cell mediated immunity:** Naïve mature B cells produce both IgM and IgD. After activation by antigen, these B cells proliferate and begin to produce high levels of IgM and IgD. If these activated B cells are also activated via their CD40 and IL-4 receptors (both modulated by T helper cells), they undergo antibody class switching to produce IgG, IgA or IgE antibodies. During class switching, the constant region portion of the antibody heavy chain is changed, but the variable region of the heavy chain stays the same. Since the variable region does **not**

change, class switching does **not** affect antigen specificity. Instead, the antibody retains affinity for the same antigens, but can interact with different effector molecules.]

- **Concept:** IgM is the **only Ab** where there is **NO** class switching required. So If **thymus (T-cells)** is <u>not</u> involved, there is <u>no</u> class switching & **only IgM is produced**
- <u>When organisms are presented to **CD8 cells**</u>, they kill organisms directly by perforins, granzymes, **gamma interferon** and Fas & Fas ligand (which induce apoptosis). [**Cell mediated immunity, T-cell mediated immunity**]
- When <u>Neutrophils</u> engulf organism, they kill them directly. Killing occurs through two pathway, oxygen dependent and oxygen independent.
- <u>Oxygen Dependent:</u> Killing occurs by producing H_2O_2, superoxide anion, Hydroxyl radicals, HOCl. This involve **NADPH oxidase** [produce superoxide anion] & **Myeloperoxidase** enzymes [produce HOCl]
- <u>Oxygen Independent:</u> Killing occur by lysozymes, defensins, lactoferins, hydrolytic enzymes
- **Concept:** Oxygen independent killing is still working in patient with NADPH oxidase [Chronic Granulomatous Disease] and Myeloperoxidase disease
- **Concept:** In Myeloperoxidase deficiency, H_2O_2 is still produce so organisms which lack catalase enzyme can be still killed by neutrophils. [<u>Example:</u> **Streptococci** are still **killed** but **not staphylococci** which produce catalase]

2. **Important CD markers on different cells**

CD Markers	Different Cells	Functions
▪ CD 3	▪ All T-cells	▪ TCR associated signal transduction molecule ▪ TCR = T-cell receptor
▪ CD 2	▪ All T-cells	▪ Adherence to other cells, bind to LFA-3 ▪ LFA-3 = Lymphocyte Function associated Antigen
▪ CD 4	▪ Helper T-cells	▪ Interaction with MHC class 2 cells
▪ **CD 28**	▪ Helper T-cells ▪ Most CD 8 cells	▪ Co-stimulatory molecule needed for activation of T-cells ▪ Binds on B-cells, Macrophage, Dendritic cells
▪ **CD 40 ligand**	▪ Activated Helper T-cells	▪ Binds to CD 40 on B-cells ▪ **Essential for class switching (from IgM to IgG, IgA or IgE)**
▪ CD 14	▪ Macrophage	
▪ CD 16, CD 56, CD 2	▪ NK cells ▪ Lymphokine Activated Killer (LAK)	▪ **NO** CD 3,4,8,19 on NK cells
▪ CD 19, CD 20, **CD 21, CD 40**	▪ B-cells	▪ CD 40: Require for class switching ▪ CD 21: Serve as receptor for EBV (Ebstein-Bar Virus)

▪ CD 15, CD 30	▪ Reed – Sternberg Cells	

3. Important antigen receptors on different cells
- TCR: γδ [T-cells in Skin & Mucosal surface], αβ [T-cells at other sites]
- BCR: Ig M, Ig D
- MHC-1: **α** 1,2,3 **β₂**
- MHC-2: **αβ**

4. Receptors through which signal transduction occur in B & T cells
- B-cells – α, β, CD 19,20,21
- T-cells – CD 3

5. **Human leukocyte antigens and different classes:**
- The human leukocyte antigen system (**HLA**) is the name of the **major histocompatibility complex** (MHC) in humans. It is **located on chromosome 6**. Two different classes.
- HLA class 1 [MHC-1]: **HLA-A, HLA-B, HLA-C**
- HLA class 2 [MHC-2]: **HLA-DP, HLA-DQ, HLA-DR**

  ∗ **Location of MHC-1 & MHC-2 antigens:**
- MHC-1: All nucleated cells & platelets (**NO** MHC on RBC)
- MHC-2: Antigen Presenting cells (Dendritic cells, langerhans cells, activated macrophage, B-cells, activated T-cells & activated endothelial cells)

  ∗ **Importance:**
- MHC-1 is necessary for antigen recognition by **CD8+ T-cells**
- MHC-2 is necessary for antigen recognition by **CD4+ T-cells**

  ∗ **Difference:**
- **MHC-1:** React with **ENDOGENOUSLY** produce peptides by virus, intracellular bacteria, intracellular parasites and tumor cells
- **MHC-2:** React with **EXOGENOUSLY PROCESSED** antigens

  ∗ **Handling of organisms:**
- MHC-1: It works with intracellular organisms *so after reacting with endogenously processed antigen*, **β₂** microglobulin transports MHC class-1 molecules to the cell surface where it can be recognized by CD 8 T-cells and organisms are then killed by CD8 T-cells
- MHC-2: It works with Extracellular organisms so once organisms engulfed, MHC class-2 molecule *fuse with vacuole containing exogenously processed antigen*, invariant chain is released and MHC-2-peptide complex is then transported to the cell surface where it can be recognized by CD 4 T-cells. **Invariant chain** prevents interaction b/w endogenously produced peptide and MHC-2 molecules intracellularly

6. How does ADCC [Antibody Dependent Cellular Cytotoxicity] and NK cells mediated cytotoxicity differed?
   - ADCC: **IgG** + NK cells → use CD 16 molecule (Fc receptor) to identify target cells.
   - NK cells mediated cytotoxicity: use CD 56 (**No** antibody involve Ex.- **lysis of infected RBC**)

7. **Complement system:**
   - **Classical Pathway:** activated by antigen-Ab reaction (IgG & IgM, IgM most efficient) [start point C1] [C1 - C4 - C2 - C3] [C4bC2a is C3-convertase] [C4bC2aC3b (C5-convertase) splits C5 into C5a & C5b which then form C5b,6,7,8,9]
   - **Alternative Pathway:** C3 hydrolyze *spontaneously* in our body into C3a & C3b. If there is a pathogenic membrane surface nearby, C3b binds to it. If not, both C3a & C3b rejoin. Upon binding with a cellular membrane, C3b is bound by factor B to form C3bB. This complex in presence of factor D will be cleaved into Ba and Bb. Bb will remain covalently bonded to C3b to form C3bBb which is the alternative pathway C3-convertase. Alternative pathway is also activated by simple presence of organism in body (LPS of cell wall of gram (-) bacteria), it *doesn't require antibody*. [**start point C3b**] [C3b splits C5 into C5a & C5b which then form C5b,6,7,8,9]

   - **Important Products of Complement Pathways:** C3a,C4a,C5a; C3b and C5b6789

   * **Function of complement system:**
   - C3b – Opsonization of pathogen
   - C3a,C4a,C5a – Play role in Chemotaxis
   - C5b,6,7,8,9 – Membrane attack complex – kill pathogen

   * **How to determine complements are working:**
   - ↓C2/C4 – classical pathway is working
   - ↓Factor B – alternate pathway is working
   - ↓C3 – both pathways are working

   - C3-convertase can be inhibited by Decay accelerating factor (DAF)
   - C5a and C3a are known to trigger mast cell degranulation
   - The inhibition of C1-complex is controlled by C1-inhibitor (C1 esterase). [C1-esterase also inhibits proteinases of the fibrinolytic, clotting, and kinin pathways. The kinin-kallikrein system makes bradykinin. Deficiency of C1-inhibitors leads to activation of plasma kallikrein which produce bradykinin which is a potent vasodilator responsible for angioedema.]

8. Important points to remember about **different immunoglobulins:**
   - **IgG:** Main Ab in Secondary immune response – highest concentration in the body – **only Ab** that can **cross placenta** – remain up to 4-6-months in the newborn – capable of **Opsonization**

   - **IgM:** Main Ab in Primary immune response – **largest Ab** in the body, has five Fc regions (circulates as a pentamer) – presence on IgM in newborn suggest recent infection

– **first Ab to appear** in the serum **after exposure to antigen** – effective in complement fixation – Isohemagglutinins, rheumatoid factors, and heterophile antibodies are all IgM

- **IgA:** present in secretions [**Breast milk (colostrum)**, GI secretions, saliva, tears] – deficiency of IgA causes **repetitive upper respiratory tract infections, <u>transfusion reaction</u>**

- **IgD:** functions as a cell surface antigen receptor on **undifferentiated B cells.**

- **IgE:** involved in **allergic response and immediate type of HS** (type-1) – Fc region of IgE binds to basophils and mast cells – binding of antigen to two IgE molecules leads to mast cells degranulation and release of leukotrines, Histamines, eosinophils, hemotactic factors and Heparin – IgE is also involved in killing of parasites [IgE + eosinophils mediated cytotoxic reaction – type-2 HS].

9. What is the difference b/w papain & pepsin?
   - **Papain:** If Ab reacts with papain & then Ag is added – Ag will be unaffected
   - **Pepsin:** If Ab reacts with pepsin & then Ag is added – Ag will agglutinate / precipitate

10. **<u>Antigen Specificity</u>:** Variable region of both heavy & light chain. **Class switching doesn't affect Variable region of both heavy & light chain** therefore class switching doesn't affect specificity of antibody to that antigen

11. What are Allotype & Idiotype?
    - **Allotype:** A genetically determined difference in molecule b/w two members of the **SAME SPECIES**
    - **Idiotype:** The <u>individual, unique</u> differences b/w antibodies of different <u>antigen-binding specificities</u>

12. **Important interleukins, other immune system cells & their functions:**
    - IL-4 – class switch to **<u>IgE</u>**
    - IL-5 – class switch to IgA & ↑**<u>Eosinophils</u>**
    - Macrophage – IL-1, IL-6, IL-8, TNF-α
    - **IL-10** – Downregulate CMI (cell mediated immunity), Th1 [helper T-cell 1]
    - **γ interferon** – Downregulate Th2
    - **Th1 – Delayed Type Hypersensitivity** (DTH) (type-IV HS)
    - Th2 – Antibody mediated immunity
    - IL-1 – Pyrogenic (**fever inducing**)
    - IL-6 – Stimulate Acute phase proteins
    - IL-3 – Stimulate Bone marrow stem cells (granulocyte & monocytes)
    - IL-7 – Stimulate Pre-B & Pre-T cells (lymphoid cell development)
    - IL-2 – stimulate B-cells to produce antibody and self stimulation of T-cells. IL-2 is produced by Th1, NK and Tc

13. Important points to remember about **Hypersensitivities & their examples:**
  - **Type I Hypersensitivity reaction (HS):** Anaphylaxis [**bee stung**, severe allergic reaction due to peanut]; mast cells and Basophils degranulation (release of Histamines) – Bronchospasm, vasodilation, etc – <u>Tx</u>: Epinephrine [SC, 1:1,000] [prevents mast cell degranulation by increasing cyclic AMP levels; relax smooth muscle of respiratory tract]
  - **Type II HS: Antibody to receptor** [eg. Myasthenia gravis, Good-Pasture's, Grave's disease] and **Cytotoxic reaction** [Ab binds to antigen which activate complements causing cell destruction, eg. IgG + complement mediated platelet destruction in **ITP**, IgE + eosinophils and complements mediated cytotoxic lysis of filaria, complement mediated lysis of RBCs, **Rheumatic fever, Erythroblastosis fetalis**]
  - **Type III HS:** deposition of circulating Immune complexes in different tissues and then activate complement system which produce damage [eg. Vasculitis, **Rheumatoid arthritis, SLE**, Arthus reaction] [Blockage of C3b by Ab helps in patient with disease due to Type-3 HS]
  - **Type IV HS:** CD4 cells mediated HS [eg. **Tuberculosis, poison Ivy, latex gloves**]

  - * Which *HS reaction* is responsible for symptoms of nematodes infection and destruction of filaria?
  - In **Nematodes infection**, larva migrates to lung and produce cough, wheezing, etc. These symptoms are due to ***Type-1 HS*** reaction
  - In **Filarial Infection,** destruction of microfilaria is **IgE dependent Cytotoxicity (*Type-2 HS*)**

  - * How does destruction of Toxoplasma occur?
  - Usually IgE involved in parasite destruction but Toxoplasma is intracellular parasite and IgE is **not** involved in its destruction. *Th1, Tc, NK, ADCC involve in killing of Toxoplasma*

---

14. Different types of graft:
  - Allograft – transplant b/w different genetic make-up within the same species
  - **Isograft** – transplant b/w genetically identical (monozygotic twins)
  - Autograft – transplant from one site to another on the same individual
  - Xenograft – transplant across species barriers (transplant a heart from baboon to human)

15. Graft-vs-Host Disease: when immunocompetent tissue (fresh whole blood, thymus, bone marrow) is transplanted into an immunocompromised host
  - **Important point: T-cells from transplant tissue attack host tissues.** (*Type-4 Hypersensitivity(HS) reaction*)

16. Different type of rejections:
  - **Hyperacute** Rejection: **Mins. To Hrs.** – preformed antidoner antibody.(*Type-2 HS*)
  - **Acute** Rejection: **Days to Weeks** – primary activation of T-cells. (*Type-4 HS*)
  - **Chronic** Rejection: **Months to Years** – causes unclear. (*Type-4 HS*)

- **Accelerated** Rejection: **Days (3-5)** – reactivation of sensitized T-cells. Ex. If 1 kidney is rejected, then you transplant another kidney. If it is rejected second time, then it rejects faster than first time.

17. Important HLA association with different diseases:
- HLA-A3 – Hemochromatosis
- HLA-B27 – Ankylosing Spondylitis
- HLA-DR2 – Multiple Sclerosis, Goodpasture , Narcolepsy, Hay fever
- HLA-DR2,DR3 – SLE
- HLA-DR3 – Celiac Sprue, Dermatitis herpatiformis
- HLA-DR3,DR4 – Type-1 DM
- HLA-DR4 – Rheumatoid Arthritis(RA), Pemphigus Vulgaris
- HLA-DR5 – Pernicious Anemia, Juvenile RA
- HLA-DR7 – Steroid-responsive Nephrotic Syndrome

18. <u>Important syndromes / diseases due to deficiency of different immune components:</u>

- **Phagocyte Dysfunction (CGD, Chediak-Higashi Syndrome)** – *Extracellular Bacteria* (Staph. Aureus) + *Fungi* (Aspergillosis) [**CGD** – negative NBT (nitro-blue tetrazolium test)]
- **T-Cells Deficiency (DiGeorge Syndrome)** – *Intracellular Organisms* (Virus, **Candida,** TB) but **NOT** Extracellular; **3rd&4th pouch defect**, <u>absent thymus</u>; **Hypocalcaemia** due to <u>absent parathyroid glands</u>
- **B-cells Deficiency (Bruton's Agammaglobulinemia)** – *Extracellular Pyogenic Bacteria* but **NOT** intracellular
- **SCID (severe combined immune deficiency)** – *Bacteria, Virus, Fungus* (*extracellular + intracellular*); **Adenosine Deaminase deficiency**; Neutrophils - ↑ or N, **B&T cells - ↓↓↓**

- **Bruton's Agammaglobulinemia** – *tyrosine kinase deficiency* – arrest of B-cell maturation – virtually ***absent B-cell*** but pre-B cells present and **low circulating immunoglobulins**
- **Wiskott-Aldrich Syndrome** – *deletion of <u>T & B cells</u>* – Eczema, **Thrombocytopenia** and **Low IgM**, association with *Non-Hodgkin Lymphoma*
- **Bruton's Agammaglobulinemia & Wiskott-Aldrich Syndrome** are the only **X-linked recessive** immune deficiency syndromes. [Both have **LOW** circulating immunoglobulins but Wiskott-Aldrich has low T cells too]

- Hereditary Angioedema – **C1 esterase deficiency**
- **C3 deficiency** – Pyogenic Bacteria
- **C1,C4 or C2 deficiency** – Opsonization not efficient
- **C5-8 deficiency** – Neisseria Infections
- **Paroxysmal Nocturnal Hemoglobinuria (PNH):** Defect in molecule anchoring decay accelerating factor(DAF) which normally degrade C3&C5 convertase on hematopoetic cell membranes therefore in the absence of DAF, complement mediated Intravascular lysis of RBC occur (Hemoglobinuria) [<u>**Clue:**</u> Red urine in the morning]
- ↑**IgM** but **deficient IgG & IgA** – CD40 ligand deficiency on activated T-cells

- <u>**How to assess different Immunodeficiency Syndromes in exam**</u>: **look at the organisms in question**

  If <u>recurrent infection with only Staph Aureus</u> then you are most probably dealing with **phagocyte dysfunction** [CGD & Chediak-Higashi syndrome] **or** <u>C3 deficiency</u>. If you find word **neutrophil inclusions** in questions then go with **Chediak-Higashi** but if you find word **negative NBT** (Nitro-blue tetrazolium) test in question then go with **CGD** (chronic granulomatous disease).

  If **<u>no</u>** Staph Aureus infection in question but **infection with** <u>intracellular</u> **(virus, TB, <u>Candida</u>) organisms <u>&/or</u>** sign & symptoms of **hypocalcemia** (tetany) then go with **DiGeorge Syndrome.**

  If Intracellular (Virus, TB) + Extracellular (staph, Aspergillosis) organisms then go with **SCID**

  If **<u>Low</u> immunoglobulins** then **either Bruton's <u>or</u> Wiskott-Aldrich. If low IgM, Thrombocytopenia & Eczema** present then go with **Wiskott-Aldrich**

  If staph (Extracellular) infection & ask about which complement then **C3 deficiency**

  If **deficient Opsonization** (recurrent **<u>encapsulated</u>** organism infection) and ask about which complement then go with **C1, C4 or C2 deficiency.** But if they ask **which complement is responsible for opsonization**, then remember it is **C3b.**

  If disseminated **Neisseria infection (meningococcal and gonococcal)** then go with **C5-8 deficiency**

<u>Important Clinical Scenarios</u>

1. A 9-month-old child is hospitalized for a **severe yeast infection** that does not respond to therapy. The patient has a history of **multiple, acute pyogenic infections**. A differential WBC count shows 90% neutrophils, 2% lymphocytes, and 3% monocytes. A bone marrow biopsy contains **no plasma cells or lymphocytes**. A chest x-ray reveals the **absence of a thymic shadow**. These findings are most consistent with
a) Wiskott-Aldrich syndrome
b) chronic granulomatous disease
c) **severe combined immunodeficiency**
d) DiGeorge Syndrome
e) Waldenström's macroglobulinemia

2. A 7-month-old boy baby is evaluated because of **repeated infections with encapsulated bacteria**. Serum studies demonstrate **very low levels of all immunoglobulin**. Which of the following is the most likely diagnosis in this patient?
a) Wiskott-Aldrich syndrome
b) DiGeorge syndrome

---

c) Bruton's agammaglobulinemia
d) Chronic granulomatous disease

[Understand the concept in questions 1 and 2. In **SCID**, there is deficiency of *both B & T cells* so you will get <u>no</u> plasma cells and <u>no</u> lymphocytes on bone marrow biopsy and patient will get infection from *both intracellular and extracellular organism*. In **Bruton's agammaglobulinemia**, *only B cells* are deficient (B cells do not mature in Bruton's) so only antibody mediated defense is <u>not</u> working so patient will get recurrent infection from *extracellular, encapsulated infection*]

3. A 5-yo boy comes to the office for c/o intense **itching**. His past medical history is significant for **recurrent bacterial and viral infection**. An **uncle had similar problems**. Physical examination is remarkable for multiple petechial lesions on the skin and mucous membranes. Lab results are remarkable for **increased IgE** and **low platelets**. Which of the following is the most likely diagnosis?
a) **Wiskott-Aldrich syndrome**
b) Ataxia telangiectasia
c) DiGeorge syndrome
d) Atopic dermatitis

4. A 5-yo boy comes to the office with c/o productive cough. Past history is significant for **recurrent fungal infections**. He didn't show reaction to PPD. CXR showed active TB lesion. Evaluation of his serum electrolytes reveals **hypocalcemia**. Which of the following is the most likely diagnosis?
a) Wiskott-Aldrich syndrome
b) DiGeorge syndrome
c) Bruton's agammaglobulinemia
d) Chronic granulomatous disease

5. A 5-yo boy is brought to the office for **recurrent boils** on his body. Her mother denies any history of eczema or typical childhood illnesses such as measles or chicken pox. Lab results show normal CBC, immunoglobulin levels, B cell & T cell counts, complement levels, serum calcium and parathyroid hormone level. **The NBT (nitro blue tetrazolium) test is negative**. Which of the following is the most likely diagnoses?
a) Wiskott-Aldrich syndrome
b) Chronic granulomatous disease
c) DiGeorge syndrome
d) SCID (severe combined immunodeficiency disease)

6. A 30-yo male patient is being evaluated for **recurrent infections with encapsulated bacterial organisms**. Lab study shows normal immunoglobulin levels and NBT test positive. Which of the following is the correct diagnosis?
a) Selective IgA deficiency
b) C3 deficiency
c) X-linked hypogammaglobulinemia
d) Wiskott-Aldrich syndrome

7. A 30-yo male patient is being evaluated for **recurrent infections with encapsulated bacterial organisms**. Lab study shows normal immunoglobulin levels and NBT test positive. Which of the following is the correct diagnosis?
a) Selective IgA deficiency
b) **C1, C4 or C2 deficiency**
c) X-linked hypogammaglobulinemia
d) Wiskott-Aldrich syndrome

8. A 23-yo college student presents with the wrist pain and knee pain. On examination, you found red line along the tendons of the forearm muscles. She had **two similar previous episodes. She just had her menstrual period during the previous week.** These symptoms are most likely due to deficiency of
a) C1 esterase inhibitor
b) C3
c) **C5-C8**
d) C1, C4 or C2

9. A 20-yo woman brought to the ER with profuse internal bleeding due to car accident. She underwent abdominal surgery and required blood transfusion. She is transfused with **appropriate blood group match with her blood group**. But as the transfusion begins, she rapidly becomes hypotensive and **developed anaphylaxis**. Review of system shows **h/o recurrent sinusitis**. Which of the following is the most likely reason for developing these symptoms?
a) DiGeorge syndrome
b) **Selective IgA deficiency**
c) Wiskott-Aldrich syndrome

19. "Clue" to diagnose leukocyte adhesion defect
- Delayed separation of placental cord in newborn – **Leukocyte Adhesion Defect**

20. How does CD8 & CD4 T-cells differentiate in thymus?
- **In thymus,** cells with **LOW** affinity for MHC-1 molecule differentiate into CD 8 T-cells. (no affinity/high affinity cells are eliminated) Cells with **LOW** affinity for MHC-2 molecule differentiate into CD 4 T-cells

21. What are first & last events in maturation of B-cells?
- **1st event in Pre B-cells** – gene rearrangement of heavy chain
- **Last event in mature B-cells – IgM & IgD molecule on the surface of B-cells**

22. What is normal ratio for T-cells to B-cells?
- **T-cells to B-**cells ratio in the body – Three to One

23. **Primary & Secondary Immune Responses:**
- **Primary Immune response** – when antigen presented to our immune system **first** time – IgM

- **Secondary Immune response** – when same antigen presented to our immune system **second** time – IgG

24. <u>Active and Passive Immunities:</u>
- **Natural Active Immunity** – Chickenpox
- **Natural Passive Immunity** – Mother IgG protects her baby

- **Acquired Active Immunity** – Chickenpox vaccine
- **Acquired Passive Immunity** – Hepatitis B immunoglobulins

25. How does Superantigen work?
- **Superantigen binds** to **β chain of TCR** & MHC-II molecule of APC (antigen presenting cells) **stimulating T-cell activation**

26. What is responsible for killing of pathogen intra-macrophage?
- **γ interferon**

27. Which T-cells are involved in T-cells mediated cytotoxicity & Type-4 HS?
- **T-cell mediated cytotoxicity** – CD8 cells
- **Type-4 HS** – CD4 cells

28. How does destruction occur in TB?
- **TB** → macrophage → Th → secrete IL-2 & activate macrophage via γ interferon to become epitheloid cells & multinucleated giant cell → epitheloid cells secrete IL-1 & TNF-α (acute phase response), macrophage release large number of inflammatory mediators which are responsible for tissue damage → Fibrosis. So in TB damage occur by immune system (DTH), but **<u>NO</u>** endotoxin/exotoxin

29. What do we check in HIV screening & confirmatory test?
- We **check antibodies** in patient, **<u>NOT</u>** antigen

30. When do we consider western blot test positive?
- The **HIV Western blot** is considered **positive** when the patient demonstrates the **presence of antibody to <u>at least two of three</u> important HIV antigens**, which are gp120, gp41, and p24.

31. Important autoantibodies in different diseases:

Autoantibodies	Disease
Antiacetylcholine receptor	Myasthenia gravis
Anti-basement membrane	Goodpasture syndrome
Anticentromere	CREST syndrome
Antiendomysial & Antigliadin	Celiac disease
Anti-insulin,Anti-islet cell	Type-1 DM
Anti-intrinsic factor, Anti-parietal cell	Pernicious anemia
Antimicrosomal	Hashimoto's thyroiditis
Antimitochondreal	Primary billiary cirrhosis
p-ANCA	**P**olyarteritis nadosa (microscopic polyangitis)
c-ANCA	Wegener's granulomatosis
Antiribonucleoprotein	Mixed connective tissue disease
Anti-TSH receptor	Grave's disease
Anti-Scl-70	Scleroderma
Anti-SS-A, Anti-SS-B	Sjogren syndrome
Anti-smith, Anti-ds-DNA, ANA (antinuclear antibody)	Systemic Lupus Erythematous (SLE)
Anti-histone antibody	Drug induced lupus

BIOSTATISTICS

- **Incidence Rate** $=$ $\dfrac{\text{\textbf{New} cases of disease}}{\text{\textbf{Total} Persons \textbf{exposed} to Risk factor for that disease}}$ **X** Multiplier

- **Prevalence Rate** $=$ $\dfrac{\text{\textbf{Total} cases of disease at a given place \textbf{at a given time}}}{\text{\textbf{Total} Persons \textbf{exposed} to Risk factor for that disease at a place at a given time}}$ **X** Multiplier

- **Prevalence = Incidence X Duration**

- **True positive:** Sick people correctly diagnosed as sick
- **False positive:** Healthy people wrongly identified as sick
- **True negative:** Healthy people correctly identified as healthy
- **False negative:** Sick people wrongly identified as healthy

- **Sensitivity:** "True Positive rate" (All disease People)

$$= \frac{TP}{TP + FN}$$

- **Specificity:** "True Negative rate" (All healthy People)

$$= \frac{TN}{TN + FP}$$

- **Positive Predictive Value:** "Predictive value of positive test" (Only disease People)

$$PPV = \frac{TP}{TP + FP}$$

- **Negative Predictive Value** → "Predictive value of Negative test" (Only healthy People)

$$NPV = \frac{TN}{TN + FN}$$

S.S.Patel , M.D.

$\uparrow$ **Sensitivity** $\propto$ $\uparrow$ **NPV**	$\uparrow$ **Specificity** $\propto$ $\uparrow$ **PPV**

- Decrease ($\downarrow$) upper limit of test reference $\rightarrow$ Increase ($\uparrow$) test sensitivity. e.g. cut down reference range for DM from 140 mg / dl to 126 mg / dl will $\uparrow$ test sensitivity $\rightarrow$ $\uparrow$ test NPV

$\uparrow$ **Prevalence** $\propto$ $\uparrow$ **PPV**	$\uparrow$ **Prevalence** $\propto$ $\downarrow$ **NPV**

$\uparrow$ **Prevalence – <u>No Change</u> in sensitivity**

- **<u>Cross – Sectional Study</u>:**
- we get **Prevalence**
- Analysis done by Chi – square (x^2) test

- **<u>Case – Control Study</u>:**

- Retrospective Study
- We get **<u>Causal relationship</u>**
- Analysis done by **Odds Ratio (OR) = AD / BC**

A	B
C	D

- Always try to find (**A**) cell first
- **<u>A = Disease + Exposure</u>** to risk factor

- **<u>Cohort Study</u>:**

- Prospective Study
- We get **<u>Incidence</u>** and **<u>Causal relationship</u>**
- Analysis done by **<u>Relative Risk (RR)</u>** and **<u>Attributable Risk (AR)</u>**

- **RR = Incidence Rate (exposed) / Incidence Rate (None exposed)**

- **AR = Incidence Rate (exposed) - Incidence Rate (None exposed)**

PSYCHIATRY

- **IQ :** Average(90 – 109) (50 % of population)

- Add 10 for High average , Superior , Very Superior (2.5 % population)
    (110-119)   (120-129)   (over 130)

- Autistic children → IQ less than 70

- **Commonly used IQ test:**

- **WAIS – R – Adult (> 17 yrs)**

- **WPPSI – Pre – School & Primary (4 – 6 yrs)**

- **Stanford – Binet Scale – children (2 – 6 yrs)**

- **WISC – R – children (6 –17 yrs)**

- **Mood Disorders:** Depression or Mania (hyper)

- **Dysthymia** (non-psychotic depression) → chronic **(atleast 2 yrs)**

- **Unipolar (Major depression)** → Symptoms for **atleast 2 weeks**
- Early morning waking, **pseudodementia** in elderly

- **Cyclothymia** (non-psychotic bipolar) → chronic **(atleast 2 yrs)**
- ego-syntonic

- **Bipolar** – **Manic Symptoms** +   Major depression
    (bipolar-1)   **(bipolar-2)**

- **Schizophrenia:** Delusion, illusion, hallucination (Auditory 75 %), Blunted affect, loose associations.

- **Differential:** Schizophrenia - > 6 month of symptoms
    Schizopheniform - < 6 month of symptoms
    Brief Psychotic - < 1 month of symptoms
    Schizoid Personality – life long pattern of social withdrawal seen by
        others as eccentric, isolated
    Schizotypal personality – **Magical thinking**, illusions, ideas of
        Reference, very odd, strange, weird
    Schizoaffective – **Alteration in mood** is present during substantial
        Portion of illness + Sx of Schizophrenia

- **Subtypes of Schizophrenia:**
- **Paranoid** – Delusions of persecution (or) grandeur, hallucinations (voice)
- **Catatonic** – <u>Rigidity of posture</u>, Complete stupor, may be mute
- **Disorganized** – uninhibited, unrecognized (disorganized) behavior & speech, poor personal appearance, little contact with reality.
- **Undifferentiated** – psychotic symptoms **but** doesn't fit in above three category.
- **Residual** – Previous episode **but** no prominent psychotic symptoms at evaluation, some negative symptoms.
- **Positive Symptoms:** Delusion, hallucination, bizarre behavior (dopamine)
- **Negative Symptoms:** Flat affect, apathy, mutism (muscarinic receptor)
- **Brain structural and Anatomic abnormalities:**
- Large ventricle size, cortical atrophy, smaller volume of left hippocampus and amygdala, Atrophy of temporal lobe.
- Limbic system seen as the primary pathology site for schizophrenia.
* **Delusional Disorders: No** hallucination, Delusions are **not** bizarre (like I'm a millionaire (believable - could be possible) whereas in Schizophrenia bizarre delusion like I'm a king of Moon (not believable) and patient is not functioning.

- **Somatoform Disorder:** Production of **somatic symptoms** (like abdominal pain, headache, etc) – <u>extensive diagnostic procedures fail to show any pathology</u> – constantly change their primary physicians – unconscious symptom production
- **Factitious Disorder:** intentional symptoms production but there is no motivation to produce symptoms means symptom production is not for any gain
- **Malingering:** Intentional symptoms production for gaining something

- **Munchausen Syndrome:** Factitious disorder – usually medical field person (nurse)
- **Munchausen Syndrome by proxy:** mother produce symptoms in her baby

7. **Conversion Disorder:** One (or) more **NEUROLOGIC symptoms** (eg. paralysis of half of the body) **without** any real organic cause.
- **Loss of functioning is real & unfeigned**

* **Post-Traumatic Stress Disorder: Flashback**, Avoidance of associated stimuli – Symptoms must be exhibited for **> 1 month after passing few months** of traumatic event

- **Acute stress Disorder:** symptoms for **< 1 month soon after** traumatic event.

- **Adjustment disorder** – Symptoms must occur **within 3 months of <u>stressors</u>** and must **not** last more than 6 months – **Tx:** Supportive Psychotherapy

- **Substance Abuse:**
  - Cocaine, amphetamine, cannabis, hallucinogens and PCP (phencyclidine) → **paranoia (Schizopheniform delusion disorder)**
  - Cannabis, inhalants, hallucinogens and PCP do **not** have withdrawal reactions.

- **Cocaine** – Intoxication → **Paranoia, arrhythmias**
  Withdrawal → Depression
- **Amphetamine** – Intoxication → **Paranoia, pupillary dilatation**
  Withdrawal → Depression
- **Cannabis** – Slowed reaction time, social withdrawal, **injected conjunctiva**
- **Hallucinogens** – Ideas of reference, **brilliant color hallucination**, pupillary dilatation.
  Withdrawal – flash back (feels same as they are on drug without drug)
- **Opiates** – Intoxication → **pupillary constriction**, respiratory arrest
  Withdrawal → **flu-like symptoms Tx:** Clonidine, methadone
- **PCP – violence, vertical nystagmus**
- **Benzodiazepines** – Intoxication → inappropriate sexual / aggressive behavior
  Withdrawal → **seizures**

- **Sleep:**   Sleep cycle is regulated by super chiasmatic nucleus.
  - Non-REM → 1st half, REM → 2nd half (REM cycle → 90 mins)
  - Adults wake out of REM / 2nd stage of non-REM
  - REM → Rapid eye movement – eye is a part of brain so brain is active & body is inactive (↑ eye movement, ↓ muscle tone)
  - NREM → Opposite to REM means brain is inactive & body is active (↑ muscle tone)
  - REM sleep is requiring for memory
  - Melatonin → inhibited by Daylight (responsible for jetlag)
  - **Elderly** → REM – 20 % (constant) , stage - 4 (delta) – Vanish (↓)

- **Neurotransmitters:**
  - Serotonin – initial sleep
  - ACh – REM sleep
  - Norepinephrine - ↓ in REM sleep
  - Dopamine – Arousal & wakefulness

- **Sleep Waves:**
  - Awake → low-voltage fast waves – Beta waves
  - Drowsy →**Alpha waves** (8-12 cps) (closing the eyes)
  - Stage -1→Theta waves (3-7 cps)
  - Stage -2→ Sleep spindles **& K complexes.** (12-14 cps)
  - Delta sleep →Delta waves (1/2 –2 cps) [Delta – D means Deep sleep]
  - REM sleep →low-voltage fast with **saw tooth waves.**

- **Somnambulism:** sleep walking –occur during stage-4 (Delta sleep).

- **Nightmare:** REM sleep – person often awake – dreaming (dreams of frightening nature) – **can recall**
- **Night terror:** NREM sleep (stage 4) – person often **impossible to fully awaken** can't remember the episode

- **Narcolepsy:** excessive daytime sleepiness and abnormalities of REM sleep greater than 3 months.
  - REM sleep **occurs in less than 10 mins**
  - **Cataplexy** → Sudden loss of muscle tone
  - **Sleep paralysis**
  - **Falling asleep quickly at night**
  - **Tx:** Psychostimulant; If cataplexy present → Antidepressants

- **Modeling / Observational Learning (Social Learning):**
  - victim of abuse is now abusing his/her own child

- **Defense Mechanisms:**

* **Projection** – Paranoid behavior [Do not trust anyone!]

- **Introjection** – try to act like someone
* **eg:** Students act like the resident

* **Denial** – denies every thing
  - **eg:** I know I don't have cancer [even though patient have cancer]

- **Isolation of Affect** – no reaction on their face!
- Blunted affect (Schizophrenia)

- **Splitting** – split their behavior! Sometime very good Sometimes very bad
  - **Borderline personality**

- **Blocking** – Transient block on our memory!
  - **eg:** Oh! What's his name? I can't seem to remember his name

- **Repression** – **nonretrievable forgetting**
  - **eg:** sexually abuse girl in her childhood doesn't remember anything in her adulthood

- **Suppression** – **Forgetting is reversible**
  - **eg:** I went out for movie before the day of my anatomy exam but after coming back I again started my reading [remembered that I have exam tomorrow!]

- **Regression** – Returning to an earlier stage of development
  - **eg:** Enuresis in previously toilet train child after birth of another baby

- **Somatization** – productions of somatic symptoms [somatoform disorder]
  - **eg:** Just thinking of six flag I get Butterflies in my stomach

- **Displacement** – source stays the same, target changes
  - **eg:** My elder brother angry at me and I angry at my younger one

- **Acting out** – doing something to hide emotion!
- **eg:** Whistling in dark who is afraid of going in darkness

- **Rationalization** – Explanations are used to justify unacceptable behavior
- **eg:** USMLE step 1 exam was hard that's why I failed [Not coz he / she didn't read!]

- **Reaction formation** – Unacceptable transformed into its opposite
- **eg:** Feel love but show hate

- **Undoing** – Action to symbolically reverse the unacceptable
- **eg:** I need to wash my hands whenever I touch something
- Obsessive- compulsive behavior

- **Dissociation** – Separating self form one's own experience
- **eg:** Raped victim describe event as she is watching whole things form the roof
- Fugue, depersonalization

- **Humor** – A pleasant release from anxiety
- **eg:** Laughter hides the pain

- **Sublimation** – Unacceptable action transform into acceptable action
- **eg:** person who likes pornography becomes director of sensor board

- **Altruism** – Individual provides a helpful, gratifying service to others as a means of quelling their own anxiety. Eg: Alcoholic cirrhotic patient works as a volunteer for a non profit organization that assist patient with alcoholic cirrhosis

- **Personality Disorders:**

- **Paranoid Personality** – suspicious in nature
- Coldness & distance in most relationship
- Very hostile reaction to other people's innocent or even positive act.
- Their reaction to others may then perpetuate their problems, since other may driven away by the paranoid person's reaction

- **Narcissistic personality** – Person feels "entitled" to recognition. They often believe they are so special that others are envious of their talents. They **do not tolerate perceived rejection well.**

- **Histrionic Personality** – excessive emotion and attention seeking
- Seductive behavior - Women > Men

- **Borderline Personality** – mood swings, unstable relationship, recurrent suicidal behavior - Women > Men

- **Anti–social Personality** – continuous antisocial (or) criminal acts.
  - Usually behavior
  - Men > Women

- **Avoidant Personality** – Social inhibition, **fear of rejection, shy**

- **Dependent Personality** – Submissive, gets others to assume responsibility, can't express disagreement.

- **Obsessive–Compulsive Personality** – Perfectionist, orderly, rigid, inflexible

- **Obsessive-Compulsive anxiety disorder (OCD)** – has Obsession (persistent thoughts) and Compulsion (repetitive acts). Obsession and compulsion that are focal and acquired and have functional impairment whereas obsessive-compulsive personality disorder is life- long and less functional impairment

- ■ **Impulse Control Disorders:**

- **Intermittent Explosive Disorder** – Failure to resist aggressive impulses that result in serious assaultive acts

- **Kleptomania** – Failure to resist impulses to steal objects that the patients does not need
  - Associated with Eating disorder, mood disorders, OCD

- **Pyromania** – characterized by deliberate fire setting on more than one occasion

- **Trichotillomania** – characterized by pulling one's own hair, resulting in hair loss patient may eat hair, resulting in bezoars stomach, obstruction & malnutrition

- **Oppositional defiant disorder** – frequently loss their temper, disobey their elders, deliberately annoy others, **no** violation of rules

- **Conduct Disorders** – disregard rights and rules of the society, **< 18 yrs of age**

- **Anti-Social** – disregard rights and rules of the society, **> 18 yrs of age**

- **Selective Mutism** – speak normally in other situation **or** at home

- **Autism** – **<3 yrs of age**, repetitive behavior, marked hearing impairment

- **Undetected hearing impairment** – hereditary, repeated ear infection, symptoms are same as autism but detected at later age compare to autism

- **Childhood disintegrative disorder** – period of normal development for atleast 2 yrs followed by loss of previously acquired skills like expressive or receptive language, social skill, play & motor skills.

- **Kubler-Ross Stage of adjustment in dying patient** :

  - **D**enial
  - **A**nger
  - **B**argaining
  - **D**epression
  - **A**cceptance

  (**D A B D A**)

  • Any stage can occur first. (this order is not necessary)

- **Fuge:** Person has an abrupt change of geographic location (or) identity without alteration in consciousness (or) memory change

- **Delirium** – Acute onset, impaired cognitive functioning, fluctuating & brief
  - **Reversible**
  - **Tx:** Benzodiazepine for 3-5 days

- Suicide rate is high in native American adolescence

- **Reactive attachment disorder of infancy:** caused by sever interruption in the parent - child bond, with the parent being unable to supply the nurturing needed for adequate development of the infant.

- **Anorexia Nervosa** – **distorted body image (perception** problem – even with very thin body patient looks herself as a fatty person), 15-20 % loss of body weight – **Complication:** osteoporosis (Ca^{+2}, estrogen deficiency)**,** elevated carotene and Cholesterol, euthyroid sick syndrome, amenorrhea (estrogen deficiency), small for gestational age baby, **Cardiac arrhythmia** (due to **Hypokalemia**) (**hypomagnesemia** is another electrolyte abnormality) – First step in management of patient with Anorexia Nervosa – **Tx:** Hospitalization (weight gain & prevent complication)

- **Bulimia Nervosa** – Binge & purge – looks healthy compare to anorexia – presence dental caries, excoriation on knuckle of hand due to repeated vomiting – Level of **serotonin** is **decreased** in Bulimia that's why **SSRIs** are good choice for Bulimia.

- **Eating disorder, not otherwise specified:** features suggestive of both anorexia and bulimia, but doesn't meet the criteria for one specific eating disorder

ANTIPSYCHOTIC MEDICATIONS

- **Mood Disorders:**
- **Lithium** (DOC) (**C/I in pregnancy**), Divalproex (2nd choice)
- In pregnancy → Clonazepam, Gabapentin
- **M/A:** ↓ PIP_2 → ↓IP_3 & DAG → ↓ cAMP [renal v_2 receptor coupled to cAMP]
- **AE :** Goiter & Hypothyroidism, Teratogenic, exacerbate psoriasis
  Nephrogenic DI [Treat with Amiloride (K· sparing) **not** Thiazide]
  Low Na · → enhance toxicity
  Concentration >4 mEq/L require emergent dialysis

- **Anti- Depressants:** (Depression → Functional deficiency of **NE/5HT** in Brain)

- **MAO Inhibitors:** (Phenelezine, Tranylcypromine)
- **AE:** Hypertensive crises with Tyramine.
     Severe drug reaction with Meperidine

- **TCA s (Tricyclic Antidepressants):**
- **MA:** inhibit re-uptake of 5- HT and NE
- Amitriptyline, Imipramine, Clomipramine, Amoxepin, Doxepin .
- **USES:** Major depression, Phobic & panic anxiety state, Neuropathic pain, **Enuresis** (Imipramine), **OCD** (clomipramine).
- Similar to Phenothiazines (M block, α block, sedation, ↓ seizure threshold)
- **Cardiotoxicity** ("quinidine like"), **SIADH**

- **SSRIs:** (Fluoxitine, Sertraline, Citalopram)
- It takes 5 wks to reach steady state & 6-8 wks to show adequate response
- **Uses:** PMS, Bulimia, OCD, Alcoholism
- **AE:** Agitation (need sedatives), Weight loss (but regained after 12 months treatment), Seizure , **Sexual dysfunction** (always discuss with patient)
- **Serotonin Syndrome:** diaphoresis, rigidity, hyperthermia, ANS instability, myoclonus – occurs when it takes with MAOI.

- **Bupropion (Atypical):** block DA reuptake – **USE:** Smoking Cessation

- **Buspirone:** partial agonist at $5HT_{1A}$ - **USE:** Generalize Anxiety Disorder

- **Trazadone:** block 5HT reuptake, $5HT_2$ antagonist – **AE:** Priapism

- **Nefazodone:** block both NE & 5HT reuptake

- **Venlafaxime:** similar to SSRI

- **Mirtazapine:** similar to TCAs

- **Anti-Psychotic Drugs:**
- **Phenothiazines (Typical):** DA (dopamine) receptor antagonist
- Chlorpromazine (rarely use now), Fluphenazine, Thioridazine.
- M block, α-block, H1 receptors block, Sedation, ↓Seizure threshold.
- Quinidine **like cardiotoxicity** (Thioridazine)
- Tardive dyskinesia (TD) → Extrapyramidal dysfunction
- Fluphenazine can cause **hypothermia**

- **Butyrophenone (Typical):** DA receptor antagonist
- **Haloperidol**
- Dystonia (torticolis – spasm of sternocleidomastoid, Occulogyric crisis – eyes rolled upwards) (**Within first few day**) [Tx: **Benztropine** / Diphenhydramine]

- TD [involuntary movement of upper extremity, lip smacking, tongue protrusion, etc] **(after long term use)** [Tx: discontinue drug and start atypical antipsychotic]
- **↑ Prolactin** → gynecomastia
- Reversible **pseudo-parkinsonism**
- **Neuroleptic Malignant Syndrome** [Tx: Dentroline] [**Benztropine** is C/I because anti-cholinergic drugs retain heat]

- **Clozapine, Olanzepine, Risperidone [Atypical Anti-Psychotics]** :
- Improve negative symptoms.
- Block $5HT_2$ receptors. (not DA receptor)
- **Agranulocytosis** (**clozapine** – that's why it is not used as first-line drug)
- TD **has not** reported with clozapine and olanzapine.
- Side effect of Risperidone – movement problem likes EPS and Parkinsonism
- Side effect of Olanzepine – Obesity

- **Pimozide:** DOC for Tourette's Syndrome

- Alternative drug for bipolar – Valproic acid & Carbamazapine

- Treatment of choice for **acute management of mania, psychosis or extreme agitation** – Haloperidol (rapid onset of action) **or** Lorazepam. Lithium takes 4-10 days to exert its effect.

- Drugs should be avoided in post-traumatic stress disorder? – Benzodiazepines. **Treatment** of post-traumatic stress disorder – SSRIs, exposure or cognitive therapy.

- Personality disorders – Individual Psychotherapy
- Anxiety disorders – Behavioral Therapy (breathing exercise, exposure therapy)
- Schizophrenia – Supportive Therapy (build up trust so they talk more with you)
- Drug addiction – Group Therapy

- Treatment of **Catatonic Schizophrenia** – Benzodiazepam (Lorazepam)

- Acute Treatment of Panic Attack – Alprazolam
- Chronic Treatment of Panic Attack – SSRIs

Pharmacology

* **General Pharmacology:**

1. Which form of the drug contributes to concentration gradient?
   - Only **free drug forms** contribute to the concentration gradient

2. Which form of the drug can cross cell membranes?
   - Only **non-ionized** (**uncharged**) form of a drug crosses biomembranes

3. How P^H and P^{Ka} will affect drugs?
   - P^H and P^{Ka} will help us determine if drugs are in non-ionized form or ionized form. If $P^H – P^{Ka}$ value is **negative, weak acid** acids are **in non-ionized form** and can absorb better. For example, if $P^H – P^{Ka}$ value is -2, 99% of weak acids are in non-ionized form means they can cross cell membrane easily. If value is 0, 50% of drugs are in non-ionized form and 50% of drugs are in ionized form.
   - If $P^H – P^{Ka}$ value is **positive, weak bases** are **in non-ionized form** and can absorb better.

4. In which medium weak acid will cross cell membrane?
   - In acidic medium [means weak acid absorb better in stomach]

5. In which medium weak base will cross cell membrane?
   - In basic medium, weak base will cross cell membrane

6. Which drug form is reabsorbed from the kidney?
   - only non-ionized form reabsorb [Both ionized & non-ionized form filtered through glomerulus]

7. How acidification and alkalization of urine will affect elimination of drug?
   - **Acidification of urine** causes increase ionization of weak bases means **increase elimination of weak bases**
   - **Alkalization of urine** causes increase ionization of weak acids means **increase elimination of weak acids**

8. What are the things we use to acidify and alkalize urine?
   - NH_4Cl, Vit- C, Cranberry juice to acidify urine
   - $NaHCO_3$, Acetazolamide to alkalize urine

9. Which route has 100% bioavailability (f)?
   - IV route

10. What is the relationship b/w distribution of drug (V_d) and plasma concentration of drug?
    - Increase V_d – decrease plasma concentration of drugs
    - Increase plasma protein binding – decrease V_d

11. What should I remember for drug with high V_d?

- Drugs with **high V_d** value raise the possibility of **displacement** by other agents and therefore change in pharmacologic activities

12. What is loading dose? How will it affected by bioavailability?

- Variables are used to calculate the loading dose:
  Cp = desired peak concentration of drug
  Vd = volume of distribution of drug
  F = bioavailability
- The required loading dose may then be calculated as
  LD = Cp x Vd / F
- Bioavailability (f) is affect LD in following way
- **If f = 0.5** then **LD should double** (×2)
- **If f = 0.25** then **LD should quadruple** (×4)

13. What is the renal clearance of drug?

- $K = Cu \times Q / C_P$ [Cu = concentration in urine, Q = urine flow, Cp = plasma concentration]

14. What is infusion rate?

- Drug $_{\text{Infusion rate}}$ = steady state concentration (C_{ss}) x Clearance

15. What is maintenance rate?

- Drug $_{\text{maintenance rate}}$ = steady state concentration (C_{ss}) x Clearance x dosing interval

16. What is elimination constant?

- Ke (elimination constant) = $0.7/ T_{1/2}$ = Clearance / Vd

17. What is elimination half life?

- $T_{1/2}$ = 0.7 / Ke

18. What is steady state and on what it depends?

- Steady state: rate in = rate out. It depends on $T_{1/2}$

19. At which half life we attain clinically significant steady state?

- 4-5 times $T_{1/2}$

20. What is zero order elimination? Give 2 important examples

- There are circumstances where sufficient quantity of drug is ingested which saturate the metabolic enzymes in the liver, and so is **eliminated** from the body **at an approximately constant rate (amount)**
- Examples: large amount of Ethanol, Salicylates (Aspirin) at toxic dose

21. What is first order elimination? How it differs from zero order?

- **constant proportion (percentage)** of the drug is **eliminated** per unit time

- Difference: Amount of drug eliminate in per unit time is same in zero-order means if 50 mg is eliminated in one hour then 50 mg will be eliminated after each hour. If 200 mg in the body zero-order will follow like this: 200 – 150 – 100 – 50 – 0. Percentage of drug eliminate in per unit time is same in first-order means if 50% of drug is eliminated in one hour then 50% will be eliminated after each hour. If 200 mg in the body first-order will follow like this: 200 – 100 – 50 – 25 – 12.5

22. What happen to elimination when you increase drug dose in first order elimination?
- **Increase drug dose** in first-order will **increase elimination** [that's not happen in zero-order]

23. What is potency? What is efficacy?
- Efficacy: ability of a drug to induce a **biological response** in its molecular target. [there is no matter how much amount require]
- Potency: **amount** of drug require to achieve maximal response
- Example: If 100 mg of drug X produce maximal effect and 10 mg of drug Y produce same maximal effect, then both drug X & Y have same efficacy but drug Y is more potent then drug X

24. What is full agonist? What is partial agonist?
- Full agonist: bind and activate receptors and show full efficacy at that receptor
- Partial agonist: bind and activate receptor but show partial efficacy at that receptor compare to full agonist
- Inverse agonist: bind and activate receptor but show reverse the action of that receptor

25. What happen if partial agonist is given to the patient who already received full agonist?
- Response will decrease b/c partial agonist displace full agonist from receptor. Here it will work as Antagonist

26. What is antagonist? Competitive, Non-competitive?
- Antagonist: binds to the receptor but doesn't provoke any response, but block or decrease the agonist-mediated response
- Competitive: **reversibly** bind to receptors at the **same binding site** as the endogenous **agonist bind**, but **without activating the receptor** [Increase level of agonist may replace competitive antagonist and reverse its action]
- Example: Atropine for ACh receptors
- Non-competitive: bind to a distinctly **separate binding site** from the agonist on the receptor and exert their action to that receptor [Increase level of agonist doesn't have any effect on non-competitive antagonist]
- Example: Phenoxybenzamine at alpha-receptors
- [learn how to identify effect of agonist, antagonist and partial agonist on graph]

27. What are the difference b/w physiological antagonist and pharmacological antagonist?

- Physiological antagonist works on different receptors [example: ACh causes decrease in heart rate through M2 receptor where as Epinephrine causes increase in heart rate through beta-receptors. ACh & Epinephrine are antagonist to each other's action and both work at different receptors]
- Pharmacological antagonist works on same receptors as endogenous agonist works. [example: Atropine binds to same receptor where ACh binds but exert opposite effect than ACh]

28. What is therapeutic index (TI)? Importance of it? Give 2 examples of drugs with low TI

- It is the ratio given by the toxic dose divided by the therapeutic dose
- Importance: drugs with narrow TI should monitor more frequently as slight fluctuation in their level can produce toxic effect
- Examples: Lithium, Warfarin, Theophylline

29. How intracellular receptors differ from membrane bounded receptors?

- Intracellular receptors act via modifying gene expression so it takes time for them to exert their effect
- Example: Steroids, Hormones

30. Give examples of receptors that directly couple with ion channels

- N_N (Ach) in ANS ganglia, CNS $\rightarrow$ Directly coupled to Na / K ion channel
- N_M (Ach) in skeletal muscle $\rightarrow$ Directly coupled to Na / K ion channel
- GABA $_A$ in CNS $\rightarrow$ Directly couple to Cl$^-$ ion channel

31. Give examples of receptors that linked via protein to ion channels

- α, beta, Dopamine, Histamine, Glucagon, M, Angiotensin-2, opioid, serotonin receptors

32. What is the difference b/w Gs & Gi protein? Give examples of both

- **Gs:** stimulate Proteinkinase A causes $\uparrow$ cAMP – exert **stimulating effect** on organs; Examples: **Beta**, D_1, H_2, **Glucagon**
  Gi: $\downarrow$ cAMP – exert **inhibitory effect** on organs; Examples: α_2, M_2, D_2

33. How Gq protein works? Give examples of receptors that use this pathway

- **Gq:** produce IP3 & DAG; IP3 increases $\uparrow Ca^{+2}$ and DAG stimulates Proteinkinase C; Examples: α_1, M_1 & M_3, **Angiotensin-2** (AG-II)

34. Give examples of receptors that use cGMP

- **H_1, M_3, NO (nitrous oxide)** [cGMP is present in vascular smooth muscles. It relaxes smooth muscles and **produce vasodilation**]

35. Give examples of receptors that work through transmembrane enzymes. How?
- Insulin, EGF, PDGF, ANF; they stimulate tyrosine kinase domain in cytoplasm to exert their action

36. How cytokines work?
- Erythropoietin, Somatotropin, Interferon; they stimulate tyrosine kinase domain in cytoplasm to exert their action

* **ANS (Autonomic Nervous System):**
37. What are the ANS receptors and neurotransmitters? Where are they located?
- Nicotinic, Muscarinic, Alpha & Beta receptors
- <u>Neurotransmitters</u>: ACh (act on nicotinic and muscarinic receptors), Epinephrine & Norepinephrine (act on alpha and beta receptors)
- N_N – Cell bodies in ganglia of both PANS & SANS & in the **adrenal Medulla**
- N_M - Skeletal muscles
- M_{1-3} – Located on the organ & tissues innervated by PANS & **on thermoregulatory sweat glands which are innervated by <u>SANS</u>**
- Alpha & Beta – Located on the organ & tissues innervated by SANS
- <u>Easy way to remember</u> **important** <u>Muscarinic location</u>: only Heart has M_2, all other places have M_3, GI glands have M_1;
- Now remember M_2 is operated through Gi so it has inhibitory effect on the organ. So whenever ACh stimulate M_2 it causes decrease in heart rate and decrease in conduction velocity (AV block); M_{1-3} operated through Gq so they have stimulating effect whenever they are stimulated through ACh [<u>Location of M_3</u> – **Eye**: Miosis (constriction of pupils) through contraction of <u>sphincter muscles</u> of pupil and Accommodation for near vision through contraction of <u>Ciliary muscles</u>; **Bladder:** voiding of urine through contraction of detrusor muscles; **Sphincters:** contraction of all sphincters in the body except LES (lower esophageal sphincter) which relax; **Blood vessels:** dilation of blood vessels through nitrous oxide and EDRF; **GIT:** increase motility of stomach, increase secretions of GI glands
- <u>Easy way to remember</u> **important** <u>Alpha receptors location</u>: α_2 present at only three locations 3P [Platelets, Pancreas & Pre-junctional nerve terminal] All other places have α_1
- Now remember α_2 works through Gi so whenever they stimulate they have inhibitory effects. So they decrease norepinephrine secretion at pre-junctional nerve terminals, decrease release of pancreas and causes aggregation of platelets
- α_1 receptors works opposite to ACh so they produce Mydriasis (dilatation of pupils), vasoconstrictions and urinary retention; other important location vas deference in male
- <u>Easy way to remember</u> **important** <u>Beta receptors location</u>: β_1 presents on heart and kidney; all other places have β_2
- Now remember both beta receptors work through Gs so they have stimulatory effect on the organ whenever they are stimulated; β_1 increases every thing means it increases heart rate, conduction velocity, force of contraction and release of renin

- Stimulation of β_2 receptors causes vasodilation, relaxation of uterus, bronchial dilation; other important location skeletal muscles (increase contractility – **tremors**), liver (increase glyconeogenesis) and pancreas (increase insulin secretion)

Cholinergic	Anti-Ch	α_1 Receptor	α_2 Receptor	β_1 Receptor	β_2 Receptor
Miosis (all cholinergic action occur through M_3 except in heart where it is M_2)	**Mydriasis** Atropine enter in CNS will produce confusion, hallucination	**Mydriasis**	↓ **insulin secretion**	**Increase everything** (HR, force of contraction, conduction velocity Renin secretion.)	↑ insulin secretion
AV block (M_2)	Urinary retention	Urinary retention	↓ **NE**		Dilation of bronchi
Vasodilation		**Constriction of vessels**			vasodilation
Voiding of urine	Dry mouth				Relaxation of uterus

- **Agonist** of above receptors produce **same effect as above** receptors
- **Indirect agonist** produce same effect as agonist but different mechanism
- **Antagonist** of above receptors produce **opposite effects than above** receptors

38. What is an important thing about thermoregulatory gland and which ANS receptors are present there?
- Thermoregulatory glands contain muscarinic receptors but they are innervated by SANS

39. Which neurotransmitter is present at pre-ganglionic fibers of both PANS & SANS?
- ACh (acetylcholine)

40. What are the neurotransmitters for post-ganglionic fibers of PANS & SANS?
- Post-ganglionic PANS – ACh
- Post-ganglionic SANS – NE, E, DA

41. Which is dominant in the tissue with dual innervation? (PANS & SANS) What is an exception to this rule?
- For effector tissues **with Dual innervation, PANS is dominant**
- Exception: Blood vessels – **only SANS** → produce vasoconstriction

42. Synthesis & Degradation of ACh
- Choline + Acetyl Co-A → choline acetyltransferases → ACh
- Choline acetyltransferases is found in neurons
- ACh → acetylcholinesterase → Choline + Acetate
- Choline is taken up for reuse

- Acetylcholinesterase is found in synaptic cleft

43. Which drug inhibits choline uptake?
- Hemicholinum [decrease ACh formation]

44. Which drug inhibits Ach release?
- Botulinum toxin

45. Give the name of drugs which directly stimulates Ach receptors
- Pilocarpine, Bethanechol, Methacholine

46. Give the name of indirectly acting cholinomimetics drugs
- Neostigmine, Physostigmine, Edrophonium, Pyridostigmine, Donepezil [by <u>reversibly</u> inhibiting acetylcholinesterase, they increase effect of ACh]
- Echothiophate, Organophosphate insecticides [by <u>irreversibly</u> inhibiting acetylcholinesterase, they increase effect of ACh]

47. Give the name of Muscarinic receptor antagonist
- Atropine, Ipratropium, Scopolamine (Hyoscine)

48. Give the name of Nicotinic receptor antagonist (Ganglion blockers)
- Mecamylamine, Hexamethonium

49. Give the name of Neuromuscular blockers
- Succinylcholine, Atracurium, Tubocurarine, Vecuronium

50. Difference b/w succinylcholine and other neuromuscular blockers
- **Succinylcholine** is **Depolarizing** neuromuscular blocker
- Others are non-depolarizing neuromuscular blockers

51. Why do we use pilocarpine in acute angle closure glaucoma?
- It causes constriction of pupils by which it pulls Ciliary process and increase aqueous drainage so it decrease IOP fast

52. Use of drugs that directly stimulate Ach receptors
- <u>Pilocarpine</u>: acute glaucoma, sweat test for diagnosis of Cystic Fibrosis
- <u>Bethanechol</u>: urinary retention, post-op Ileus
- <u>Methacholine</u>: diagnosis bronchial hyperactivity in COPD

53. Use of drugs that indirectly stimulate Ach receptors (AchE inhibitors)
- <u>Physostigmine</u>: glaucoma, anticholinergic overdose (atropine)
- <u>Neostigmine</u>, <u>Pyridostigmine</u>: myasthenia gravis
- <u>Edrophonium</u>: to differentiate myasthenia from cholinergic crisis
- <u>Donepezil</u>, <u>Tacrine</u> (enter in CNS): Alzheimer's disease

54. Use of anti-cholinergic drugs
  - Atropine (enter in CNS): Anti-AchE inhibitors overdose, Bradycardia, Heart block, pupillary dilation with cycloplegia
  - Ipratropium: COPD
  - Scopolamine: motion sickness

55. Use of neuromuscular blockers
  - Endotracheal intubation

56. Important side effects of succinylcholine
  - Malignant hyperthermia [Tx: Dantrolene – inhibits release of Ca^{++} from sarcoplasmic reticulum – relax all muscles], Hyperkalemia

57. Important side effects of Atracurium
  - It releases histamine [vasodilation, rash, bronchial constriction]

58. Treatment of overdose of non-depolarizing neuromuscular blockers
  - Physostigmine, Neostigmine

59. Difference b/w Physostigmine & Neostigmine, Pyridostigmine
  - **Physostigmine** can **enter in CNS** that's why it is used in anticholinergic overdose

60. Treatment of AchE Inhibitors poisoning.
  - Atropine & Pralidoxime (2-PAM) (as early as possible) (2-PAM will reactivate acetylcholinesterase)

61. How anti-cholinergic drugs are helpful in Parkinsonism? Which symptom is not improved by anti-cholinergic drugs?
  - In Parkinsonism, there is imbalance b/w ACh & DA (dopamine). There is increase in ACh so giving anti-cholinergic will reduce tremors and rigidity symptoms of Parkinsonism. It has **no effect on Bradykinesia**

62. What is the difference b/w Atropine and Phenylephrine when it comes to use for eye dilatation?
  - Atropine - **Mydriasis & Cycloplegia** (spasm of accommodation)
  - Phenylephrine (α_1 – agonist) $\rightarrow$ Mydriasis **without** Cycloplegia

63. How ANS work to control BP
  - ($\uparrow\alpha_1$) $\uparrow$ TPR $\rightarrow$ **$\uparrow$ BP $\rightarrow$ reflex bradycardia**
  - ($\uparrow\beta_1$) $\downarrow$ TPR $\rightarrow$ **$\downarrow$ BP $\rightarrow$ reflex Tachycardia**

64. Difference b/w Norepinephrine & Epinephrine
  - Norepinephrine (NE) – $\alpha_1 \alpha_2 \beta_1$ [**No** β_2 action]
  - Epinephrine (E) – $\alpha_1 \alpha_2 \beta_1 \beta_2$ [act on all adrenergic receptors] [**Low dose** of E – **beta action** is predominant] [**High dose** of E – **alpha** action is predominant]

65. What is Epinephrine reversal
- High dose epinephrine ($\uparrow$ BP through α **action**)
  $$\downarrow$$
  Then if α Blocker given
  $$\downarrow$$
  Fall in BP occur ($\downarrow$ BP) (Because α activity block but β activity remains)

66. Use of epinephrine
- Anaphylaxis, Cardiac arrest, Laryngospasm, Status asthmatics

67. Give Name of Alpha & Beta receptors agonist
- α_1 agonist: Methoxamine, Phenylephrine
- α_2 agonist: Clonidine (mixed α_1 & α_2 actions), Methyldopa
- β_2 agonist: Salmeterol, Salbutamol, Terbutaline, Metaproterenol, Dobutamine ($\beta_1 > \beta_2$), Dopamine

68. Give Name of Alpha & Beta receptors antagonist
- α_1 antagonist: Prazosin, Terazosin, Doxazosin
- α_2 antagonist: Yohimbine, benzylpiperazine
- Non-selective α antagonist: Phenoxybenzamine (non-competitive), Phentolamine (competitive)
- Non-selective β antagonist: Propranolol, Timolol, Pindolol (ISA), Sotalol
- Selective β_1 antagonist: Acebutolol (ISA), Metoprolol, Atenolol, Esmolol

69. Use of Alpha agonists:
- Methoxamine: paroxysmal supraventricular tachycardia
- Phenylephrine: nasal decongestant
- Clonidine: antihypertensive, opioid detoxification, also use in conjunction with methylphenidate in ADHD
- Methyldopa (alpha methylnorepinephrine is an active form of methyldopa which act centrally): gestational hypertension

70. Use of Alpha antagonist:
- Phenoxybenzamine: As an anti-HTN in Pheochromocytoma
- Doxazosin: BPH (benign prostatic hypertrophy), Anti-HTN
- Yohimbine: postural hypotension, impotence

71. Use of Beta agonist:
- Salmeterol, Salbutamol: bronchial asthma
- Terbutaline, Ritodrine: pre-mature labour
72. Use of Beta antagonist:
- HTN, CHF, MI, Angina, Arrhythmia, **Migraine prophylaxis**, Glaucoma, **Essential tremor**, **Portal HTN**, **Social anxiety**

73. Important side effect of Clonidine
- Rebound HTN on abrupt withdrawal

74. Important side effect of alpha blocker
- First dose syncope

75. Important contraindications of beta blockers
- Bronchial Asthma, COPD, PVD

76. Important side effects of non-selective beta blockers
- Sexual dysfunction, delayed hypoglycemia, alter plasma lipids, fatigue, heart block, depression

77. Dopamine receptor locations:
- D_1 (Peripheral): Renal, Mesenteric, coronary vessels
- D_2: Central Nervous System

78. Difference b/w Dopamine & Dobutamine
- Dopamine has effect on renal vasculature which is advantage over Dobutamine

79. What is an important thing to remember about indirect acting adrenoceptor agonist?
- Indirect agonist act only on effector tissues innervated by SANS. Denervated tissues are non-responsive. (e.g. If Heart is transplanted , then SANS fibers are not present their , so in that pt. indirect acting adrenoceptor agonist give **no** response)

80. What is tachyphylaxis?
- Tachyphylaxis means a rapid loss of pharmacologic activity; Chronic use of decongestant produce tachyphylaxis b/c NE store may become depleted

81. What is the main difference b/w Phenoxybenzamine & Phentolamine?
- Phenoxybenzamine (non-competitive), Phentolamine (competitive)

82. Name of non-selective beta blockers with ISA (intrinsic Sympathomimetic action)
- Pindolol

83. Name of selective beta-1 antagonist with ISA
- Acebutolol

84. Usefulness of beta-blockers with ISA
- Less bradycardia & minimal change in plasma lipids

85. Drugs with both alpha-1 & beta blocking activity
- Labetalol, Carvedilol

* **CVS (Cardiovascular System):**
  86. Mechanism of different classes of Antiarrhythmic drugs
  - Class 1: Block Na^+ channels [increase action potential duration by decreasing Vmax]
  - Class 2: beta blockers [AV block so useful in supraventricular tachycardia]

- Class 3: Block K$^+$ channels [Prolong repolarization and refractory period so useful in re-entrant tachycardia]
- Class 4: Block Ca^{++} channels [decrease conduction through AV node and shorten phase-2 (plateau) – decrease contractility]

87. Name of drugs according to different classes [class 1 to 4]
- Class 1a: Quinidine, Procainamide
- Class 1b: Lidocaine, Phenytoin
- Class 1c: Flecainide, Propafenone
- Class 2: Propranolol, Esmolol, Sotalol
- Calss 3: Amiodarone, Sotalol
- Class 4: Verapamil, Diltiazem

88. What are important characteristics of quinidine?
- Also block K$^+$ channel, M$_2$ receptors and alpha-1 receptors

89. Use of quinidine
- Atrial fibrillation (AF) [Quinidine itself increase risk of arrhythmia therefore prior digitalization is required], Also used in malaria

90. Important AE (adverse effects) of quinidine
- Immune thrombocytopenia, **Immune hemolysis**, Cinchonism [quinidine intoxication: tinnitus (characteristic), occular dysfunction], **Torsade de pointes** [increase QT interval]

91. Important use of **Procainamide**
- **WPW syndrome** [Wolff-Parkinson-White]

92. What is the characteristic of Lidocaine?
- Not useful orally due to rapid first-pass metabolism

93. Use & AE of Lidocaine
- Use: Post-MI ventricular arrhythmia, arrhythmia due to digoxin
- AE: **Seizures** in overdose

94. Anti-arrhythmic use of Phenytoin
- Arrhythmia due to Digoxin overdose

95. What are important things I should remember about Amiodarone?
- Mimic all 4 classes, long half lives
- AE: Interstitial lung disease (**pulmonary fibrosis**), **Thyroid dysfunction** (hypothyroidism / hyperthyroidism), Increase LDL, Torsade de pointes

96. What is an important thing I should remember about Sotalol?
- Mimic both class 2 & 3

97. What is the main difference b/w Verapamil and Nifedepine
- Verapamil is more cardio selective

98. Different Class of Calcium Channel Blockers (CCB)
- **Dihydropyridine:** Nifedepine, Amlodepine, Felodepine – less cardio selective – more effect on vasculature so useful in HTN – <u>SE</u>: vasodilation & hypotension causes reflex tachycardia
- **Phenylalkylamine:** Verapamil – more cardio selective – reverse cardiospasm so use in treating angina
- **Benzothiazepine:** Diltiazem – intermediate – both cardio selective & vasodilator – use in controlling HR in atrial arrhythmias – less reflex tachycardia due to both effects.
- **Effect of cardio selective CCB on Heart:** reduce heart rate (cardio depressant!!) mainly through AV block that's why used in atrial arrhythmias

99. Where shouldn't we use calcium channel blockers (CCB)?
- WPW syndrome [Digoxin is C/I too], CHF

100. Mechanism & Use of Adenosine
- <u>Mechanism</u>: Inhibits adenyl cyclase by which it **reduces cAMP** and so it causes **cell hyperpolarization** by increasing outward K+ flux. It is a **potent coronary vasodilator**
- <u>Use</u>: DOC for paroxysmal supraventricular tachycardia (**PSVT**)

101. Drugs causing Torsade. **Treatment of Torsade**
- Drugs that block K^+ ion channel produce Torsade like quinidine, Procainamide, Amiodarone, Sotalol
- <u>Tx</u>: **Magnesium**

102. Safe anti-hypertensive drug in Pregnancy & renal dysfunction
- **Methyldopa**

103. Anti-hypertensive (HTN) drug that is contraindicated in pregnancy
- Angiotensin converting enzyme inhibitors (ACEI)

104. Mechanism of water retention when we use anti-HTN drugs
- Water retention ($\downarrow$ BP → increase in ADH release & Renin-Angiotensin system activity → Na & water retention)

105. Between alpha & beta blockers which affect plasma lipid level
- Beta blockers [Alpha blockers have no effect on plasma lipid]

106. Name & Mechanism of vasodilators
- <u>Hydralazine, Nitroprusside</u>: Increase cGMP via release of nitrous oxide
- <u>Minoxidil</u>: K^+ channel agonist; chemical structure similar to nitrous oxide so may be nitrous oxide agonist

107.   Drugs for **HTN emergency**
- Nitroprusside, Labetalol

108.   Side effect of Hydralazine
- Drug induced lupus erythematous

109.   Side effects of Nitroprusside
- Rebound HTN, Cyanide poisoning

110.   Side effect of Minoxidil for which this drug is used clinically
- Hypertrichosis (used clinically in hair loss)

111.   Side effect of Diazoxide for which this drug is used clinically
- Insulinoma [decrease insulin release]

112.   Which CCB is used in subarachnoid hemorrhage?
- Nimodipine (produce constriction of cerebral vasculature)

113.   Name of ACEI and AT-1 receptor blockers
- ACEI: Captopril, Enalapril, Lisinopril
- AT-1 antagonist: Losartan

114.   Which are the most important side effects of ACE inhibitors?
- Dry cough (increase bradykinin), Hyperkalemia

115.   Contraindication of ACEI
- Anaphylaxis (Angioedema)
- Renal artery stenosis

116.   What is the difference b/w ACEI and AT-1 receptor blocker?
- Dry cough is not seen with AT-1 receptor blockers

117.   What are the side effects of Loop & Thiazide diuretics in regards to pH & Potassium?
- Both Loop & thiazide diuretics produce **Alkalosis & Hypokalemia**

118.   What are the side effects of Carbonic anhydrase (CA) diuretics in regards to pH & Potassium?
- CA inhibitors diuretics produce **Acidosis & Hypokalemia**

119.   What are the side effects of K+ sparing diuretics in regards to pH & Potassium?
- K^+ sparing diuretics produce **Acidosis & Hyperkalemia**

120.   What is the mechanism of action of Mannitol? Important uses
- M/A: filtered but do <u>not</u> reabsorbed; It draws more water with it in urine

- Use: to decrease intracranial pressure, to decrease occular pressure in acute glaucoma, to prevent renal failure in hemolysis and rhabdomyolysis

121. In which condition Mannitol is C/I?
- Pulmonary edema

122. What is the site of action of CA inhibitors? Important uses & AE
- M/A: block formation of H_2CO_3; indirectly block Na/H transporter in PCT
- Use: glaucoma, benign intracranial hypertension (pseudotumor cerebri), high altitude sickness
- AE: **Renal stone**, numbness & tingling in fingers and toes

123. What is the mechanism and site of action of Loop diuretics? Important AE
- M/A: Inhibits Na^+- K^+-2Cl^- symporter in thick ascending loop of Henle
- A/E: Ototoxicity (ethacrynate), Hypomagnesemia, Hypocalcemia (increase Ca loss in urine)

124. What is the mechanism and site of action of Thiazide diuretics?
- M/A: Inhibits Na^+- K^+-2Cl^- symporter in DCT
- AE: hyperglycemia, hyperlipidemia, Hypercalcemia (decrease Ca in urine)

125. What is the relationship b/w GFR & thiazide diuretic?
- ↓ GFR α ↓ activity

126. How will I identify loop & thiazide diuretics from urine analysis?
- loop causes **Hypocalcemia** by loosing more Ca^{++} in urine where as **Thiazide causes Hypercalcemia** by ↑ Ca^{++} Absorption & is the **only** diuretics which absorb Ca^{++}. Therefore thiazide is **given in Pt with h/o Ca^{++} stone**

127. What is the mechanism and site of action of K+ sparing diuretics? Important AE of Spironolactone
- Spironolactone: competitive antagonist of aldosterone; prevent potassium and hydrogen secretion
- Amiloride, Triamterene: directly block epithelial Na channel in DCT
- A/E: Gynacomastia, hirsutism, sexual dysfunction (Spironolactone), renal stones

128. What is the main difference b/w mechanism of action of Reserpine & Guanethidine?
- Reserpine: **block** the vesicular monoamine transporter (VMT) [decrease NE in sympathetic neurons by **decreasing** its **uptake** which leads to ↓ **CO** & ↓ **PVR**]
- Guanethidine: **blocks** the **release** of norepinephrine in response to arrival of an action potential so decrease NE in synaptic cleft which leads to ↓ **CO** & ↓ **PVR**]

129. Important side effect of Reserpine
- **Severe depression**, hypotension, Hyperprolactinemia

130. Important side effect of Guanethidine
- Hypotension, Sexual dysfunction

131. What is the MA of ACEI in CHF?
- ↓ Preload & ↓ afterload

132. What is the mechanism of action (MA) of digitalis?
- **Inhibits Na / K ATPase**

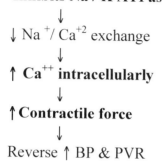

↓ Na$^+$/ Ca^{+2} exchange
↓
↑ Ca^{++} **intracellularly**
↓
↑ **Contractile force**
↓
Reverse ↑ BP & PVR

133. Is digitalis prolongs survival of patient with CHF?
- No. [ACEI prolongs survival of patient with CHF]

134. Uses of digitalis. (Vagomimetic effect)
- In reentrant cardiac arrhythmias and to slow ventricular rate in atrial fibrillation

135. Symptoms of digitalis toxicity; treatment of the same
- Nausea, vomiting, anorexia, diarrhea, abdominal pain, hallucinations, heart block, bradycardia, tachycardia
- Tx: Lidocaine, Phenytoin, Digitalis Fab antibodies, cardioversion

136. What increases digitalis toxicity?
- Hypokalemia [K$^+$ and Digitalis both competes for Na-K ATPase], Hypomagnesemia [Most diuretics causes hypokalemia and hypomagnesemia so electrolyte should be monitored frequently for those who are on diuretics and digitalis]

137. In which condition CCB & digitalis should avoid?
- WPW syndrome

138. Which drug has shown to reduce mortality in patient with CHF when use in conjunction with ACEI?
- Spironolactone

139. What is the MA of Nitrates? What is the MA of Sildenafil (Viagra)?
- Nitrates: venous and arterial vasodilation through NO
- Sildenafil: inhibits cGMP specific phosphodiesterase 5 (PDE-5) – increase in cGMP which causes vasodilation

140. What happen if we use Viagra and Nitrates together?
- Excessive fall in BP occurs

141. Use of Sildenafil besides erectile dysfunction
- Pulmonary HTN

142. What is the half life of Nitrates?
- Around 5-hrs

143. Are beta-blockers helpful in Prinzmetal angina?
- No. [Prinzmetal angina is caused by spasm of coronary vessels and beta blockers doesn't relieve spasm]

144. What is the MA of CCB in angina?
- Decrease contractility, decrease preload & afterload (vasodilation), decrease vasospasm

145. Which drugs are useful in hyper-TGs?
- Niacin, Atrovastatin, Gemfibrozil

146. Which is the only "statins" lower TG?
- Atrovastatin

147. What is the MA & side effect of bile acid sequesters?
- M/A: They serve as ion exchange resins so they bind with bile acids and prevent its reabsorption to enter in enterohepatic circulation
- AE: Decrease absorption of fat soluble vitamins (A,D,E,K)

148. What are the main AE of HMG-CoA reductase inhibitors?
- Myositis, Myopathies and Rhabdomyolysis (increase risk with fibrates)

149. What are the important effects of Nicotinic acid? Important AE
- It blocks breakdown of fats in adipose tissue by which it decreases level of VLDL (a precursor of LDL)
- AE: facial flushing and itching, dyspepsia, hyperglycemia

150. What are the MA & important AE of gemfibrozil?
- MA: increase activity of peroxisome proliferators-activated receptor alpha which is involved in metabolism of carbohydrates and fat; also **increase lipoprotein lipase synthesis** – decrease VLDL, LDL and TGs
- AE: Gallstones, Hypokalemia, Rhabdomyolysis with statins

* **CNS (Central Nervous System):**
  151. MA of Barbiturates and Benzodiazepines
  - <u>MA</u>: Both binds to GABA$_A$ receptors at different sites and potentiate its effect. GABA$_A$ receptor is potential CNS inhibitors. **Barbiturates** produce their pharmacological effects by **increasing the length of time the chloride ion channel remains open** at the GABA$_A$ receptor whereas **benzodiazepines increase the opening frequency of the chloride ion channel** at the GABA$_A$ receptor

  152. Which benzodiazepines metabolized outside of liver (means doesn't require phase-1 metabolism)? What's the advantage of it?
  - Lorazepam, Oxazepam
  - <u>Advantage</u>: can be used safely in liver dysfunction and elderly people

  153. Non-benzodiazepine drugs that activate benzodiazepine receptors
  - Zolpidem

  154. Drug use in barbiturates withdrawal
  - Diazepam

  155. DOC for status epileptics
  - Lorazepam

  156. Important C/I of barbiturates
  - Porphyria

  157. M/A of Buspirone and **Indication**
  - 5 HT1A pre-synaptic receptor partial agonist
  - **No** action on GABA
  - <u>Indication</u>: Generalized anxiety disorder (GAD)

  158. DOC for social and performance anxiety
  - Propranolol

  159. **DOC for alcohol overdose**. M/A of it
  - Fomepizole
  - <u>MA</u>: long acting inhibitors of alcoholic dehydrogenase (ADH)

  160. Reason for giving Ethanol in Methanol poisoning
  - Ethanol inhibits formation of formaldehyde which form formic acid (toxic to eyes)

  161. M/A of Disulfiram. Use of it. Drug causing Disulfiram like reaction when use with alcohol
  - Normally alcohol is converted into acetaldehyde by alcohol dehydrogenase which is then convert into acetic acid by acetaldehyde dehydrogenase; Disulfiram

inhibits acetaldehyde dehydrogenase by which it increase level of acetaldehyde which produce unpleasant symptoms after drinking alcohol

- Use: alcohol detoxification
- Drugs causing Disulfiram like effects with alcohol: Metronidazole, Cephalosporins, Oral anti-diabetic agents

162. M/A of different anti-epileptic drugs
- MA: The major molecular targets of anticonvulsant drugs are 1) voltage-gated sodium channels [carbamazapine, phenytoin, Valproic acid]; 2) components of the GABA system, including GABA$_A$ receptors [Benzodiazepines, Barbiturates]; and 3) voltage-gated calcium channel [Ethosuximide, Valproic acid]

163. Safe anti-epileptic drug during pregnancy
- Phenobarbital

164. DOC for Absence (Petitmal) seizure
- Ethosuximide

165. Usually a DOC for all other seizure
- Valproic acid

166. Important drug interaction of all anticonvulsants
- Decrease efficacy of oral contraceptives

167. Important AE of all anticonvulsants
- Phenytoin: horizontal nystagmus, gingival overgrowth, Megaloblastic anemia (folic acid depletion), Fetal hydantoin syndrome (teratogenic)
- Carbamazapine: SIADH, teratogenic (supply folic acid)
- Valproic acid: thrombocytopenia
- Ethosuximide: GI distress

168. DOC for trigeminal neuralgia
- Carbamazapine, Gabapentin

169. M/A of newer anticonvulsants
- Block AMPA receptor – lamotrigine, topiramate
- Block NMDA receptor – felbamate

170. M/A of general anesthetics
- MA: Inhibits excitatory function of some CNS receptors [glutamate, 5-HT receptors], some stimulate inhibitory receptors [GABA$_A$]

171. Importance of Blood-gas ratio for inhaled anesthetics
- High blood-gas ratio – quick redistribution in adipose tissue
- Quick redistribution in fat – require high dose to maintain blood level
- High dose – late recovery

- Importance: High blood-gas ratio – late recovery, Low blood-gas ratio – fast recovery

172. **Important AE of Halothane** and Tx of that adverse reaction. M/A of drug that used to Tx adverse reaction of Halothane
- **Malignant hyperthermia** in genetically susceptible individuals [Tx: Dantrolene – inhibits release of Ca^{++} from sarcoplasmic reticulum – relax all muscles]

173. Which inhaled anesthetic produce dose related depression of myocardial contractility?
- Enflurane [Another side effect – lower threshold for seizure so it should not be used in patient with h/o epilepsy]

174. Name and uses of IV anesthetics
- Thiopental: ultra short acting barbiturate used as IV in general anesthesia; **Rapid recovery** b/c redistribution from CNS to Peripheral tissues [exhibits zero-order kinetics]
- Propofol: rapid onset and recovery, produce amnesia, Useful for minor out-patient procedure like colonoscopy, AE: Dystonia

175. What is a neuroleptic anesthesia?
- Droperidol and Fentanyl combination is used to achieve pain control for minor procedure which is called neuroleptic anesthesia. Sometimes N_2O ["laughing gas"] is also added in this combination

176. Which drug produce "dissociative anesthesia"?
- Ketamine [block NMDA receptors, also bind opioid μ (mu) and σ (sigma) receptors]

177. M/A of local anesthetics. Two groups of local anesthetics
- MA: reversibly decrease the rate of depolarization and repolarization by **inhibiting Na influx** through sodium channels in neuronal cells
- Amino Amide: Lidocaine, Bupivacaine
- Amino Esters: Procaine, Cocaine

178. **How pH affect action of local anesthetics**
- **Acidosis** such as caused by inflammation at wound reduce the action of local anesthetics

179. What is the main AE of amino ester group of local anesthetic
- Amino Ester group of anesthetics metabolized to PABA through pseudocholinesterase; **Allergic reaction** to PABA is the most important side effect

180. **C/I of Morphine**
- Raised intracranial pressure so head trauma
- Asthma (bronchial constriction)

- Renal failure (accumulate metabolite morphine-6-glucuronide)
- Billiary colic (contract billiary apparatus)

181. Important characteristic of Morphine
- Predominantly act on μ receptors (agonist)
- **Miosis** (constriction of pupils), constipation

182. Name of **partial opioid agonist**
- Nalbuphine, Pentazocin

183. Which drug is an exception to all opioids? How?
- **Meperidine** [it causes muscarinic receptor block so useful in billiary colic, it causes Mydriasis whereas all other produce miosis]

184. DOC for opioid overdose
- Naloxone

* **Anti-Microbial Drugs:**
185. Best initial antibiotics for different microorganisms
- Staph Aureus: Dicloxacillin, Oxacillin [Penicillins] / Cefadroxil, Cefalaxin [1st generation Cephalosporins]
- If patient is allergic to above groups – Macrolide, newer fluoroquinolone
- If patient has MRSA – Vancomycin / Linezolid
- Streptococcus: **Penicillin (if sensitive)** / Ceftriaxone / levofloxacin
- Strep Pneumonia: Penicillin G / Ceftriaxone / levofloxacin
- Strep Viridans: Penicillin G / Ceftriaxone
- Strep Pyogens: Ampicillin / Ampicillin + Sulbactam
- Strep Meningitis: **Ceftriaxone**
- Listeria Monocytogens: Ampicillin
- Legionella Pneumonia: Erythromycin
- Rickettsia in children: Chloramphenicol, Erythromycin
- Rickettsia in adults: Doxycycline
- Lyme disease in children < 9yrs of age: Amoxicillin
- Lyme disease in children >9 yrs of age and adults: Doxycycline
- Lyme disease in Pregnant women: Amoxicillin
- Disseminated Lyme disease [Bell's palsy, Cardiac involvement, CNS involvement]: Ceftriaxone
- Syphilis: Penicillin G
- Gonococcus: Ceftriaxone
- Chlamydia, Mycoplasma: Macrolides / Doxycycline
- C.Jejunii: Erythromycin
- H Influenzae: 2nd or 3rd generation cephalosporin
- E coli: Ciprofloxacin / Ampicillin
- Pseudomonas: Piperacillin, Ticarcillin [Anti-pseudomonal penicillin]
- Klebsiella: 2nd or 3rd generation cephalosporin
- Cryptococcus: Amphotericin B (severe), Fluconazole (prophylaxis)

- Candida: Fluconazole
- Dermatophytes: Terfinabine (oral) / Meconazole (local)
- PCP: Trimethoprim + Sulfamethoxazole
- Actinomycetes: Penicillin
- Nocardia: Sulfonamides
- Anaerobes: Metronidazole / Clindamycin
- Penicillin and Aminoglycosides have **synergistic effects** so combination of both (Penicillin + Aminoglycosides) is used in Enterobacteraceae and Pseudomonas infections

186. M/A of Penicillins
- **Inhibit** formation of peptidoglycans cross-link in **cell wall synthesis** which weakens the cell wall and death occurs due to osmotic pressure

187. Mechanism of resistance to Penicillins
- Enzymatic hydrolysis of beta lactam ring by beta lactamase (penicillinase) enzyme
- Due to possession of altered penicillin-binding proteins [this mode is seen in MRSA and penicillin resistant in streptococci]

188. Difference b/w Benzathine penicillin and Benzylpenicillin (Penicillin G)
- Benzathine Penicillin: slowly absorbed into the circulation, IM use, prolonged antibiotic action over 2–4 weeks after a single IM dose, useful in prophylaxis of rheumatic fever
- Benzylpenicillin (Penicillin G): IV use, achieve high concentration quickly, Increased antibacterial activity

189. Important AE of Penicillins. What is Jarisch–Herxheimer Reaction?
- AE: Allergic reactions, Interstitial nephritis [Methicillin]
- Jarisch-Herxheimer reaction: occurs most often in secondary syphilis and with penicillin therapy, characterized by fever, fatigue, and transient worsening of any mucocutaneous symptoms, and usually subsides within 24 hours, Tx: Acetaminophen

190. Name of beta lactamase resistant penicillin
- Dicloxacillin, Oxacillin, Methicillin

191. Name of cephalosporins according to different generation
- First Generation: Cefadroxil, Cefalexin, Cefazolin
- Second Generation: Cefaclor, Cefuroxime
- Third Generation: Cefdinir, Cefotaxime, Ceftriaxone, Ceftizoxime
- Fourth Generation: Cefepime

192. Coverage of all generation of cephalosporin
- First: penicillinase-producing staph, E.coli, Klebsiella, Proteus
- Second: increase activity against gram negative organism

- Third: hospital acquired infections, anti-pseudomonal activity (cefoparazone, ceftazidime), less gram positive activity
- Fourth: same gram positive as first generation, greater resistance to penicillinase, anti-pseudomonal

193. M/A of Cephalosporin / Mechanism of resistance
- Same as penicillin

194. Important AE of Cephalosporin
- Allergic reaction, **Hypoprothrombinemia**, Disulfiram-like reaction

195. Which drug group should we use in patient allergic to Penicillins and Cephalosporins
- For Gram (+) infection – give Macrolides
- For Gram (-) infection – give Imipenem (Carbapenem)

196. Reason for using Cilastatin with Imipenem. AE of Imipenem
- Imipenem is hydrolysed by a dehydropeptidase enzyme in the Kidney. This enzyme is inhibited by Cilastatin by which it increases the activity of Imipenem
- AE: **Seizure**

197. M/A of Vancomycin. Mechanism of resistance to Vancomycin
- MA: It prevents incorporation of N-acetylmuramic acid (NAM)- and N-acetylglucosamine (NAG)-peptide subunits into the peptidoglycans (**early stage** of wall synthesis) [It is **not** active against gram negative organisms]
- Mechanism of resistance: alteration to the terminal amino acid residue of NAM and NAG;

198. Can Vancomycin penetrate CNS?
- No

199. Important use & AE of Vancomycin
- Use: MRSA, Pseudomembranous colitis
- AE: Red man syndrome [non-specific mast cell degradation – Tx: antihistamines], **Ototoxicity**, Nephrotoxicity

200. Is cephalosporin & Penicillins has cross-allergenicity?
- Yes

201. What is an important feature of **Aztreonam**?
- **No cross-allergenicity with penicillin and cephalosporins**

202. M/A of Macrolides / Mechanism of resistance of macrolies
- MA: Inhibition of protein synthesis by binding to 50S subunit of ribosome. It prevents peptidyl translocation of t-RNA (**Same for Clindamycin**)

- Mechanism of resistance: (1) post-transcriptional methylation of 23S ribosomal RNA (2) production of drug-inactivating enzymes (3) active ATP-dependent efflux proteins that transport the drug outside of the cell

203. Should erythromycin dose be reduced in patient with renal dysfunction?
- **No**

204. Is Macrolide has any effect on P450 metabolism system?
- **Yes**

205. Important AE of Macrolide
- QT prolongation (Torsade de pointes)

206. Name of important antimicrobial agents that should be avoided in pregnancy
- Aminoglycosides
- Fluoroquinolones (ciprofloxacin)
- Tetracyclines
- Erythromycin & Clarithromycin [Azithromycin is safe in pregnancy]

207. M/A of Tetracycline / Mechanism of resistance
- MA: Inhibits protein synthesis by binding 30S ribosomes by which it inhibits binding of aminoacyl t-RNA to mRNA-ribosome complex
- Mechanism of resistance: (1) enzymatic inactivation, (2) active efflux of drug and (3) ribosomal protection

208. Important organism **coverage of tetracycline**
- Brucella, Vibrio, Lyme disease, Rickettsia, Chlamydia, Tularemia, Plague, Anthrax

209. Important use of **Demeclocycline**
- **SIADH**

210. Effect of antacid on absorption of tetracycline
- Tetracycline binds to Aluminum, Magnesium, Iron and Calcium which reduce its absorption

211. Which tetracycline can use safely in renal dysfunction?
- Doxycycline

212. Important AE of tetracyclines
- Teeth discoloration, Steatosis, **Phototoxicity**, pseudotumor cerebri, Ototoxicity (Minocycline)

213. Important AE of Clindamycin
- **Pseudomembranous colitis** [Tx: Metronidazole (DOC), Vancomycin]

214. Important use of clindamycin
- Acne, malaria, MRSA, bacterial vaginosis in early stage of pregnancy

215. M/A and resistance of Aminoglycosides
- MA: Inhibits protein synthesis by binding 30S ribosome, it prevents translocation of the peptidyl-tRNA from the A-site to the P-site
- Resistance: enzymatic inactivation

216. Why anaerobes are resistant to Aminoglycosides?
- It requires more energy for uptake and anaerobes doesn't have much energy (no oxygen!!!)

217. Use of neomycin. Is it useful systemically?
- Neomycin is used orally in Hepatic encephalopathy to ↓ NH3 production by intestinal bacteria otherwise it has no systemic use. It is used locally

218. Name important **Nephrotoxic antimicrobial drugs**
- Aminoglycosides
- Amphotericin B
- Foscarnet

219. Use of Aminoglycosides
- TB, Plague, Infective endocarditis

220. M/A and resistance of Chloramphenicol
- MA: It inhibits peptidyl transferase and binds to 23S rRNA of 50S subunit and prevent peptide bond formation
- Resistance: reduced membrane permeability, mutation of the 50S ribosomal subunit and elaboration of Chloramphenicol acetyltransferase

221. AE of Chloramphenicol. Is dose reduction required in LIVER dysfunction
- **Aplastic anemia**, Bone marrow suppression [reversible once drug is stopped], **Gray baby syndrome** in newborns [hypotension, cyanosis]

222. Drugs use for **Vancomycin resistant organisms**
- **Linezolid**, Daptomycin

223. M/A of sulfa drugs
- MA: Inhibits folic acid synthesis by competitively inhibiting Dihydropteroate synthesis [prevent formation of PABA to dihyropteroate]

224. Uses & Important AE of Sulfa drugs
- Use: PCP [Pneumocystis Carinii Pneumonia], UTI, Inflammatory bowel disease [Sulfasalazine], Nocardia infection, Trachoma (sulfacetamide), Burn patient (silver sulfadiazine), Toxoplasmosis (Sulfadiazine + Pyrimethamine), Whipple's disease (Sulfamethoxazole + Trimethoprim)

- AE: **Allergies**, known to **increase level of Warfarin** (Sulfamethoxazole/Trimethoprim), **Steven Johnson syndrome**, Agranulocytosis, **Kernicterus in the newborn** if used during last 6 weeks of pregnancy

225. Which other drugs have sulfa component?
- Thiazide diuretics, Celecoxib and Glipizide/Glyburide

226. M/A of Trimethoprim & Pyrimethamine
- Both inhibit folic acid synthesis by inhibiting Dihydrofolate reductase

227. M/A of Fluoroquinolones
- Inhibits DNA gyrase, topoisomerase II and topoisomerase IV. These enzymes are necessary to separate replicated DNA. By inhibiting them, it prevent cell division

228. Important side effect in adults
- Achilles tendon rupture (tendonitis); Delirium in elderly patient

229. Effect of antacid on absorption
- Aluminum, Iron, Calcium bind with it and prevent its absorption

230. M/A of Amphotericin B and Nystatin
- It binds with Ergosterol (important substance in fungal cell wall) and form pores in the fungal cell wall leads to leakage of K^+ and fungal death

231. How can we prevent AE of Amphotericin
- Important AE of Amphotericin B are fever, chills, hypotension, nausea, vomiting. It occur due to release of histamine and increase prostaglandin synthesis so it can be **prevented by Acetaminophen, Aspirin, diphenhydramine and/or hydrocortisone**

232. M/A of Azoles
- Inhibits synthesis of Ergosterol

233. AE of Ketoconazole
- **Inhibit synthesis of testosterone** (useful in prostate cancer) (also useful in androgenic alopecia), **glucocorticoids** (useful in Cushing's disease), **Gynacomastia**

234. Important use of **Fluconazole**
- **DOC for Candidiasis**, **Prophylaxis of cryptococcal meningitis**; first-line drug for coccidioidomycosis and Histoplasmosis

235. Which is the only azole that can penetrate in CNS?
- Fluconazole

236. Drug use for **topical fungal infection**
- Miconazole and Clotrimazole

237. What is the M/A of Flucytosin?
- <u>MA</u>: It is a fluorinated pyrimidine analog. (1) It intrafungally converted into the cytostatic fluorouracil and interacts as 5-fluorouridinetriphosphate with RNA synthesis (2) It inhibits fungal DNA synthesis by conversion into 5-flourodeoxyuridinemonophosphate

238. AE of Flucytosin
- **Bone marrow suppression**, GI toxicity

239. What are M/A and AE of Gresiofulvin?
- <u>MA</u>: It inhibits mitosis by binding to tubulin and interfering with microtubule function
- <u>AE</u>: Disulfiram-like reaction with ethanol, Phototoxicity

240. What is the M/A of Terbinafine?
- It inhibits synthesis of Ergosterol by inhibiting squalene epoxide enzyme

241. M/A and **Uses of Metronidazole**
- <u>MA</u>: It **inhibits nucleic acid synthesis**. [It is converted in anaerobic organisms by the redox enzyme Pyruvate-ferredoxin oxidoreductase. The nitro group of metronidazole is chemically reduced by ferredoxin (or a ferredoxin-linked metabolic process) and the products are responsible for disrupting the DNA helical structure, thus inhibiting nucleic acid synthesis]
- <u>Use</u>: Amoebic dysentery, Bacterial vaginosis, Trichomonas Vaginitis (give Metronidazole to <u>both</u> partners), diarrhea due to Giardia, H.Pylori regimen, anaerobic infections

242. Important **AE of anti-tubercular drugs**
- <u>Rifampin</u>: Thrombocytopenia, **Orange color body fluids**, Hepatitis
- <u>INH</u>: **Neuropathy** [prevented by Vit-B6 (pyridoxine)], **Hemolysis** in G6PD patients, **Drug induced lupus**, Hepatitis
- <u>Ethambutol</u>: **Optic neuritis**
- <u>Pyrazinamide</u>: **Hepatitis**, Arthralgia

243. M/A anti-tubercular drugs
- <u>Rifampin</u>: inhibits RNA transcription by inhibiting DNA dependent RNA polymerase
- <u>INH</u>: activated by catalase-peroxidase enzyme KatG to form isonicotinic acyl anion or radical which binds with NADH radical and **inhibit mycolic acid synthesis** [Mutations of the catalase gene is the reason of resistance]
- <u>Pyrazinamide</u>: Pyrazinamidase enzyme in M.tuberculosis convert it into pyrazinoic acid which inhibits fatty acid synthesis [Mutations of the pyrazinamidase gene is the reason of resistance]

- Ethambutol: Inhibits formation of cell wall

244. M/A and use of acyclovir
- MA: It is selectively **converted into acyclo-guanosine monophosphate** (acyclo-GMP) **by viral thymidine kinase**. Subsequently, the monophosphate form is further phosphorylated **into the active triphosphate form**, acyclo- guanosine triphosphate (acyclo-GTP), **by cellular kinase of host cell**. Acyclo-GTP is a **very potent inhibitor of viral DNA polymerase; it has approximately 100 times greater affinity for viral than host cellular polymerase**. As a substrate, acyclo-GMP is incorporated into viral DNA, **resulting in chain termination**.
- Use: **HSV and VZV infections**

245. Is acyclovir has any effect on post herpetic neuralgia?
- <u>No</u>. It reduce the severity and duration of herpes zoster, but do **not** reliably prevent post-herpetic neuralgia

246. Drugs use in **shingles**
- **Famciclovir & Valacyclovir**

247. M/A of **ganciclovir**
- MA: It competitively inhibits the incorporation of dGTP by viral DNA polymerase, resulting in the termination of elongation of viral DNA
- Use: **CMV infections (cytomegalovirus)**

248. What are the characteristics of Foscarnet?
- MA: selectively inhibits the pyrophosphate binding site on viral DNA polymerase at concentration that do not affect human DNA polymerases
- Use: **Acyclovir and Ganciclovir resistant viruses**

249. Important AE of Foscarnet when it is used with Pentamidine
- Hypocalcemia

250. Difference b/w NRTI & Non-NRTI
- NRTI must be activated by cell kinase to act

251. Important **AE of Zidovudine**
- Hematotoxicity (anemia, bone marrow suppression)

252. Drugs that increase Zidovudine toxicity
- Aspirin, Trimethoprim, Cimitidine

253. Use of Lamivudin
- Hepatitis B

254. M/A and Important **AE of protease inhibitors**
- MA: Inhibits viral replication by inhibiting HIV-1 protease

- AE: Nephrolithiasis, hyperlipidemia, Bizarre alterations in body shape

255. **Only teratogenic anti-HIV drug name**
- **Efavirenz**

256. M/A of Amantadine. Other use of Amantadine. Is Amantadine useful against Influenza B? AE of Amantadine
- MA: Amantadine interferes with a viral protein, M2 (an ion channel), which is required for the viral particle to become "uncoated" once it is taken inside the cell by endocytosis
- Other use: Parkinsonism
- No. It is **not useful against Influenza B**
- AE: Livedo reticularis (reaction that results in skin mottling and purpurish mesh network of blood vessels) (also seen with atropine)

257. **Difference b/w Amantadine & Zenamivir**, Oseltamivir
- Oseltamivir & Zenamivir are active against both Influenza A & B viruses
- Both are neuraminidase inhibitor

258. M/A and Use of Ribavirin. **Is it used in Hep C?**
- MA: inhibit RNA dependent replication in RNA viruses
- Use: RSV (respiratory syncytial virus)
- Yes. It is used in conjunction with α-interferon

259. Important Anti-Protozoal drugs
- **Mebendazole, Albendazole:** by selectively and irreversibly block uptake of glucose and it is a spindle poison which induce chromosomes; Use: pinworm, whip worm, tapeworm hookworm, roundworm
- **Pyrantel Pamoate:** acts as a depolarizing neuromuscular blocking agent, thereby causing sudden contraction, followed by paralysis, of the helminths; Use: hookworm, roundworm
- **Anti-Leishmaniasis:** meglumine antimoniate and sodium stibogluconate
- **Praziquantel:** Praziquantel increases the permeability of the membranes of parasite cells for calcium ions and thereby induces contraction of the parasites resulting in paralysis in the contracted state; Use: liver fluke, Schistosomiasis
- **Anti-malarial drugs:** Quinine, Chloroquine, Pyrimethamine, Mefloquine, Proguanil, Sulphdoxine, Primaquine, Atovaquone; Prophylaxis: Mefloquine and Chloroquine

* **Anticoagulants, Thrombolytics & Anti-platelets:**
260. M/A and important AE of Heparin
- MA: binds to antithrombin III which inactivate thrombin and factor Xa
- AE: **thrombocytopenia**, osteoporosis

261. Drug use in heparin induced thrombocytopenia
- Bivalirudin (direct inhibitor of thrombin)

- Fondaparinux (Xa inhibitor) (it has no affinity to PF-4)

262. Can heparin be used in pregnancy?
- **Yes**

263. How we monitor patient on Heparin / Warfarin
- Heparin – aPTT
- Warfarin – PT

264. Antagonist of Heparin & Warfarin
- Heparin: Protamine sulfate
- Warfarin: Vit-K, Fresh frozen plasma

265. M/A of Warfarin
- <u>MA</u>: It inhibits Vit-K epoxide reductase by which it reduces synthesis of Vit-K dependent factors (2,7,9 and 10)

266. Most important AE to keep in mind when we give Warfarin
- Warfarin necrosis (skin necrosis occurs due to deficiency of protein C), Teratogenic (contraindicated in pregnancy)

267. M/A of thrombolytics. Difference b/w Streptokinase & Alteplase
- <u>MA</u>: Activate plasminogen which clears the cross-linked fibrin mesh.
- <u>Difference</u>: Streptokinase is **not clot specific**, can cause allergic reaction, activity may decrease if recently used or recent strep infection

268. Antagonist of thrombolytics
- Aminocaproic Acid, Tranexamic acid

269. Difference b/w Aspirin, Clopidogrel and Abciximab
- <u>Aspirin</u>: **irreversible** inactivation of the cyclooxygenase (COX); Low-dose aspirin use irreversibly blocks the formation of thromboxane A_2 in platelets, producing an inhibitory effect on platelet aggregation.
- <u>Clopidogrel</u>: an irreversible blockade of the ADP receptor on platelet cell membranes
- <u>Abciximab</u>: block glycoprotein IIb/IIIa receptor on the platelet

* **Endocrine Pharmacology:**
270. M/A of Propyl thiouracil (PTU) & Methimazole?
- <u>MA</u>: PTU inhibits the enzyme thyroperoxidase, which normally acts in thyroid hormone synthesis. Also acts by inhibiting the enzyme 5'-deiodinase, which converts T_4 to the active form T_3.

271. Which one is **safe in pregnancy** out of above two drugs?
- **PTU** (extensively plasma protein bound)

272. AE of PTU
- Agranulocytosis

273. Use of Propranolol in hyperthyroidism
- Propranolol treats symptoms of hyperthyroidism like palpitations, trembling, and anxiety which are mediated by beta adrenergic receptors

274. M/A and important AE of ^{131}I
- MA: The radioactive iodine is picked up by the active cells in the thyroid and destroys them. Since iodine is only picked up by thyroid cells
- AE: Hypothyroidism

275. Name & use of GH agonist
- Somato**tropin**: short stature

276. Name & use of Somato**statin**
- Octreotide: more potent inhibitor of GH, Glucagon, and insulin; Use: Acromegaly, Carcinoid syndrome, VIPomas, Esophageal varices

277. Name & use of ACTH agonist
- Cosyntropin: used in ACTH stimulation test to evaluate and diagnose cortisol disorder, infantile spam

278. Name & use of GNRH agonist
- Leuprolide, Nafarelin: Prostate cancer, Endometriosis, fibroids, precocious puberty, Breast cancer

279. Name & use of Prolactin inhibiting hormones (Dopamine agonist)
- Bromocriptine: Hyperprolactinemia

280. Use of oxytocin
- Labor induction, lactation

281. Use of Vasopressin
- Desmopressin (analog): binds V2 receptors in renal CD which increase water reabsorption, also stimulate release of factor VIII through V1a receptor; Use: Bed wetting, Central DI, vWD, Hemophilia

282. M/A and use of Cyproheptadine
- MA: 5–HT$_2$ antagonist, H1 blocking action too
- Use: Carcinoid, GI tumors, Post-gastractomy, Anorexia nervosa

283. Use of Megestrol acetate
- Use in cachexic patient to improve appetite

284. Name of drugs that block steroid receptors
   ▪ Spironolactone, Mifepristone

285. Name of drugs that inhibit steroid synthesis
   ▪ Metyrapone, Ketoconazole

286. Important AE of Estrogen, Progesterone & Androgens
   ▪ <u>Estrogen</u>: Endometrial Hyperplasia, ↑ **gall bladder diseases, Cholestasis,** ↑ Blood coagulation (↓ antithrombin III)
   ▪ <u>Progesterone</u>: ↓ HDL & ↑ LDL , Glucose intolerance
   ▪ <u>Androgen</u>: Premature closer of Epiphysis, **cholestatic jaundice**

287. Name & M/A of anti-androgens
   ▪ Flutamide - Androgen receptor blocker
   ▪ **Finasteride - 5 α reductase inhibitor;** <u>Use</u>: BPH, male type baldness
   ▪ Ketoconazole - Synthesis inhibitor

288. M/A & use of Anastrozole, Danazol, Clomiphen citrate, Tamoxifen and Raloxifen. Difference b/w Tamoxifen & Raloxifen
   ▪ <u>Anastrozole</u>: inhibits aromatase enzyme which convert androgens to estrogen; <u>Use</u>: Breast CA
   ▪ <u>Tamoxifen</u>: competitively binds to estrogen receptors and inhibits estrogen effects [<u>antagonist</u> in <u>breast tissue</u> and <u>partial agonist</u> in <u>Endometrium</u>]; <u>Use</u>: **Breast CA**, Anovulatory infertility, Gynacomastia
   ▪ <u>Raloxifene</u>: Estrogen **agonist at bone** and **antagonist on breast & uterus** <u>Use</u>: to prevent osteoporosis in post-menopausal women [<u>Can be used in patient with h/o breast CA in family</u>]
   ▪ <u>Difference b/w Tamoxifen & Raloxifene</u>: Raloxifene has antiestrogenic effect on uterus
   ▪ <u>Danazol</u>: inhibits ovarian steroidgenesis resulting in decreased secretion of estradiol; also has weak androgenic activity; <u>Use</u>: Endometriosis, fibrocystic breast disease [C/I in pregnancy]
   ▪ <u>Clomiphen citrate</u>: inhibiting the action of estrogen on the gonadotrope cells in the anterior pituitary gland which leads to increase FSH leading to increase ovulation; <u>Use</u>: infertility ("pregnancy drug")

289. Insulin forms that can be used as IV
   ▪ Regular insulin

290. M/A of Sulfonylureas
   ▪ <u>MA</u>: Block k^+ Channel → depolarization of beta cells → Insulin Release

291. Important **AE of Chlorpropamide** (1st generation sulfonylurea)
   ▪ SIADH, Disulfiram like reaction with ethanol
   ▪ <u>C/I of sulfonylureas</u>: Sulphonylureas should be avoided where possible in severe hepatic and renal impairment and in Porphyria, Breast feeding and Pregnancy

185

292. M/A & important **AE of Metformin**
- <u>MA</u>: suppression of hepatic gluconeogenesis ["Euglycemic"] so decrease postprandial blood glucose
- <u>AE</u>: **Lactic acidosis in patient with <u>renal dysfunction</u>**

293. M/A of Acarbose
- It <u>inhibits alpha-glucosidase enzymes</u> in the brush border of the small intestines so it decreases carbohydrate digestion which leads to decrease blood glucose level

294. M/A of Thiazolidinediones
- Bind to nuclear peroxisome proliferators activating receptors (PPAR) involved in transcription of insulin–responsive gene → **Sensitization of tissues to insulin; ↓ Hepatic gluconeogenesis & TGs; increase HDL**

295. M/A of Repaglinide
- Block k^+ Channel → depolarization of beta cells → Insulin Release

---

Incretin: a group of gastrointestinal hormones includes Glucagon-like-Peptide-1 (GLP-1) & Gastric Inhibitory Peptide (GIP). It causes an increase in the amount of insulin released from pancrease, <u>even before blood glucose levels become elevated.</u> GIP inhibits gastric emptying so it also decreases absorption of food into blood.
Dipeptidyl peptidase-4 (DPP4): It inactivates incretin.

---

296. M/A of Exenatide (Byetta)
- It is an incretin mimetics so it enhances glucose-dependent insulin secretion by the pancreatic beta-cell, suppresses inappropriately elevated glucagon secretion, and slows gastric emptying.
- The only disadvantage is it must be administered by SC injection!

297. M/A of Sitagliptin (Januvia)
- It inhibits DPP-4 so enhance incretin activities.
- Its advantage over exenatide is it can be used orally.

298. M/A of Bisphosphonates
- They inhibit osteoclast action and the resorption of bone so useful in osteoporosis

299. Important AE of Alendronate / why do we ask patient to take alendronate with full glass of water
- Esophageal ulcers [Esophagitis]

* **Anti-cancer Drugs:**
  300. Is anticancer drugs kill fix percentage of tumor cells or fix number of tumor cells?
  - Anticancer drugs kill a fixed percentage of tumor cells

301. Drugs known as spindle poisons
- Vincristine, Vinblastine [Both act on M-phase of cell cycle]

302. **AE of Methotraxate, Cyclophosphamide and Doxorubicin**. How can we prevent it?
- Methotraxate: Nephrotoxicity [Hydrate well to prevent it], Folate deficiency [give **Folinic acid** to prevent it]
- Cyclophosphamide: Hemorrhagic cystitis [give Mesna, a sulfhydryl donor and binds acrolein, to prevent it]
- Doxorubicin: Dilated cardiomyopathy [give Dexrazoxane to prevent it]

303. M/A of Azathioprine, 6-MP & 5-FU
- **Azathioprine** → 6MP (Purine antimetabolite) → bioactivated by HPGR transferase [6MP is used in ALL]
- **5–FU** (Pyrimidine antimetabolite) bioactivated to inhibits thymidylate synthase [used in basal cell CA & Keratosis]

304. M/A of cyclosporine
- MA: It binds to cyclophilin of immunocompetent lymphocytes, especially T-lymphocytes. This complex inhibits calcineurin, which under normal circumstances is responsible for activating the transcription of IL-2. It also inhibits lymphokine production and interleukin release and therefore leads to a reduced function of effector T-cells.
- Use: to prevent rejection in organ transplant

305. M/A and **AE of Bleomycin**
- MA: It induces DNA strand breaks. DNA cleavage by bleomycin depends on oxygen and metal ions
- AE: **Pulmonary fibrosis**

* **Drugs for Gout:**
306. Give name of drugs that used in acute gouty attack (NSAID)
- **Indomethacin**, Colchicine

307. M/A & Important **AE of Colchicine**
- MA: It inhibits microtubule polymerization by binding to tubulin so it inhibits mitosis ["mitotic poison"] and also inhibits neutrophil motility and activity, leading to a net anti-inflammatory effect
- AE: Diarrhea, **Agranulocytosis**

308. Difference b/w Allopurinol and Probenecid
- Allopurinol inhibits uric acid synthesis by inhibiting xanthine oxidase whereas Probenecid increases uric acid elimination in urine.

309. **Relationship b/w Probenecid & GFR**
- It is ineffective if GFR< 50 ml/min

310. Is Allopurinol has any effect on 6-MP metabolism
- It inhibits 6MP metabolism

* **Drugs for Rheumatoid Arthritis (RA):**
311. Name of drugs that are used in treatment of RA
- Methotraxate, Sulfasalazine, Hydroxychloroquine, Steroids, Leflunomide, Anti-TNF (infliximab, etanercept), NSAIDs (best initial drug)

312. When will you start DMARD (Disease Modifying Anti-Rheumatic Drug)?
- Within 3 months for any patient with established RA and ongoing inflammation

313. Best initial DMARD
- Methotraxate

314. Important points to remember before starting Tx with anti-TNF
- Screening for Tuberculosis

* **Drugs for Asthma:**
315. Name of drugs that used in treatment of Asthma
- Beta agonists, Cromolyn, Corticosteroids, Anti-Leukotrines

316. M/A of Theophylline
- It inhibits phosphodiesterase (PDE) → ↑ cAMP → **antagonize Adenosine** (Adenosine is Bronchoconstrictor)

317. M/A of Cromolyn. **Is Cromolyn useful in acute attack of asthma?**
- Prevent degranulation of pulmonary mast cells & ↓ release of mediators (histamine) that attract inflammatory cells
- No. It is not useful for acute attack. It uses to prevent asthma attack

318. Difference b/w Zafirlukast & Ziluton.
- Zafirlukast: Leukotrines receptor antagonist. Use to prevent asthma attack
- Ziluton: Inhibits Lipoxygenase

* **Miscellaneous:**
319. Name & use of different PGs
- PGE_1: Alprostadil; treatment of erectile dysfunction, is a vasodilator
- PGE_2: Dinoprostone; as a vaginal suppository, to prepare the cervix for labour; also used as an abortificient
- $PGE_{2\alpha}$: Carboprost; used in postpartum bleeding (Atonic PPH)

320. **Difference b/w Aspirin (ASA) & other NSAID**
- Aspirin irreversibly inhibits COX

321. **Reason for using low Aspirin**
- At low dose, it irreversibly blocks **only** the formation of thromboxane A_2 in platelets

322. How Aspirin eliminate from the body at high toxic dose
- Zero order kinetics

323. Symptoms specific for Salicylism
- Tinnitus

324. Treatment of Aspirin overdose
- alkalization of urine facilitate its renal elimination

325. Give name of selective COX-2 inhibitor and advantage of it over other NSAID
- Celecoxib
- Advantage: It has less GI side effects

326. Difference b/w Acetaminophen & other NSAID
- Acetaminophen has **No** Peripheral COX inhibition
- Inhibits COX in CNS – **lacks anti-inflammatory effects**. But **equivalent analgesic& antipyretic activity to ASA**

327. Tx of acetaminophen overdose
- **N–acetylcystine** [give as soon as possible]

328. Name of anti-emetic drugs according to different groups
- 5-HT_3 antagonist – Ondansetron
- DA antagonist – Prochlorperazine, Metoclopramide
- H_1 antagonist – Meclizine, Promethazine
- M antagonist – Scopolamine (motion sickness)

329. Use of Cisapride. Why is it withdrawn from market?
- Prokinetic drugs, used in GERD
- Due to arrhythmias, it was withdrawn from the market

330. M/A of Sucralfate. Important things to remember about it
- MA: coat stomach surface and prevent it from acid exposure
- **Never use with antacid / PPI** [antacid & PPI inhibits action of sucralfate]

PATHOLOGY

Systemic Pathology

CARDIOLOGY

- **Myocardial Ischemia / Myocardial Infarction**: <u>Substernal squeezing</u> chest pain
- **Pericarditis**: chest pain <u>relieve by leaning forward</u>
- **Costochondritis**: chest pain <u>reproduce by palpation</u>
- **Dissecting aortic aneurism**: <u>tearing</u> chest pain <u>radiate to back</u>
- **Pneumonia**: <u>pleuritic (increase on inspiration)</u> chest pain
- **Pulmonary embolism**: pleuritic chest pain, <u>dyspnea, tachypnea</u>
- **Esophageal spam ("nut cracker disease")**: <u>past h/o GERD, gastritis</u>, pain occur after eating, <u>normal EKG</u>

- **Stable angina**: chest pain **after** exertion
- **Unstable angina**: chest pain **at rest** [ST **D**epression] [**D** → **E**]
- **Myocardial Infarction**: chest pain **at rest** [ST **E**levation]
- **Prinzmetal angina**: chest pain **at rest** [ST elevation – **Transmural Ischemia**] [due to coronary artery spam. Pain may relieve by little exercise like patient gets up and walking and pain relieve because exercise causes **increase in Adenosine** which is a potent coronary vasodilator]

* **Complication of MI :** Ventricular Arrhythmia (MCC of Death)

- Rupture (Ant. Wall, Papillary muscles, Interventricular Septum) – **3-7 days**
- Autoimmune Pericarditis (Dressler's Syndrome) – **6-8 weeks** Post–MI

- **EKG changes in Acute MI**: Peak tall T-wave → ST elevation → T-wave inversion → Q-wave
- **Inferior wall MI [RC]**: II, III, aVF
- **Anterior wall MI [LAD]**: $V_2 - V_4$
- **Anteroseptal [LAD]**: $V_1 - V_3$
- **Lateral wall MI [LAD / Circumflex]**: I, aVL, $V_4 - V_6$
- **Posterior wall MI [Posterior Descending]**: $V_1 - V_2$

Congestive Heart Failure

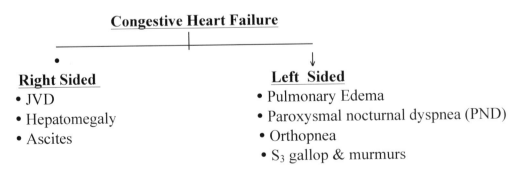

Right Sided
- JVD
- Hepatomegaly
- Ascites

Left Sided
- Pulmonary Edema
- Paroxysmal nocturnal dyspnea (PND)
- Orthopnea
- S_3 gallop & murmurs

- Chronic CHF – "nutmeg liver" – variegated mottled appearance to liver

S.S.Patel , M.D.

- ■ **Mitral valve Prolapse:** Mid-late Systolic **Click**
- • Presentation → Asymptomatic, **Palpitation**, Chest pain, Syncope, Sudden death
- • **Marfan Syndrome**

- ■ **Infective Endocarditis:** Splinter hemorrhages, Roth's spot in eye, Janeway lesions, **Valve regurgitation**
- - Strep. Viridians → <u>most common</u> overall cause (previously damage valve)
- - Staph. Aureus → **IV drug abuse** (Normal / Previously damage valve) **Tricuspid Valve**
- - Staph Epidermidis → Prosthetic devices
- - **Strep bovis → ulcerative colitis / colorectal cancer patient**
- - Loeffler Endocarditis – prominent **Eosinophil infiltrates**

- ■ **Valvular Heart Disease:**
- • <u>**Stenosis**</u> → Problem in opening of valve therefore murmur occurs during opening of the valve
- • <u>**Regurgitation**</u> → Problem in closing of valve therefore murmur occurs during closing of the valve
- • **Austin Flint murmur**: regurgitant stream from incompetent Aortic valve hits anterior mitral valve leaflet producing a diastolic murmur

- • **Right sided murmur increase in intensity with Inspiration**

Mitral Stenosis	Aortic Regurgitation	Mitral Regurgitation	Aortic Stenosis
• <u>**Diastolic**</u> murmur	• **Diastolic** decrescendo	• <u>**Holosystolic**</u> radiate to the <u>**Axilla**</u>	• <u>**Systolic**</u> ejection radiate to **carotid**
• Opening **snap**	• Austin Flint murmur		• **Chest pain / Syncope during exercise in elders**
• **CXR** → double density Right heart Border	• <u>**Endocarditis Prophylaxis**</u>		• <u>**Endocarditis Prophylaxis**</u>

- • **Hypertrophic Cardiomyopathy:** Autosomal Dominant (AD), chromosome 14 – **disproportionate thickening of interventricular septum** – conductance disturbance is responsible for **sudden death in athletes**

- • **Valsalva / Standing -** ↓ preload → ↑ obstruction → ↑ murmur
- • **Squatting / Hand grip -** ↑ preload → ↓ obstruction → ↓ murmur

- • Increase in Pre-load – decrease murmur in Mitral valve prolapse and Hypertrophic cardiomyopathy.

Acute Pericarditis	Cardiac Temponade	Constrictive Pericarditis
• **Chest pain** which is **relieved by leaning forward**	• **Pulsus paradoxus** ($\downarrow$ SBP more than 10 mmHg on normal inspiration)	• **Kussmaul's Sign** ($\uparrow$ jugular venous distension with inspiration)
• **Pericardial friction rub** (Diagnostic)	• **Neck vein distension** with clear lung	• **Pericardial knock**
• **EKG** – **diffuse** ST segment elevation (**In MI** – ST elevation is in different leads according to involvement of heart and it is convex)	• **Shock** [Beck's triad – Hypotension, JVP, muffled heart sound]	• **EKG** – **low voltage**

- ■ Pericardial Effusion:
  - ▪ Serosanguineous → TB / neoplasm
  - ▪ **CXR** – "water-bottle" configuration of cardiac silhouette

  - ▪ **Patent ostium primum** (patent foramen ovale) – failure of septum primum to fuse with endocardial cushions
  - ▪ **Atrial Septal Defect (ASD)** – incomplete adhesion b/w septum primum & septum secondum – **Wide fixed split S2**
  - ▪ **VSD** – defect in membranous interventricular septum
  - ▪ **PDA** – machinery murmur – associated with **congenital rubella** – PGE_2 keep it open – it shunts pulmonary artery blood to aorta in fetus

- ■ **Acute Rheumatic fever:**
  - - Aschoff bodies (pathognomic) [central area of necrosis surrounded by reactive Histiocytes (Anitschkow cells)]
  - - Pericarditis, Polyarthritis, Chorea, Erythema marginatum and subcutaneous Nodules (Jones criteria)
  - - Usually occur **1-3 weeks after a preceding Strep. Pyogens pharyngitis**
  - - $\uparrow\uparrow\uparrow$ ASO titers
  - - Treatment of acute infection and **monthly Penicillin prophylaxis then after**.

Location of Murmur	Conditions
Upper Rt sternal border	AS, IHSS
Upper Lt sternal border	PS, PDA
Lower Lt sternal border	VSD
Apex	MVP

- ▪ **Cardiac Myxoma** – left atria – mesenchymal tumor – embolic episode, syncopal episode – **adult**
- ▪ **Rhabdomyoma** – **children** – associated with tuberous sclerosis – hemartoma

DERMATOLOGY

- **Urticaria:** Type – 1 HS – I_gE & mast cell mediated – wheals & hives

- **Morbilliform rashes:** rash resembles measles – " typical " type of drug reaction – lymphocyte mediated – maculopapular eruption that blanches with pressure

- **Erythema multiforme:** Mycoplasma / Herpes Simplex – **target- like lesions** that occur on the palms & soles ("iris-like")

- **Stevens – Johnson Syndrome**: (**Erythema multiforme major**) – usually involve < 10-15 % of the total body surface area – **target-like lesions** – **mucous membrane involvement** oral cavity , conjunctiva , respiratory tract – Hypersensitivity reaction to drugs

- **Toxic epidermal necrolysis:** Cutaneous hypersensitivity reaction to drugs – (+) Nikolsky sign – **skin** easily sloughs off – 40-50 % mortality rate

- **Staphylococcal scalded skin syndrome:** loss of the **superficial layers** of the epidermis – Toxin mediated – (+) Nikolsky sign

- **Fixed drug reaction:** localized allergic drug reaction that recurs at precisely the same anatomic site on the skin with repeated drug exposure – round , sharply demarcated lesions that leave a hyperpigmented spot at the site after they resolved

- **Erythema nodosum:** multiple **painful**, red, raised **nodules on the anterior surface of the lower extremities** – recent streptococcal infection, Celiac Sprue

* **Toxic Shock Syndrome:** toxin produced from **staphylococcal** attached to a foreign body (tampon use in female during menstruation) – **fever , Hypotension** , desquamating rash , vomiting , involvement of mucous membrane – **Hypocalcemia** due to capillary leak leads to ↓ albumin level

- **Impetigo**: superficial bacterial infection – up to epidermis – **honey colored crusted lesions** (Strep Pyogens) & Staph Aureus (bullous impetigo)

- **Erysipeals:** both dermis & epidermis involve – shiny red, edematous, tender lesion, fever, chills, bacteremia – Strep Pyogens

- **Folliculitis , Furuncles , Carbuncles:** Staphylococcus
- Folliculitis → infection of hair follicle
- Furuncles → collection of infected material around hair follicle
- Carbuncles → several furuncles become confluent in to a single lesion
- Hot tub Folliculitis → Pseudomonas

- **Necrotizing Fasciitis:** Very high fever, portal of entry into skin, pain out of proportion to the superficial appearance, presence of bullae, **palpable crepitus** – Group A strep (strep Pyogens) – X-ray will show air in the tissue

- **Dermatophyte Infection:** Microsporum, Trichophyton, Epidermophyton
- Microsporum – Skin , Hair , Nail
- Trichophyton - Hair , Nail
- Epidermophyton – Skin , Nail
- Usually annular lesions expand peripherally and clear centrally

- **Tinea Versicolor:** Malassezia furfur (Pityrosporum orbiculare) – white, scaling lesions that tend to coalesce

- **Pityriasis rosea:** "herald patch" Christmas tree pattern –self-limited – looks like secondary syphilis **except** it spares palm & sole – VDRL / RPR → negative .

- **Pediculosis: lice** - Dx → direct examination of hear-bearing area

- **Telogen effluvium:** loss of hair in response to excessive physiological stress . (eg. cancer, malnutrition) – **Tx:** correct underlying stress

- **Alopecia areata:** autoimmune – **Tx:** localized steroid injection

- **Solar lentigo: Freckles** – sun exposed area in elderly

- **Seborrheic keratosis: verrucoid** lesion with **"stuck on appearance"** – **no** malignant potential

- **Actinic keratosis: Precancerous lesion** – sun exposed area – can progress to squamous cell CA

- **Acanthosis nigricans: Verrucoid** pigmented skin lesion usually located in **Axilla** – Stomach adenocarcinoma, MEN II b, insulin resistance (DM, Obese)

- **Nevocellular nevus (Mole):** nevus cells are modified melanocytes
- Junctional nevus → basal cell layer (childhood)
- Compound nevus → extend into superficial dermis (adolescents)
- **Intradermal nevus** → compound nevus loses its junctional component (**Adult**)
- Dysplastic nevus (Atypical mole) → ↑ risk for malignant melanoma – yearly dermatologic examination require

* **Melanoma:** Most common **type of** malignancy – sun exposed area - ↑ risk in dysplastic nevus syndrome, xeroderma pigmentosa – **asymmetry, borders irregular, color changes, diameter increased** – **depth of invasion – best prognostic factor** [< 0.76 mm – do not metastasize, > 1.7 mm – potential for metastasis]

- **Basal cell CA :** Most common <u>**skin**</u> cancer – sun exposed area – <u>**upper lip** Raised</u> <u>**papule**</u> , shiny (or) <u>**"Pearly " appearance**</u>

- **Squamous cell CA :** <u>**Lower lip**</u> – sun exposed area, tobacco use, scar tissue in 3rd degree burn, <u>Actinic keratosis</u> – <u>**ulcerated lesion**</u>

- **Pemphigus vulgaris** – IgG against **desmosomes** (intracellular attachment)
- Suprabasal, **(+) Nikolsky sign, Oral lesions**
- **Acantholysis** of karatinocytes in the vesicle fluid

- **Bullous Pemphigoid** – IgG against **basement membrane**
- Subepidermal vesicle, (**–**) Nikolsky sign
- **No** Acantholysis of karatinocytes in the vesicle fluid

- **Dermatitis Herpetiformis** – IgA-anti-IgA complex deposit at the tips of the dermal papillae
- Subepidermal vesicle with Neutrophils, microscopic blisters
- **Strong association with Celiac disease**

* **Psoriasis** – coin-shaped lesions cover with **silvery-scale** – on **extensor surface** – **nail pitting** – development of lesion in area of trauma (<u>Koebner phenomenon</u>) – bleeding occur when scale is scraped off (<u>Auspitz sign</u>) – neutrophil collection in stratum corneum (<u>Munro microabscesses</u>)

* **Atopic Dermatitis** – extreme pruritus – **flexor** surface - ↑ IgE – avoid scratching – **Type-1 HS**

* **Contact Dermatitis** – linear, streaked vesicles (**weeping lesion**) – **Type-4 HS**

* **Seborrheic Dermatitis (dandruff)** – scaly, **greasy, flaky skin** – pityrosporum ovale

* **Stasis Dermatitis** – hyperpigmentation built up from hemosiderin in the tissue – varicose veins for long time.

* **Xerosis (Asteotic Dermatitis)** – dry skin – elderly (due to decrease in lipid)

* **Keratoacanthoma**: rapidly growing, benign crateriform tumor with a central keratin plug – sun exposed area. Regress spontaneously with scarring

* **Nummular Dermatitis:** coin-shaped lesions (discoid lesions) .

* **Pompholyx:** deep-seated vesicles on the palms, fingers and soles

ENDOCRINOLOGY

- Hyperprolactinemia: Non-functioning Pituitary adenoma – Microadenoma (**women** – amenorrhea, galactorrhea) – Macroadenoma (**men** – visual field defect – heteronymous hemianopsia) – **dopamine antagonist** (Phenothiazine, metoclopramide) – **dopamine depleting agents** (methyldopa, Reserpine) – **primary hypothyroidism** (increase TRH-activated dopamine which overcome the normal dopamine inhibition) – **Diagnosis** – Prolactin level > 100 ng/ml suggest pituitary adenoma

- Acromegaly: ↑↑ GH (gigantism in children) – pituitary adenoma – b/w 3rd and 5th decade – **c/o unable to wear wedding ring, increase in shoe size** – entrapment neuropathy, osteoarthritis, hypertension, impaired glucose tolerance, **CHF** (late) – symptoms for an average of 9 yrs before diagnosis – **Diagnosis**: GH level remains > 5 ng/ml after giving 100gm of glucose orally
- Laron Dwarfism – **congenital absent** of **GH receptor** - ↑ GH, ↓ IGF-1 & undetectable GH binding protein in blood

- Hypopituitarism: loss of function of anterior pituitary – loss of FSH, LH, GH, TSH and ACTH – Causes: Hypothalamic tumors (Craniopharyngioma, meningioma, gliomas), Pituitary apoplexy (acute h'ge in preexisting pituitary adenoma - **emergency**) – **Sheehan syndrome** [postpartum necrosis of pituitary due to loss of blood intrapartum – inability to lactate (1st sign)]

- CT head – **No** pituitary + **normal** hormone level – **Empty sella Syndrome**

- Diabetes Insipidus: excessive thirst, polyuria (form **dilute urine** in the presence of **Hypernatremia**) - **central** (insufficient ADH) & **Nephrogenic** (unresponsiveness of kidney to ADH) – **Diagnosis**: 1. **increase** in Urine Osm **after** giving vasopressin – **central DI**. 2. **increase** Urine Osm **after dehydration** – **psychogenic polyuria**

- SIADH: cancers (small cell CA of lung), Drugs (Chlorpropamide, carbamazapine) – continuously form **concentrated** urine in the presence of **hyponatremia**

- Conn's Syndrome: Primary Hyperaldosteronism – adenoma of zona glomerulosa (adrenal gland) – hypertension(sodium retention), hypokalamia (muscle weakness) – **Tx**: resection [Renal artery stenosis – BUN:Cr >20:1, abdominal bruits, hypokalamia is less severe than Conn's syndrome; For example if Hypokalamia in Conn's is in 2.something range, hypokalamia in renal artery stenosis is in 3.something range but less than 3.5; (3.5 – 5.0 normal range)]

- Hyperthyroidism: ↑↑ T3 & T4, ↓↓ TSH – heat intolerance, weight loss, diarrhea, tremor, arrhythmias; **Exophthalmos & dermatopathies** (only in **Grave's disease**) – **Grave's disease** - ↑ RAIU (radioactive iodine uptake), anti-TSH receptor antibodies. **Toxic nodular goiter** (single / multiple) - ↑ RAIU. **de Quarian Thyroiditis** (subacute granulomatous, giant cell) – ↓ RAIU – **painful** (transient hyperthyroidism). **Subacute**

lymphocytic Thyroiditis - ↓ RAIU – **painless** (transient hyperthyroidism). Ectopic thyroid tissue – struma ovarii

- Hypothyroidism: ↓↓ T3 & T4, ↑↑ TSH (primary) but normal / ↓ TSH (secondary / tertiary) – cold intolerance, weight gain, amenorrhea, carpal tunnel syndrome, **slow deep tendon reflexes with prolonged relaxation phase**, myxedema – **Hashimoto Thyroiditis**: anti-microsomal antibody, anti-thyroglobulin antibody, lymphocytic infiltration – associated with lymphoma in thyroid gland – **Tx:** levothyroxine(T4), in secondary & tertiary first give hydrocortisone then replace thyroid hormone.

- Reidle Thyroiditis: intense fibrosis of thyroid gland and surrounding structure.

- Papillary CA: most common thyroid CA – **h/o radiation exposure**

- Follicular CA: elderly – **spread hematogenously**

- Medullary CA: parafollicular cell of thyroid gland - ↑↑↑ Calcitonin – association with MEN type-2b – more malignant then follicular

- Anaplastic CA: elderly – highly malignant with rapid and painful enlargement of thyroid gland – poor prognosis

- Parathyroid Hormone: stimulates Osteoclasts & 1-α-hydroxylase (increase production of active form of Vit-D → 1-25-(OH)2-D) – increase Ca+2 level by bone resorption (osteoclast) & by absorption of Ca+2 from gut and kidney (Vit-D).

- Vit-D: increase absorption of **both** Ca+2 & Phosphorus (PO4) **from intestine** and increase absorption of Ca+2 and **decrease** absorption of **PO4 from kidney**.

- Magnesium: cofactor for adenylate cyclase – cAMP is require for PTH activation – therefore hypomagnesemia can cause hypocalcemia (hypomagnesemia is the most common pathologic cause of hypocalcemia in the hospital)

- Calcitonin: inhibit bone resorption

- Primary Hypo- / Hyperparathyroidism: plasma calcium & phosphate levels are **changing in opposite direction EXCEPT** CRF which causes secondary hyperparathyroidism but in CRF there is hypocalcemia & hyperparathyroidism (moves in opposite direction)

- Secondary Hyperparathyroidism: **Increase PTH**, decrease Ca+2 level & its excretion and decrease PO4 level & normal/increase its excretion

- Secondary Hypoparathyroidism: **Decrease PTH**, increase Ca+2 level & its excretion and increase PO4 level & normal/decrease its excretion.

- <u>Hypercalcemia</u>: primary hyperparathyroidism (one gland hyperplasia), PTH-like substance secretion from CA – Osteitis fibrosa cystica, lytic lesions on x-rays – serum Ca+2 level more than 10.2 mg/dl

- <u>Hypocalcemia</u>: **tetany**, muscle cramps / spasm, Chovestic sign (percussion of Facial N. leads to contraction of facial muscles), **Trousseau's sign** (inflation of BP cuff on the arm of patient above SBP for more than 3 mins leads to flexion of metacarpophalangeal joints and extension of interphalangeal joint), **QT prolongation on EKG** – always check for albumin level (1 gm/dl drop in albumin → calcium level drop by 0.8 mg/dl)

- <u>Diagnosis of DM</u>: symptomatic patient (polyuria, ploydipsia, polyphagia) with random blood glucose level › 200 mg/dl <u>or</u> fasting blood glucose › 126 mg/dl on two occasion <u>or</u> blood glucose › 200 mg/dl at 2 hrs on two occasions

- <u>HbA1c</u>: used to follow compliance of the treatment and glucose control in patient with diabetes.

- <u>Insulinoma</u>: increase in both plasma insulin and C peptide

- <u>Exogenous insulin administration</u>: very high insulin level but **low** C peptide

- <u>Sulfonylureas</u>: increase in both plasma insulin and C peptide, plasma/urine sulfonylurea (+)

- **Primary Hypercortisolism** (<u>Adrenal Tumor</u>) - ↑ cortisol, ↓ ACTH
- **Pituitary Cushing** (<u>Cushing's disease</u>) - ↑ cortisol, ↑ ACTH. **High dose Dexamethasone test - ↓cortisol, ↓ ACTH by 50%**
- **Ectopic ACTH secretion** - ↑ cortisol, ↑ ACTH. High dose Dexamethasone test – **No** suppression of ACTH
- **Sign & Symptoms:** buffalo hump, purple striae on abdomen, moon face

- <u>17 α Hydroxylase Deficiency</u>: ↓ cortisol and androgen but ↑ **11 deoxycorticosterone** (weak mineralocorticoid due to which retention of sodium occur and hypertension develop)
- <u>21 β Hydroxylase Deficiency</u>: ↓ cortisol and mineralocorticoid but ↑ **androgens**
- <u>11 β Hydroxylase Deficiency</u>: ↓ cortisol but ↑ **androgens and mineralocorticoid**

- Increase ACTH in all of 3 enzymes deficiency (above)
- Male ambiguous genitalia (male pseudohermaphrodite) – 17 α Hydroxylase
- Female ambiguous genitalia (female pseudohermaphrodite) – 21 & 11 β Hydroxylase
- Female Hypogonadism – 17 α Hydroxylase
- Precocious puberty in male – 21 & 11 β Hydroxylase

- <u>MEN 1</u> (Wermer) – Pancreas (ZE syndrome), Pituitary, **Hyperparathyroidism** (3P)
- <u>MEN 2a</u> (Sipple) – **Hyperparathyroidism**, <u>Pheochromocytoma</u>, <u>Medullary CA of Thyroid</u>

- MEN 2b (3) – Pheochromocytoma, Medullary CA of Thyroid, mucosal neuroma (lips/tongue)

- Presence of Y chromosome – germinal tissue differentiate in to Testes.
- **hCG + LH → leyding cells** → testosterone → **wallfian duct** (epididymis, ductus deference, ejaculatory duct) → 5 α reductase convert testosterone in dihydrotestosteron (DHT) which induce urogenital sinus & genital tubercle to form penis, prostate & scrotum.
- **Sertoli cells** → secrete MIF (mullerian inhibiting factor) which inhibit **paramesonephric duct** (uterus, uterine tubes, cervix & upper part of vagina)
- **If MIF absent** – uterus (paramesonephric duct structure) develop with normal male structure
- **If Testosterone absent** – wallfian duct regress (male internal structure **not** develop)
- **If 5 α reductase absent** – DHT **not** formed. Therefore **male external structures not develop** but female external structures develop.
- Absence of Y chromosome – germinal tissue differentiate in to Ovaries. Wallfian (mesonephric duct) regress and female genitalia develop.
- Testicular Feminization – **androgen receptor insensitivity**, Mullerian duct structure develop in the presence of testes. (No effect of testosterone & DHT)

GESTROENTEROLOGY

- ▪ **M**idline to Lateral – Sublingual (**M**ucous) – Submandibular (mix) – Parotid (serous)

* **Dysphagia:**
- Dysphagia for solids **not** liquid → **Obstruction** – stricture, esophageal CA
  Plummer–Vinson Syndrome
- Dysphagia for solids **and** liquid → **Peristalsis problem** – Achalasia , Systemic
  Sclerosis, CREST, Polymyositis

- ■ **Achalasia** – normal amplitude contraction with **high tone of lower sphincter** (failure to relax) – Absent myenteric ganglion
- ■ **Esophageal spasm** – **high amplitude contraction** with normal relaxation of lower esophageal sphincter
- ■ **Scleroderma** – absence peristalsis wave with very low tone of lower esophageal sphincter

* **Ring & Webs :**
- **Schatzki's ring** – more distal & located at the squamocolumnar junction
- **Plummer-Vinson** - more proximal & located in the hypopharynx

* **Esophageal CA** : Tobacco + Alcohol → SCC →Upper 2/3
- GERD & Barrett esophagus → Adenocarcinoma → lower 1/3

* **Zenker's Diverticulum**: out pocketing of the posterior pharyngeal Constrictor muscles at the back of the pharynx
- **Bad breath, aspiration pneumonia / lung abscess (anaerobic)**

* **Gastroesophageal Reflux Disease (GERD):**
- Epigastric pain going under sternum , <u>non-productive cough at night</u> (it can cause worsening of asthma at night by irritating bronchus), bad taste in mouth
- **Sliding Hernia of esophagus** – GE junction displaced & reach above
- **Paraesophageal Hernia** – GE junction not displaced

* **Barrett Esophagus:** Metaplasia (squamous → columnar)

* **Mallory Weiss Tear** → **continuous retching** followed by large **painless bloody vomiting** (mucosal tear)

* **Boerhaave Syndrome** → **continuous retching followed by severe chest pain**, Crepitation in the neck, air in mediastinum on CXR [Esophageal rupture – usually in distal third, posterolateral segment (where there is **no** serosa) is the most common site]

- ■ **Stomach Histology:**
- Parietal cells → HCL & IF

- Chief cells $\rightarrow$ Pepsinogen $\xrightarrow{H+}$ Pepsin
- Mucous cells $\rightarrow$ mucous, HCO_3
- G cells $\rightarrow$ gastrin
- Vagal stimulation $\rightarrow$ Ach, gastrin–releasing peptide
- Histamine $\rightarrow$ Enterochromaffin-like cells

* **<u>Zollinger–Ellison Syndrome (ZE syndrome):</u>**
- Multiple recurrent ulcers (usually duodenum) , Steatorrhea
- Associated with MEN – I (Parathyroid, Pituitary, Pancreas)
- **<u>Diagnosis:</u>** Elevated gastrin level

* **<u>Gastritis:</u>**
- **<u>Type – A</u>** $\rightarrow$ Atrophic gastritis (Autoimmune) , Vit-B_{12} deficiency , $\uparrow\uparrow\uparrow$ gastrin
- **<u>Type – B</u>** $\rightarrow$ NSAID, H. Pylori, Alcohol
- Increase chance of gastric CA in patient with Type-A gastritis

- **<u>Protein loosing enteropathy</u>: Enlarge rugal folds** – hypertrophy of mucous cells (Menetrier disease, ZES, lymphoma)

- **Inflammatory Bowel Disease:**
* **<u>Crohn's Disease: Oral / Perianal involvement</u>** , palpable Abdominal mass (**<u>granuloma</u>** – characteristic of Crohn), **Transmural involvement**, Skip lesions, Fistula formation
* **<u>Ulcerative colitis</u>: rectum involvement**, bloody diarrhea , **<u>exclusive mucosal disease</u>**
* CD $\rightarrow$ Vit–B_{12}, Vit–K, Ca^{+2}, iron deficiency $\rightarrow$ elevated PT, kidney stones, Megaloblastic anemia

* **<u>Lactose Intolerance:</u>** lactase deficiency
- Diarrhea associated with gas & bloating **after drinking milk**
- **<u>Never</u>** has blood / WBC in stool
- **<u>Diagnosis:</u>** stool osmolarity > expected osmolarity

* **<u>Irritable Bowel Syndrome:</u>**
- Abdominal pain relieved by bowel movement
- Diarrhea alternating with constipation

- **<u>Carcinoid Syndrome:</u>** tumors of the neuroendocrine syndrome
- Tip of vermiform appendix (most common site) but carcinoid tumors of terminal ileum most commonly metastasize (liver)
- Diarrhea, Flushing, Tachycardia and Hypotension
- <u>Niacin deficiency</u> (Serotonin & Niacin $\rightarrow$ Tryptophan)
- Endocardial fibrosis, Tricuspid Regurgitation, Pulmonic stenosis
- **<u>Diagnosis:</u>** <u>urinary 5 – HIAA</u> (5- hydroxyindolacetic acid)

- **<u>Celiac Disease:</u>**
- Anti-gliadin, Anti-endomysial, Anti-transglutaminase antibodies

- Loss of intestinal villi (malabsorption – diarrhea, abd distension, abd pain)
- **Celiac disease** affect **PROXIMAL** small bowel.
- Function returns if patient is on gluten free diet
- Dermatitis herpetiformis → strong association with celiac disease
- **No** wheat, rye, oat [contains gluten]

* **Whipple's Disease:** Tropheryma whippeli bacilli
- **PAS–positive macrophage** obstruct lymphatic & reabsorption of chylomicrons
- Chronic diarrhea and weight loss

* **Diverticulosis:**
- Lack of fibers in the diet
- Right sided bleed / Left sided obstruct
- Most common cause of lower GI bleed. (Angiodysplasia – 2nd MCC)

* **Diverticulitis:** (left sided appendicitis)

- **Sigmoid colon:** most common site for diverticulosis, diverticulitis and polyp
- **Rectosigmoid colon:** most common site for colon CA

- **Volvulus of Sigmoid colon** → Elderly patient → distended abdomen, similar episodes in past which resolve itself → Parrot's beak appearance (coffee bean sign / omega sign) of large gas shadow on X-ray

- **Mesenteric Ischemia** → Patient with **h/o AF / atherosclerotic disease** present with acute abdomen (**pain out of proportion to physical findings** like absent rebound tenderness, guarding, rigidity, etc) & **blood in stool**

- **Mechanical Intestinal Obstruction** → Abdominal pain, constipation, distension & vomiting (cardinal features of obstruction) → Adhesion / Indirect Inguinal Hernia
- Fever, leukocytosis, rebound tenderness in patient with indirect inguinal hernia suggest **strangulation**

* **Meckle's Diverticulum** → **painless** large bloody bowel movement in child (**brick red stool**) → **Technetium scan** (^{99m}Tc scan) to identify ectopic gastric mucosa [rule of 2's – 2 ft from ileocecal valve, 2 inches long, 2 yrs of age, 2% of population; remnant of Vitelline duct (Omphalomesenteric duct)]

- **Gastroschisis** → Normal cord, **no** protecting membrane (sac) and bowel protruding from this defect
- **Omphalocele** → shiny, thin, membranous **sac** at the base of the umbilical cord, cord goes to the defect, **not** to the baby → can have multiple defects

- **Meconium ileu** → **cystic fibrosis** → ground glass appearance on abd x-ray

- **Hirschsprung Disease (aganglionic megacolon)** → Rectal exam may lead to explosive expulsion of stool & flatus → **X-ray**: distended proximal colon (normal) and "normal looking" distal colon (aganglionic).

- **Intussception** → **sausage shaped mass** on the right side of the abdomen, "empty" looking right lower quadrant (Dancing sign), **"currant jelly stool"**

- Classic presentation of **Acute Appendicitis** [pain start in mid epigastric region and then shifted to RLQ, positive rebound tenderness]

* **Colon Cancer**: colonoscopy
- Hyperplastic polyp, Juvenile polyp, Peutz –Jeghers → **No** malignant potential
- Tubular polyp (most common neoplastic polyp), villous polyp, Familial Polyposis, Turcot syndrome, Gardner syndrome → **malignant potential**

* **Hereditary Non-Polyposis Syndrome (HNPCC) (Lynch Syndrome):**
- Mis-match base repair defect
- Colonoscopy every 1-2 yrs start at age of 25 yrs
- Very high incidence of **ovarian and endometrial cancer**

* **Familial Adenomatous Polyposis:**
- APC gene confers 100 % penetrance for the development of adenomas by the age of 35 & colon cancer by the age of 50

* **Cowden Syndrome:**
- Hemartomas, rectal bleeding in a **child**

* **Gardner Syndrome:**
- Colon CA + multiple soft – tissue tumors (osteoma, lipoma, fibrosarcoma)

* **Turcot Syndrome:**
- Colon CA + CNS malignancy

* **Peutz – Jeghers Syndrome:**
- Hemartomatous polyp + Hyperpigmented spots (lips, buccal mucosa, skin)

* **Acute Pancreatitis:**
- Mid epigastric pain classically **radiates straight to the back**.
- Amylase & **lipase (most specific)** are extremely elevated

■ **Pancreatic head cancer:** Palpable gallbladder **without** significant **tenderness**

▪ **Billirubin:** Senescent RBC → Heme → unconjugated Bilirubin (lipid soluble – can accumulate in tissue so large amt in blood can cause problem) → bind with albumin and goes to liver → conjugated in liver [water soluble – easy for our body to excrete] →

secreted in bile → 80% excreted in feces & 20% extrahepatic circulation [90% liver and 10% renal (in urine)]

- **Jaundice:** ↑ **unconjugated** [more hemolysis, liver unable to pick up (Gilbert syndrome – jaundice with fasting), liver unable to conjugate (Crigler-Najjar syndrome – deficient enzyme)] ↑ **conjugated** [liver unable to excrete in bile (Dubin-Johnson syndrome – black liver) (OCP), ↓ extrahepatic bile flow (gall stone, CA of head of pancrease)] ↑ **Both** [liver dysfunction (hepatitis)]
- Pruritus in Billiary disease is due to bile salt which deposits in skin
- For **Jaundice**, we test billirubin in urine with strip test **not** urobillinogen (UBG). UBG is normally present in urine. **UBG is absent in obstructive jaundice** but billirubin (conjugated – water soluble) is present in urine in obstructive jaundice

* **Primary Billiary Cirrhosis:**
- **Anti-mitochondrial antibody**
- Granulomatous destruction of bile ducts in portal triad
- Middle – aged women, very less elevation of bilirubin, strong association with other auto-immune diseases → Sjogren Syndrome, RA, Scleroderma
- **Diagnosis: Transaminase** are often **normal**
  ↑↑ **Alkaline Phosphatase & γ - glutamyl transpeptidase**
- ↑ risk for hepatocellular carcinoma [HCC]

- **Primary Sclerosing Cholangitis:**
- Obliterative fibrosis of intrahepatic & extrahepatic bile ducts
- Strong association with Ulcerative colitis
- Sx – same as primary billiary cirrhosis (Pruritus; etc)
- Anti-mitochondrial Antibody → negative
- ↑ risk for cholangiocarcinoma (CA of bile duct)

* **Hemochromatosis:**
- Most common inherited genetic disease
- Over absorption of iron [Ferritin (major storage protein) store iron in macrophage in bone marrow and hepatocytes, circulate in small amt in serum (↓ in iron deficiency anemia); Hemosiderin degradation product of Ferritin **in cell**, (doesn't circulate) golden brown granules in tissue & blue with Prussian blue]
- Intracellular iron produce hydroxyl ions which damage **parenchymal cells**
- **Cirrhosis, Restrictive cardiomyopathy**, Arthralgia, skin hyperpigmentation, **diabetes**, Hypogonadism
- ↑ infection with Vibrio vulnificus, Yersinia & L.monocytogens

- **Wilson Disease:**
- Autosomal recessive disease present with choreoathetoid movements
- ↓ copper transport into bile and ↓ ceruloplasmin synthesis leads to ↓ excretion of copper from body & ↑ free Cu^{+2} in the body which deposited in various tissue and produce damage

- Basal ganglia dysfunction, **Kayser-Fleischer ring** (**Slit – lamp Examination**), Fanconi Syndrome

- **Ruptured Hepatic Adenoma** → young woman on **birth control pills** present with abdominal pain, low hemoglobin, hypovolemic shock

- **Amebic liver abscess** → h/o Travel to Mexico → jaundice, weight loss, right upper quadrant pain, diarrhea

- **Liver Problem** → ↑↑↑ transaminase **Billiary Problem** → ↑↑↑ Alkaline Phosphatase **Alcoholic liver Problem** → ↑↑↑ GGT (γ–glutamyl transferase)

- **Pericentral vein zone** (zone 3) in liver contains the P450 oxidase enzyme system & is most **sensitive to Ischemic injury**
- **Periportal zone** (zone 1) in liver is most **sensitive to toxic injury**
- "Ito cells" – site of Vit-A storage, located in space of Disse

* **Choledochal cyst** – congenital benign dilatation of bile ducts
* **Caroli's Syndrome** – congenital cystic dilatation of the intrahepatic biliary tree – associated with polycystic kidney disease – Cholangitis & Cholangio CA

- **Gall stone (Cholelithiasis):**
- Cholesterol (80%) (radiolucent) - ↑cholesterol in bile and ↓bile salt & lecithin
- Pigment stone (20%) (radio-opaque) – calcium bilirubinate [Sickle cell anemia]
- **Billiary colic** → colicky right upper quadrant pain, radiate to the right shoulder, often aggravated after ingestion of fatty food / Anti-cholinergic drug → USG [presence of gall stones, **no** thickening of GB wall]
- **Acute Cholecystitis** → **F**emale , **F**orty , **F**ertile , **F**atty → colicky right upper quadrant pain, radiate to the right shoulder, often aggravated after ingestion of fatty food → **USG** [presence of gall stones, thickening of GB wall, pericholecystic fluid]

- **Gallbladder adenocarcinoma:**
- Risk factors – cholelithiasis, Caroli's disease, porcelain gallbladder [calcification of GB wall]

- Infant on **milk formula** – necrotizing enterocolitis – **transmural necrosis**

- **Diarrhea:**
- Traveler's diarrhea – E.coli
- Undercooked **hamburger** meat – E.coli 0157 : H7 (associated with **HUS**)
- Giardia lamblia – **camping**, contaminated water source
- **HIV Positive , CD4 < 50** cells , **Acid fast oocyst** – Cryptosporidium
- Ingestion of unrefrigerated meat – Cl. Difficile
- **Fired rice** – Bacillus Cerius
- Contaminate Shellfish – V. parahaemolyticus
- Severe liver disease patient – V.vulnificus

- **Reye Syndrome:**
- Encephalopathy and **microvesicular steatosis** in Liver
- Recent <u>viral URI</u>, Varicella, <u>Aspirin use</u>.
- Ammonia, Transaminases are markedly elevated
- Liver biopsy → non-inflammatory fatty infiltration, **mitochondrial injury**

HEMATOLOGY

* **Anemia:** low Hb (<13 in M & <12 in F) / low hematocrit (<40 in M & <37 in F)

Microcytic (MCV < 80)	Normocytic	Macrocytic (MCV > 96)
• Iron deficiency	• Hemolytic anemia	• B_{12} deficiency
• Thalasemia	• ACD	• Folate deficiency
• Sideroblastic		• Alcohol related
• Lead poisoning		• Liver disease
• Anemia of chronic diseases (ACD)		• Chemotherapy / Drugs

* **MCHC:** Mean corpuscular Hb concentration (Avg. Hb concentration in RBC)
  ↓ MCHC → central area of pallor – Microcytic
  ↑ MCHC → No central area of pallor – **Spherocytosis**
  <u>N</u> MCHC → **Megaloblastic** Anemia

- **Hb A - α, β Hb F - α, γ Hb A$_2$ - α, δ**

- Daily requirement of Iron – 1 mg/day in M, 2-3 mg/day in F

* **Iron Deficiency Anemia:**
- **Low** serum ferritin, serum iron **, high** TIBC
- Blood loss (menstruation), dietary deficiency

* **ACD (Anemia of Chronic Diseases):**
- **Normal / elevated** serum ferritin
- **Both** serum iron & TIBC → **Low**
- **Pathophysiology:** inflammatory cytokines increase production of hepcidin from liver. Hepcidin in turn stops ferroportin from releasing iron stores – inflammatory cytokines increase the production of white blood cells. Bone marrow produces both red blood cells and white blood cells from the same precursor stem cells. Therefore, the upregulation of white blood cells causes fewer stem cells to differentiate into red blood cells. – so decrease iron release and decrease RBC production is responsible for anemia
  [**Ferroportin:** a transmembrane protein that transports iron from the inside of a cell to the outside of it – located on the surface of Enterocytes in the duodenum, Hepatocyte and Macrophage]

*   **Sideroblastic Anemia:**
- Normal serum ferritin
- **Very high** transferrin saturation
- **High** serum iron & **Low** TIBC
- **Prussian Blue stain** of RBC in the marrow will show **ringed sideroblast**
- Vit-B_6 deficiency: ↓ Protoporphyrin & ↓ δ ALA
- Iron deficiency: ↑ Protoporphyrin & **N** δ ALA
- Lead poisoning: ↑ Protoporphyrin & ↑ δ ALA

*   **Thalassemia:**
- Underproduction of alpha/beta globin chain
- Mild – Moderate anemia with **very low MCV**
- **Target cells**, Normal serum iron & RDW

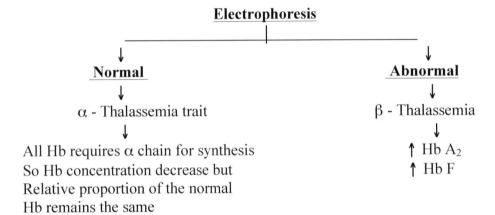

Electrophoresis

Normal

α - Thalassemia trait

All Hb requires α chain for synthesis
So Hb concentration decrease but
Relative proportion of the normal
Hb remains the same

Abnormal

β - Thalassemia

↑ Hb A_2
↑ Hb F

- ▪ **"Crew haircut"** on **skull X-ray** is distinctive radiological change seen most often in patient with **Sickle cell anemia & Thalassemia major**.

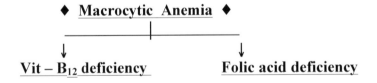

◆ **Macrocytic Anemia** ◆

Vit – B_{12} deficiency   **Folic acid deficiency**

- Peripheral Blood smear: **Hypersegmented Neutrophils** seen in <u>Both</u>

- **How to differentiate: Low** B_{12} level   **Low** RBC folic acid level
  <u>↑ Methylmalonic acid</u>
  level is seen in **only B_{12}**

- Schilling Test is occasionally used to determine etiology of B_{12} def
- **Schilling Test:** Oral Administration of Radioactive Vit – B_{12}
- Reabsorption → Pure vegan
- B_{12} + IF → Reabsorption → Pernicious Anemia
- B_{12} + Antibiotics → Reabsorption → Bacterial over growth

- B_{12} + Pancreatic extract → Reabsorption → chronic Pancreatitis.
- <u>Important</u>: Vit-B_{12} and folic acid require for DNA synthesis in all cells so their deficiency affect all bone marrow cells, not just RBC.

Hemolytic Anemia

Extravascular hemolysis
- ↑ **Unconjugated bilirubin**
- ↑ LDH
- Spherocytosis
- Sickle-cell
- Immune-hemolytic anemia

Intravascular Hemolysis
- ↑ plasma & urine Hb
- **Hemoglobinuria**
- **Hemosiderinuria**
- ↓ **Serum Haptoglobin**
- ↑ LDH
- PNH (Paroxysmal Nocturnal Hemoglobinuria)
- G6PD

- **Sickle- cell-Anemia:** Autosomal-recessive
- Substitution of Valine for glutamic acid at sixth position on β- globin chain

- ■ **Hereditary Spherocytosis:** Autosomal dominant
- RBC membrane protein defect [spectrin, ankyrin]
- **Osmotic Fragility test & ↑ MCHC**

- ■ **Autoimmune Hemolytic Anemia:**
- **Coomb's test**
- Warm – antibody (I_gG), Cold – antibody (I_gM)
- Drug – induced → Penicillin, Quinidine, α - Methyldopa

- ■ **Paroxysmal Nocturnal Hemoglobinuria (PNH):**
- Loss of anchor for DAF (Decay Accelerating Factor)
- more complements bind to RBC & intravascular hemolysis occur
- **Presentation :** Hemoglobinuria in first morning urine

- ■ **G6PD deficiency:** ↓ Synthesis of NADPH & GSH (glutathione)
- **X-linked recessive**
- Hemolysis in the presence of **Oxidant Stress**
- Oxidant Stress → Infection , **fevabeans**, **Drugs** (Sulfa, Dapsone, Primaquine, Quinidine, Nitrofurantoin, INH)
- Diagnosis → **Heinz bodies** , **bite cells** , G6PD level

- ■ **Pyruvate kinase deficiency:** ↓ Synthesis of ATP
- **Autosomal recessive**
- PK gives 2 ATPs – its deficiency produce membrane damage – RBC with **thorny projection** (echinocytes)

◆ Leukemia ◆

ALL	AML	CML	CLL
• Children (< 14 yrs)	• 15-39 yrs	• 40-60 yrs	• > 60 yrs
• Thrombocytopenia	• Thrombocytopenia	• Thrombocytopenia **Thrombocytosis in 40%**	• Thrombocytopenia
• Pre-B cells - CALLA, CD10 & TdT positive	• t (15; 17) in M_3	• **Philadelphia chromosome**, t (9 ; 22)	• **CD19 Antigen**
• T cells - CD10 & TdT negative	• **DIC in M_3**	• Basophillia	• **Predominantly B lymphocytes**.
• t (12; 21) – good prognosis	• Auer rods in M_2 & M_3		• "Smudge cells"
CALLA (common ALL antigen)	• CNS in M_4 & M_5 M_3- Premyelocytic M_4-myelomonocytic M_5- monocytic • **Vit–A** – useful in Premyelocytic (M_3)		

* **Adult T-cell lymphoma**: HTLV-1 [Human T-cell leukemia virus – 1]
- Activation of TAX gene – inhibits TP53 suppressor gene
- ↑ CD4 T-cells
- Skin infiltration and lytic bone lesion [lymphoblast release osteoclast activating factor] (hypercalcemia)
- Negative TdT

* **Hairy cell leukemia**: only leukemia without lymphadenopathy
- B-cell leukemia
- Positive TRAP stain (tartrate-resistant acid phosphate)

* **Infectious Mononucleosis**: EBV – CD21 receptor on B-cells – heterophile antibody (IgM to sheep's RBC) – danger of rupture of spleen

* **Myeloid stem cells**: RBC, granulocytes, mast cells and platelets – Polycythemia vera affect myeloid stem cells so increase everything in Polycythemia vera – myelofibosis (tear drop cells, extramedullary hematopoesis)

* **Aplastic Anemia**: Pancytopenia [Everything is decreased including RBCs, Platelets and WBCs]

◆ Plasma Cell Disorder ◆

Multiple Myeloma	Monoclonal Gammopathy of Uncertain Significance
• **Bone pain** , Infection, Anemia , Renal failure	• **No** systemic manifestation like multiple myeloma
• **Electrophoresis** – **IgG** monoclonal spike	• IgG monoclonal spike on electrophoresis
• **X-ray** – **punched out lytic lesion** (osteoclast activating factor)	• **No** lytic bone lesion on X-ray
• Hypercalcemia	• Normal lab test (creatinine, calcium)
• Bence-Jones Protein (Acidification of urine is required to test BJ protein)	
• Bone marrow biopsy – >**10% plasma cells**	• Bone marrow - < **5 % Plasma cells**

* **Waldenstrom's macroglobulinemia (Lymphoplasmatic lymphoma)**: M spike with **IgM**, BJ protein – **no** lytic lesions like multiple myeloma

- BJ proteins – kappa or lambda **light** chains

◆ Lymphomas ◆

Hodgkin Lymphoma	Non-Hodgkin Lymphoma
• **Reed-Sternberg cells**	• Reed-Sternberg cell **Absent**
• Lymphadenopathy is more common (cervical, Supraclavicular, Axillary)	• Extralymphatic involvement is more common (Spleen, liver, stomach)
• B-cells lineage involve	• **Both** B & T cell lineages involve
• Lymphocyte Predominant (Best Prognosis)	• HIV, EBV → **Burkitt lymphoma,** t (8;14)
• Mixed celluarity	• H.pylori → gastric lymphoma (mucosa associated lymphoid tissues in stomach)
• Nodular Sclerosing (**Female**) → **lacunar cells**	• CNS involvement is more common in HIV-positive patient
• Lymphocyte depletion (worst prognosis)	• **Follicular lymphoma** – t (14;18), over expression of BCL2 anti-apoptosis gene
• **RS cells** – CD15, CD 30 positive - B-lymphocyte with **somatic hypermutation**	• **Sjogren syndrome** – salivary gland & GI lymphoma
	• **Hashimoto's thyroidits** – thyroid malignant lymphoma

- **Mycosis fungoides** – cutaneous (begins in skin) T-cell lymphoma (**not** a fungal infection)

◆ <u>Bleeding Disorders</u> ◆

- ■ Tissue thromboplastin → **Factor 7** → Extrinsic Pathway (**PT**) → **Warfarin**
- ■ Subendothelial collagen, HMWK → **Factor 12** → Intrinsic Pathway (**PTT**) → **Heparin**
- ■ Common final pathway → **Factor 10 , 5 , 2 , 1** [2-Prothrombin]
- ■ **Heparin** → ⊕ **AT III** → neutralize **9 , 10 , 11 , 12 , Prothrombin & thrombin**
- ■ Thrombin → **convert fibrinogen into fibrin monomers** [fibrin monomers then aggregate which are soluble]
- ■ Thrombin → **activate fibrin stabilizing factor (13)** [once fibrin monomers aggregate, factor-13 stabilize them by making them insoluble]
- ■ Plasmin → cleaves insoluble fibrin monomers and fibrinogen into fibrin degradation products [FDP]
- ■ D-Dimers → fragments of cross-linked insoluble fibrin monomers
- ■ Protein C & S (Vit .K dependent) → inactivate **5 & 8** → enhance fibrinolysis
- ■ **tPA** – synthesized by endothelial cell , **TxA$_2$** –synthesized by Platelates
- ■ $_v$**WF** – synthesized by endothelial cell & Platelates – Func.^{n} → Platelate Adhesion & Prevent degradation of **factor VIII:C**
- ■ **Platelate Storage** → $_v$WF & Fibrinogen **(1)**
- ■ **Platelate receptors** → glycoprotein (gp) 1b – $_v$WF ; GP2b:3a – Fibrinogen
- ■ **Platelate Factors** → **PF$_3$** → Prothrombin complex (V, Xa, PF$_3$, Ca^{+2}).

  PF$_4$ → Heparin neutralizing factor

- **<u>Hemostasis in small vessel injury</u>:** injury → tissue thromboplastin (activates extrinsic pathway) & exposed collagen (activates intrinsic pathway) → Endothelial cells synthesize vWF so injury makes it expose to platelets and platelets start attaching to them and ADP from platelets help aggregating them (temporary plug) → platelets have fibrinogen at gp2b:3a → activated thrombin (by intrinsic & extrinsic pathway) convert fibrinogen to fibrin monomers which aggregate and make soluble plug → thrombin also activate factor-13 which convert soluble plug into insoluble plug → bleeding stop → tPA activates plasmin which dissolve fibrin monomer & blood flow reestablish to the tissue

- **<u>Idiopathic Thrombocytopenic Purpura</u>:**
- Sign of bleeding from superficial areas of body
- **Absent spleenomegaly,** Prolong Bleeding time
- Idiopathic **Antibody (IgG) Production to the Platelets receptors** (gp2b:3a)
- **<u>Diagnosis</u> :** Anti-platelate Antibody

  Bone-marrow → megakaryocytosis – indicate problem with platelate destruction, **not** with production

- **<u>Thrombotic Thrombocytopenic Purpura (TTP)</u>** – deficiency in vWF cleaving metalloprotease in endothelial cells leads to ↑↑vWF → more platelets attach to vWF leads to thrombosis and thrombocytopenia (due to platelet consumption in thrombosis) – microangiopathic anemia, Renal & **CNS involvement** – **schistocytes** (fragmented RBCs), Helmet-shaped cells

- **Hemolytic Uremic Syndrome (HUS)** – microangiopathic anemia, thrombocytopenia and renal involvement [**no** CNS involvement]

- Schistocytes – TTP, DIC, Aortic stenosis

- **Von Willebran Disease (VWD):** Autosomal – Dominant
- Sign of bleeding from superficial areas of body
- **Low** level of $_v$WF , factor VIII : C
- **Ristocetin Platelate Aggregation Test** : Abnormal
- **Elevated** PTT, Normal PT

- **Hemophilia:** Autosomal – recessive
- Hemophilia A – factor 8 deficiency, Hemophilia B – factor 9 deficiency
- Sign of deep bleeding → hemarthrosis, hematoma, GI bleeding
- may become apparent at the time of circumcision
- **Diagnosis** : **elevated** PTT , Normal PT
- **"Mixing Study"** : 50 % Patient's blood + 50 % Normal blood → PTT corrected → Hemophilic → If PTT is <u>not</u> corrected → Antibody inhibition of the factor
- **Treatment** : **Desmopressin,** Specific factor replacement

- **Vit–K Deficiency:** ↓ Production of **Factor 2, 7, 9, 10**
- Both **PT** & **PTT** are **elevated**
- **Diagnosis** : correction of **PT & PTT** after giving Vit-K
- **Treatment** : **Fresh Frozen Plasma** in severe bleeding

- **Liver Disease :** ↓ Production of All factors <u>except</u> $_v$WF & **Factor 8**
- **Both PT & PTT** are elevated
- **Diagnosis** : H/O liver disease & **No** correction of PT & PTT after giving Vit-K

- **DIC (Disseminated Intravascular Coagulation):**
- Platelates, ↑↑ PT & PTT, ↑ **D- dimmers** & FDP$_S$, Low fibrinogen level **schiztocytes** on peripheral blood smear
- **Treatment:** Fresh Frozen Plasma, Platelate transfusion

Joint aspiration

Cell count	Gram stain		Microscopic Polarization
▪ < 2,000 – OA, Traumatic	(+) organism	(-) organism	Needle-shaped / (-) birefringent – Monosodium Urate (**Gout**)
▪ Up to 50,000 – Inflammatory (RA, Gout, Pseudogout) ▪ >75,000 (**without crystal**) – Septic	Staph Aureus	N. Gonorrhea	Rhomboid / (+) birefringent – Calcium Pyrophosphate (**Pseudogout**)

- **Rheumatoid Arthritis (RA)**
- **Poly**articular Symmetric
- Inflammatory synovitis
- **bone erosions**
- MCP & PIP involvement
- Swan-neck deformity
- Boutonniere deformity
- radial deviation of the wrist with ulnar deviation of the digits

- **Osteo Arthritis (OA)**
- **Mono**articular Asymmetric
- Non-inflammatory
- Non-erossive
- PIP& DIP involvement
- Osteophytes & unequal joint space
- Bouchard's node (PIP)
- Heberden's node (DIP)

- ■ **Ankylosing Spondylitis:** Positive HLA B-27, M>W, 2nd - 3rd decade
  - chronic lower bake pain, morning stiffness >1 hrs improve with exercise
  - **Anterior uveitis**, Aortic insufficiency, 3rd degree heart block
  - X-ray → **sacroilitis** and eventual fusing of the sacroiliac joint, bamboo spine

- ■ **Reactive Arthritis:** infectious diarrhea (C.Jejunii) + Arthritis
  - Urethritis (Chlamydia) / conjunctivitis + Arthritis → **Reiter Syndrome**

- • **Psoriatic Arthritis:** DIP joint + **pitting of nail** + skin lesions

- • **Enteropathic Arthritis** (Ulcerative colitis/ Crohn's disease):
  - Inflammatory Bowel disease + Arthritis + Pyoderma gangrenosum + erythema nodosum

- • **Gout:** deposit of uric acid crystals in joints – most common site **first toe** (podagra) – precipitating factors are alcohol, steroid withdrawal, diuretics, Pyrazinamide, Ethambutol, following anti-cancer treatment

- **Pseudo Gout:** deposit of calcium pyrophosphate in joints – most common site knee joints – pre-existing joint damage is a precipitating factor – <u>causes:</u> Hyperparathyroidism, Hemochromatosis, Hypophosphatemia, Hypomagnesemia

- **Septic arthritis:** <u>Gonococcal:</u> migratory polyarthropathy, **Tenosynovitis** (inflammation of tendon sheath) <u>Staphylococci:</u> pre-existing joint damage (eg. RA patient)

- ■ **SLE:** anti-nuclear Ab, Anti-smith & Anti-ds-DNA Ab (most **specific**)
- **non-erosive arthritis**, **malar rash**, photosensitivity, **Renal**, CVS (Libman-Sack endocarditis – sterile vegetation on MV), CNS involvement (psychosis)
- Anti-phospholipids antibody – anticoagulant, recurrent abortion
- Anti-cardiolipin antibody – give false VDRL & RPR test

- ■ **Scleroderma:** excessive collagen deposition – Raynaud's phenomenon (blue discoloration of fingers on exposure to cold), skin thickening, dysphagia – **Anti-scl-70 Ab**

- ■ **CREST Syndrome:** Anti-centromere antibody
- **C**alcinosis, **R**aynaud's phenomena, **E**sophagus (dysphagia), **S**cleroductly (claw-like finger), **T**elangiectasia (dilated blood vessels)

- ■ **Sjogren syndrome:** anti-Ro (SS-A) & Anti-La (SS-B) Antibodies, **Dry eye** (constant sensation of foreign body in eye), dental caries, **parotid enlargement (lymphatic infiltration of glands** – lip biopsy - most **specific**) – also gives positive RA factor

- **Juvenile Rheumatoid Arthritis : salmon pink evascent rash**

- **Osteochondroma** → most common benign tumor → Metaphysis

- **Osteoma** → Facial bones → associated with Gardner's Polyposis Syndrome

- **Giant cell tumor** → Epiphysis → Females

- **Osteogenic Sarcoma** → Metaphysis of distal femur , Proximal tibia "sunburst" appearance on X-ray → Male (10-25 yrs) → Familial retinoblastoma

- **Ewing's Sarcoma** → Diaphysis & metaphysis of proximal femur, ribs, pelvic bones → "onion skin" appearance on X-ray

- **Erb's Palsy – <u>upper trunk</u>** (C_5, C_6) → Axillary N. & Musculocutaneous N. → muscles of shoulder & arm → <u>Arm:</u> medially rotated & adducted → <u>Forearm:</u> extended & pronated ("waiter's tip")

- **Klumpke's Palsy – <u>lower trunk</u>** (C_8, T_{11}) → loss of muscles of **Hand**

Nephrology

- Pre-renal Azotemia - ↑ BUN but creatinine near normal (N) (0.6 – 1.2)
- Post-renal Azotemia - ↑ BUN & ↑ creatinine
- Renal Azotemia – BUN/Cr ≤ 15 (bcoz more ↑↑ in creatinine)
- **Cortical necrosis** of both kidney sparing medulla – **DIC**
- **Sickle cell** anemia – affect **medulla** most severly – can cause Papillary necrosis
- Renal papillary necrosis (SADD) – **S**ickle cell anemia, **A**cute pyelonephritis, **D**rugs (Aspirin + acetaminophen), **D**iabetes

* **Nephritic type Glomerular Disease :** (moderate proteinuria & **RBC cast**)

- **IgA glomerulonephritis (Berger's** disease) (**Buerger's** disease – thromboangitis obliterans – male – smoking cigarettes) (both are different disease) – episodic bouts of **hematuria 1-3 days following URTI**, slow progression to CRF (40-50%), **mesangeal IgA deposit** with granular immunoflurocence
- **Post-streptococcal** – Hematuria **1-3 weeks** following group A Strep Pyogens infection
  - Skin infection - ↑ anti-DNAase B titer
  - Pharynx infection - ↑ ASO titer
  - **Diffuse proliferative** (usually resolve, CRF is uncommon)
- Diffuse Proliferative (SLE) – sub**endo**thelial Immune Complex (IC) (anti-ds DNA Ab) deposit with granular IF, "wire looping" of capillaries (CRF most common cause of death in SLE)
- Rapidly Progressive – **crescent formation,** associated with **Goodpasture** syndrome (**linear IF**) (**Lower** Resp Tract involvement, Hemoptysis followed by ARF), **Polyarteritis nodosa** (p-ANCA) (**GIT** involvement – mesenteric artery, bowel ischemia, bloody diarrhea), **Wegner's granulomatosis** (c-ANCA) (**Upper & Lower Resp Tract** involvement, perforation of nasal septum)

* **Nephrotic type Glomerular Disease:** (**proteinuria** › 3.5 g/24 hrs & **fatty cast**)

- **Minimal change disease – children** – EM show fusion of podocytes (**selective proteinuria** – Albumin **not** globulin), negative IF
- Focal Segmental – HIV, **Heroin IV abuse**, **NSAID**, Hodgkin's lymphoma – negative IF, **non-selective proteinuria**
- **Diffuse Membranous – Adults** – captopril, **HBV**, malaria, syphilis – sub**epi**thelial deposit with granular IF – "spike and dome" pattern
- Type-1 MPGN – **HCV**, HBV, cryoglobulinemia – sub**epi**thelial deposit – EM show "tram track" (progress to CRF)
- Type-2 MPGN – C3 nephritic factor (C3NeF), Ab binds to C3 convertase & prevent its degradation & sustain activation of C3 leads to very low C3 level. "dense deposit disease" (progress to CRF)
- Only in **SLE**, there is **subendothelial** deposit. In all others, there is subepithelial deposit

- Only in **Goodpasture syndrome**, there is **linear** deposit. In all others, there is granular deposit.
- Polyarteritis nodosa – p-ANCA – HbsAg (+) in 30% of cases
- Lichen planus – association with Hep. C
- Glomerular basement membrane (GBM) – type-IV collagen – heparan sulfate (negative charge to GBM) – positive charge LMW proteins are permeable – albumin has strong negative charge so it is not permeable [loss of negative charge → loss of albumin in urine]
- **Glomerular nodule** – DM / Amyloid (chronic disease) both show red on H&E stain but with Congo red stain – Amyloid – "apple-green" birefringence nodule. DM nodule is composed of Type-4 collagen & protein

- **Ethylene glycol poisoning** – Metabolic acidosis (↑ anion gap) + **oxalate crystalluria**
- **Cystinuria** – **staghorn calculi**, positive nitropruside cyanide test
- **Staghorn calculi** – Proteus infection

* Acid-Base Disturbances

- (Na + K) – (HCO3 + Cl) = 8-14 (normal anion gap)
- Only chronic acidosis/alkalosis is compensated **not** acute
- Chronic Resp. Acidosis – compensated by Metabolic Alkalosis (HCO3 – 22-28)

PCo2 - > 45 mmHg, HCO3 - ≤ 30 mEq/L – Acute Resp. Acidosis

HCO3 - > 30 mEq/L – Chronic Resp. Acidosis

- Chronic Resp. Alkalosis – compensated by Metabolic Acidosis

PCo2 - < 33 mmHg, HCO3 - ≥ 18 mEq/L – Acute Resp. Alkalosis

HCO3 - < 18 mEq/L (but >12 mEq/L) – Chronic Resp. Alkalosis

* **Renal Tubular Acidosis (Normal Anion gap Acidosis)**

- Type-1 – secondary to autoimmune diseases, Lithium, analgesics, sickle cell disease
  Inability to secrete H+ in Urine, Urine pH - > 5.4
  Patient usually gets **Renal stone**
  Acid load Test – After giving ammonium chloride, urine pH still remain elevated (normally it should be decreased)

- Type-2 – Renal threshold for absorbing HCO3 is lowered from normal of 24 mEq/L to 15 mEq/L
  Initially pH > 5.5 and then it goes back to < 5.5
  Patient usually get bone lesion (osteomalacia, rickets)

Both Type-1 & Type-2 get Hypokalamia.
- Type-4 is the only renal tubular acidosis which produce **hyperkalamia** due to destruction of JG apparatus - ↓ rennin - ↓ aldosterone
  Causes – hyaline arteriosclerosis in afferent arteriole in DM, Legionaire's disease

- Intake of salt = output of salt (95% renal & 5% sweat)
- **Hyponatremia** – Na < 135 **in the absence of hyperglycemia**
- SIADH – Oral hypoglycemic & Carbamazapine
- <u>Diagnosis</u> – Urine osm > Serum osm (Urine osm > 40 is typical)
- <u>Treatment</u> – fluid restriction, loop diuretics & normal saline, hypertonic saline, Lithium/Demeclocycline in SIADH. Rapid correction of hyponatremia results in **Central Pontine Myelinosis** – destruction of brain stem present with paraparesis, dysarthria or Dysphagia.

- **Hypernatremia** – loss of hypotonic fluids (sweating, burns, fever), central DI & Nephrogenic DI

- **Hypokalamia** – "U" wave on ECG, Alkalosis, ↑ Aldosterone

- **Hyperkalemia** – peaked T wave on ECG, Acidosis, ↓ Aldosterone

- **Hypercalcemia – Loop diuretics / Hypercalciuria – Thiazide diuretics**

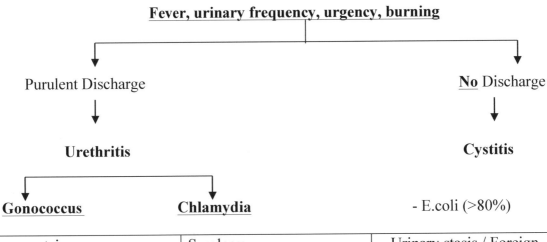

Fever, urinary frequency, urgency, burning

Purulent Discharge → **Urethritis** → **Gonococcus** / **Chlamydia**

No Discharge → **Cystitis** - E.coli (>80%)

gram stain	Serology	Urinary stasis / Foreign body Predisposes to infection
Culture	Ligase chain reaction	**Suprapubic tenderness**
Purulent discharge	**Mucopurulent** discharge	Urine Analysis - WBCs
		Nitrates → Nitrites [gram(-) organism]
		Urine culture (> **100000 colonies**)

* **Pheochromocytoma**
  - a neuroendocrine tumor of the medulla of the adrenal glands
  - Signs & Symptoms of sympathetic hyperactivity (increase HR, HTN, etc)

- Diagnosis: urinary vanillylmandelic acid (VMA)
- CT scan/MRI – to localize tumor
- Treatment – Alfa-blockade followed by surgical removal

* Important Urinary Cast
- Waxy, broad cast – signs of End Stage Renal Disease
- WBC cast – Acute pyelonephritis, acute tubulointerstitial nephritis (drug)
- Renal tubular cell cast (muddy brown granular cast) - ATN

* Juvenile Polycystic Kidney Disease
- Autosomal recessive
- Bilateral enlarged kidney **at birth**
- Maternal oligohydramnios

* Adult Polycystic Kidney Disease
- Autosomal dominant
- Bilateral enlarged kidney around 20-25 yrs of age
- Cyst also present in liver (40%)
- Intracranial berry aneurysm (10-30%) (present with subarachnoid hemorrhage), HTN, sigmoid diverticulosis, MVP

* Renal cell CA (clear cell CA, hypernephroma, Grawitz tumor)
- Derived from proximal tubule (PT)
- Risk factors – smoking, Von Hipple-Lindau syndrome, Adult polycystic kidney disease (APKD)
- Hematuria, flank mass & CVA tenderness
- Metastasize to lung [cannonball appearance on x-ray], Lt sided varicocele

* Wilms Tumor:
- Derived from mesonephric mesoderm (**unilateral flank mass**)
- **Histology:** abortive glomeruli, & tubules, primitive blastemal cells, rhabdomyoblasts
- **Hypertension in child**, Autosomal Dominant (chromosome-11)
- WAGR Syndrome (Wilms tumor, Aniridia, Genital abnormalities, Retardation)

* Neuroblastoma:
- N-myc gene amplification.
- Small blue cell tumors (Ewing sarcoma, Lymphoma, Neuroblastoma, small cell CA of Lung).
- Composed of malignant neuroblast, presence of Homer-Wright rosettes.
- Neurosecretory granules on electron microscopy.
- Hypertension in child.
- ↑↑↑ Urinary VMA (vanillylmandelic acid), HVA, metanephrines.

- **Potter's syndrome** – absent of both kidney – oligohydroamnios – **failure of ureteric buds to develop**

- **Pathogenesis of DM: Nonenzymatic glycosylation** (glucose + AA) → ↑vessel permeability to protein and ↑athrogenesis; **Osmotic damage** → Aldolase reductase (glucose → sorbitol) → sorbitol draws water into tissues causing damage (eg. retinopathy); Diabetic microangiopathy → ↑synthesis of type-IV collagen in basement membrane & mesangium

- **Alport syndrome:**
  - X - linked dominant disorder
  - Asymptomatic hematuria , Sensorineural hearing loss
  - **Renal biopsy:** Glomerular Sclerosis , thickened basement membrane tubular atrophy fibrosis and foam cells.

- **Hemolytic Uremic Syndrome (HUS):**
  - E.Coli (0157 : HS) → produce **Vero toxin** → endothelial cell injury
  - **Endothelial injury of the kidney** results in localized clotting → RBCs and intra- renal platelate damage causes **microangiopathic anemia** and **thrombocytopenia**
  - Approximately 1 week after E.Coli (0157 : H7) infection , patient develop oliguria, sign & symptoms of anemia
  - ↓ Hb level m drop in platelate count, Hematuria , proteinuria , Helmet cells on peripheral smear
  - **D/D:** TTP which involves CNS whereas HUS involves kidney.

- **Henoch – Schonlein Purpura:**
  - IgA – mediated vasculitis of small vessels
  - Non-thrombocytopenic purpura in children
  - Usually follows an URI.
  - Tetrad of **Abd. Pain, Rash, Renal involvement & Thrombocytopenia.**
  - **Palpable purpuric rash on buttocks**

NEUROLOGY

- **CSF:** Lat ventricle → foramen of Monro → 3rd ventricle → Aqueduct of Sylvius → 4th ventricle [**obstruction** to CSF flow will give **hydrocephalus**]
- Arnold-Chiari malformation – herniation of cerebellum – hydrocephalus
- Arnold-Chiari malformation type 2 – syringomyelia, myelomeningocele
- **Syringomyelia** is associated with **Arnold-Chiari** malformation in most cases.

- **Meningitis:** infection of covering of brain – fever, headache, stiff neck and **focal neurologic deficiet**
- **Causes:**
  - New born (**< 1 month**) →Group B Streptococci, E.coli, L. monocytogen
  - **1 month – 18 yrs** Old →   N.meningitides
  - **>18 yrs Old** → Strep Pneumoniae
  - Staph Aureus → recent neurosurgery
  - **L.monocytogens** → Immunocompromised (**Neonates & elderly Patients**)
  - Cryptococcus → HIV positive, CD_4^+ < 100 cells
  - **RMSF** → <u>rash</u> on wrist, ankle → <u>spread towards body</u>
  - Neisseria → <u>Petechial rash</u>
  - Cause of **viral meningitis** in pediatric population in US – Arbovirus and Enterovirus
  - **CN – 8 deficits** is more common long-term neurological deficit

- <u>CSF findings of Bacterial Meningitis</u> – **low glucose** (<40 mg/dl), **increase** WBC count [**Neutrophils**]
- <u>CSF findings of Viral Meningitis</u> – **increase** WBC (**lymphocytes**), **normal glucose**
- <u>CSF findings of Cryptococcal Meningitis</u> – **low** WBC count (**<50 cells/L**) (Lymphocytes) , **low glucose**

- **Encephalitis:** infection of parenchyma of brain – fever, headache, stiff neck and **altered mental status**
- **Causes:**
  - HSV (temporal lobe) (most common)

- * **Brain Abscess:**
- Headache, fever, **focal neurologic deficit**
- HIV positive → Toxoplasmosis / Lymphoma (90% of cases)
- * **Transverse Myelitis** – rapidly progressing lower extremity weakness following URI, accompanied by sensory loss and urinary retention – Dx: MRI
- * **Epidural abscess** – patient with h/o **IV drug abuse**

- **Subfalcine herniation:** cingulate gyrus herniates under falx cerebri [compress anterior cerebral artery]
- **Uncal herniation:** medial portion of temporal lobe herniates through tentorium cerebellli [compress midbrain & posterior cerebral artery]
- **Tonsillar herniation:** cerebellar tonsils herniates through foramen magnum [produce cardiorespiratory arrest]

■ **Guillain – Barre Syndrome:**
- Auto immune destruction of myelin
- **Begins in lower extremities and move upward**
- Patient usually c/o pain / tingling dysesthesia
- Associate with **C.Jejunii**

■ **Myasthenia Gravis:**
- Antibodies produce against Ach receptors
- **C/o diplopia , ptosis** , difficulty swallowing
- **Symptoms are improved with rest**
- Eaton – Lambert myasthenic Syndrome → increasing muscle strength on repetitive contraction. Association with malignancy, especially small cell CA
- Botulism → dilated pupils & EMG shows an incremental increase in muscular fiber contraction (opposite to Myasthenia Gravis)

■ **Huntington Disease:**
- Autosomal Dominant
- Affect Caudate nucleus
- **CAG trinucleotide repeat expansion**
- Chorea & behavioral disturbance
- Onset in 4th or 5th decade

■ **Parkinson Disease:**
- Degeneration of substantia nigra (↓ dopamine)
- Imbalance b/w dopamine (↓↓) and cholinergic (↑↑) transmitters
- Bradykinesia , Cogwheel Rigidity , Resting tremor (pill rolling) , postural instability
- **Shy-Drager Syndrome** – Parkinsonism + orthostatic hypotension

■ **Multiple Sclerosis:**
- Focal areas of demyelination
- Optic neuritis, scanning speech, intention tremor, nystagmus
- Bilateral internuclear ophthalmoplegia [demyelination of MLF] [pathognomic]
- **Blurry vision and double vision** → common initial manifestations of the disease → **resolve spontaneously**
- CSF show **oligoclonal bands** (70 –90 %)

■ **Marcus-Gunn phenomenon** – dilatation of Rt. Pupil with dilatation of Lt. Pupil occur (**Paradoxical dilatation**) in patient with Rt. Optic neuritis/ Rt. retinal detachment

■ **Alzheimer Disease:** defect in degradation of β-Amyloid protein by secretase leads to accumulation of Amyloid protein in neuron and damage neurons – mutation in Tau protein (maintain microtubule in neuron) leads to formation of neurofibrillary tangles – Microscopic [**senile plaques** (Amyloid protein) and **neurofibrillary tangles**] – Problem in memory [affect hippocampus (old brain) short term memory loss] & visuospatial abilities (early); Hallucination & Personality change (late)

- **Pick Disease:** frontotemporal dementia → Pick body (Intracytoplasmic spherules composed of paired helical filaments) → Present with **Personality change**
- **Lewy body dementia:** Lewy body (Intracytoplasmic spherules that stain brightly eosinophilic) → **fluctuating cognitive impairment** which can be confused with delirium
- **Creutzfeldt Jacob Disease (CJD):** Shorter & more **aggressive** course, present with dementia & **myoclonus**
- **Vascular Dementia:** h/o multiple strokes – multi-infarct dementia
- **Binswanger Disease:** involve subcortical white matter, slow course
- **Normal pressure hydrocephalus:** dementia, gait abnormality and Urinary incontinence

- **Krabbe's Disease:** presence of "globoid" cells (multinucleated histiocytic cells) in degenerating white matter in brain – galactocerebrosidase deficiency

- **Subacute Combined Degeneration:** Vit – B_{12} deficiency
- deficit of vibration & proprioception with Pyramidal signs like plantar extension & hyperreflexia

- **Ant. Spinal artery Infarct:**
- Acute onset of flaccid paralysis that evolves into a spastic paresis over days to weeks
- Loss of pain & temp. Sensation with Sparing of vibration and position sense.

- **Tabes Dorsalis: dorsal** column of spinal cord – **tertiary syphilis**

- **Tuberous Sclerosis:**
- Infantile spasm (**Tx :** ACTH & Prednisone)
- **Rhabdomyoma of Heart** (echocardiography)
- Ash leaf spots (Hyperpigmented lesions), shagreen patches ("orange-peel" lesions), sebaceous adenomas.
- **Angiofibroma on the face**
- **Angiolipomas in the kidney**
- Astrocyte proliferations in subependyma (Look like "candlestick drippings" in the ventricles)

- **Neurofibromatosis (NF):**
- Café au lait spots (tan/light brown flat lesion), Axillary freckling, Lisch nodules, optic nerve gliomas, Acoustic Neuroma (CN-8)(feature of NF-2)(all other NF-1).
- Association with **Pheochromocytoma, Wilms tumor**

- **Duchenne Muscular Dystrophy:**
- **Pseudohypertrophy of the calves**.
- Gower Sign (child places hands on the knees for help in standing).
- Deficiency of dystrophin.

- **Becker Muscular Dystrophy:**
- Defective dystrophin
- Less serious than Duchenne muscular dystrophy

- **Warding – Hoffman Disease:**
- Infantile spinal muscular atrophy.
- Atrophy of anterior horn cells in the spinal cord and of motor nuclei in the brainstem.
- Severe hypotonia and absent tendon reflexes.
- Legs tend to lie in a **Frog leg position**.

- **Charcot-Marie Tooth:**
- Hereditary motor–sensory neuropathy.
- **Peroneal muscular atrophy**.
- Peroneal & Tibial nerve most commonly affected.
- Wasting of the lower legs giving them stork like appearance.
- Sural nerve biopsy → "onion bulb" formation (interstitial hypertrophic neuropathy)

- **Friedreich Ataxia:**
- Expanded GAA triplet repeats
- Ataxia (before 10 yrs of age), disarthric speech, nystagmus, absent tendon reflexes (Lower extremities affected more than upper)

- **Ataxia Telangiectasia:**
- Mutation in DNA repair enzyme, thymic hypoplasia
- Cerebellar ataxia, Telangiectasia of skin & eye

- **CNS tumors:** Adult (above tentorium cerebelli) Children (below tentorium cerebelli) Most common [Adult – glioblastoma multiforme, meningioma; Children – Astrocytoma, Medulloblastoma]

  * **Oligodendroglioma** – "fried egg cell" round nuclei & clear cell – cerebral hemisphere
  * **Choroid plexus papilloma** – papillary growth in ventricle
  * **Ependymoma** – pseudorosettes & structure resembling ependymal canal
  * **Glioblastoma multiforme** – hemorrhagic tumor (multiple area of necrosis & cystic degeneration)
  * **Pilocytic Astrocytoma** – bipolar cells – cerebellum of young children
  * **Medulloblastoma** – most common in **children** – **only** CNS tumor with **both** neural & glial components – affect granular cell layer of cerebellum
  * **Meningioma** – associated with neurofibromatosis – parasagital location
  * **Craniopharyngioma** → remnant of Rathke's pouch **(Resembles to Amblioblastoma)** → calcified lesion above the sella on X-ray → bitemporal hemianopsia

- **CNS bleeds**:

  * **Epidural:** skull fracture – rupture **middle meningeal** artery
  * **Subdural: tear of bridging veins** – fluctuating levels of consciousness
  * **Atherosclerotic stroke:** usually pale infarct (since no reperfusion)
  * **Embolic stroke:** hemorrhagic infarct extends to surface of the brain

* **Intracerebral bleed:** <u>hypertension</u> most common cause – rupture of lenticulostriate Charcot-Bouchard aneurysms – **hematoma** (not an infarct) – **globus pallidus/putamen area most common sites**

* **Subarachnoid bleed: ruptured congenital berry aneurysm** [junction of communicating branch with anterior cerebral artery] – **severe occipital headache** – common in **patient with polycystic kidney disease**

PULMONOLOGY

Obstructive Pulmonary Disease	Restrictive Pulmonary Disease
• ↑ airway resistance	• ↑ in lung recoil
• ↓ expiratory flow rate	• ↓ in all lung volume
• ↑ TLC , ↓ FEV_1 / FVC	• ↑ or N FEV_1/ FVC

- A – a gradient = $150 – 1.25 \times PCO_2 – PaO_2$
- Normal → 5 –15 mmHg

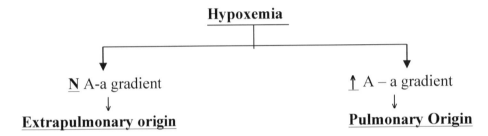

- PAO_2 = % O_2 (713) – arterial PCO_2 / 0.8

- PAO_2 = 0.21 (713) – 40 / 0.8 = 100 mmHg
- PaO_2 = 95 mmHg
- A-a gradient = 5 mmHg

- **Atelectasis** – most common cause of fever in 1st 24-hrs post operatively

- Bacterial Pneumonia → Consolidation → **dull** to percussion, ↑ **vocal framitus**
- Pneumothorax →**Hyperresonant** to percussion, ↓ Breath sound
- Pleural Effusion → dull to percussion, ↓ Breath sound, ↓ vocal framitus
- Atelectasis → dull to percussion, **Absent** Breath sound, **loss of framitus**

- **Deviation of Trachea**
  - **Pneumothorax** - opposite side
  - **Atelectasis** (upper lobe) same side

- Atelectasis (lower lobe) → elevation of diaphragm (same side)

- Trachea → Rt & Lt main bronchus → terminal bronchioles → respiratory bronchioles → alveolar duct (AD) → alveoli

- ■ **Asthma: Reversible** airway obstruction

- ■ **COPD(Emphysema & chronic Bronchitis):**
- ▪ **Non-reversible** airway obstruction

- **Emphysema:** cigarette smoking & alpha$_1$-anti-trypsin deficiency (AAT) - ↑compliance (more dilated alveoli) and ↓elasticity (failure to keep airway lumen open – essential for expiration so air trapped during expiration) – **Centriacinar** [distended respiratory bronchioles – air trapped in AD & alveoli] **Panacinar** [distended whole respiratory unit (Resp bronchioles, AD & alveoli) – air trapped in whole unit]
- **Chronic Bronchitis:** productive cough for at least 3 months for 2 consecutive years – smoking cigarette & cystic fibrosis - ↑mucus in bronchi obstruct terminal bronchioles & narrowing of lumen due to chronic inflammation and fibrosis

- **Lung Abscess**: Alcoholic, **Extremely bad odor (like decomposing dead animal)**

- **Pneumonia:**
- Following flu → Stap. Aureus (abscess)
- HIV positive (CD4+ < 200 cells) → PCP
- **C**alifornia , desert of Arizona → **C**occidiomycosis
- Young (school children) → Mycoplasma
- Alcoholics → Klebsiella
- Smoker, COPD → H. influenzae
- Elderly pt., CXR – lobar consolidation → Strep Pneumoniae
- Neutropenia , Steroid use , cavitatory lesion → Aspergillus
- Exposure to animal at the time of giving birth → Coxiella Burnetti (Q-fever)
- Birds → Chlamydia psittaci
- Elderly, smoker, Air–conditioning → Legionella

- **TB:** Alveolar macrophage → CD4$^+$ T-cells → Macrophage release IL-12 (stimulates T$_H$1 cells) and IL-1 (fever; activate T$_H$1 cells) → T$_H$1 release IL-2 (self stimulation of T$_H$1) and $_\gamma$ interferon (activate macrophage to kill tubercular bacilli) → Inflammatory mediators release from macrophage are responsible for tissue damage (**no** endotoxin or exotoxin) → Lipid from tubercular bacilli leads to caseous necrosis

- **Bronchiactasis:**
- Permanent dilation of bronchi & bronchioles.
- Chronic infection [gram(-) organisms] [destruction of cartilage & elastic tissues]
- Persistent cough with purulent **copious** sputum production, wheezes, crackles

- **Idiopathic pulmonary Fibrosis:**
- Involve only lung **except** clubbing
- Unknown etiology, occur in 5th decade
- CXR – Reticular / Reticulonodular disease
- Chest CT – ground glass appearance
- PFT- restrictive pattern

- **Sarcoidosis:**
- 20 – 40 yrs. Old women
- Presence of nonspecific **non-caseating granuloma** in the lung and other organs

- CXR – __bilateral hilar adenopathy__
- Hypercalcemia ($\uparrow$ 1-α-hydroxylase by macrophage leads to $\uparrow$ Vit–D)
- $\uparrow$ ACE (60 % of patients)
- Ophthalmoscopic examination (**uveitis** & conjunctivitis - >25% of the cases)

■ __Pneumoconiosis:__
- CXR – small irregular opacities, interstitial densities, ground glass appearance, honey combing
- **Asbestosis** → H/O exposure, usually involve lower lung fields
- **CXR** – diffuse /local pleural thickening, pleural plaques, calcification at the level of diaphragm
- Lung biopsy – barbell shaped asbestos fiber (Best diagnostic test)
- $\uparrow\uparrow\uparrow$ Risk of **Bronchogenic CA**
- $\uparrow$ Risk of pleural / peritoneal mesothelioma

■ __Coal miner's / coal worker's pneumoconiosis (CWP):__
- Usually involve upper half of lung
- Increase Levels of IgA, IgG, C3 , anti-nuclear Ab, RF
- **Caplan syndrome** – Rheumatoid nodule in the periphery of the lung in a patient with RA & CWP

■ **Silicosis** ⟶ Hyaline nodule, usually involve upper lobe
- Strong association with TB, Pt should go yearly PD & if PPD >10mm then INH for 9 months

■ **Pulmonary Thromboembolism**:
• **Sudden onset** of **dyspnea** along with **tachycardia**
• ECG ⟶ Right Axis Deviation
• H/O long term immobility

■ **Adult Respiratory Distress Syndrome (ARDS):**
- $\uparrow$Permeability of the alveolar – capillary membrane & Pul.edema
- Alveolar macrophage → cytokines → Neutrophil → damage capillary membrane
- CXR – diffuse interstitial infiltrates; whiteout of both lung fields
- Swan-Ganz Catheter – __normal__ cardiac output & capillary wedge pressure
  $\uparrow$ Pulmonary artery pressure

■ **Sleep Apnea**: Daytime Somnolence
- Obstructive sleep Apnea → floppy airway, obese patient
- Central sleep Apnea → inadequate ventilatory drive

■ __Bronchogenic Carcinoma__:
- Squamous cell CA → Centrally located → Hypercalcemia – PTH-like substance
- Small cell CA → Centrally located → SIADH, Eaton-Lambert, Venocaval obstruction Syndrome

- Large Cell CA → Peripherally located
- Adenocarcinoma → peripherally located → Pleural effusion with high hyaluronidase level in effusion fluid. Bronchoalveolar CA is subtype

- **Pancoast tumor** – Hornor's syndrome, Phrenic N involvement [Chest movement asymmetry] [a dangerous sign in patient with Pancoast tumor];

REPRODUCTIVE SYSTEM

- **Cryptorchidism:** undescended testis – usually resolve by 1 year of age – increase risk for seminoma, infertility

- **Vericocele:** "bag of worms" appearance – Lt sided most common – infertility

- **Hypospadias** → urethral opening on ventral side of the penis → **never do circumcision**

- **Epispadias** → urethral opening on dorsal side of the penis

- **Hydrocele** → usually resolve by 1 year of age. If it is not resolved by 1 year of age then surgical intervention

- **Testicular Tumors:** unilateral **painless** testicular mass in **young person**
  - Germ cell (95%) – malignant
  - Sex-cord (5%) – benign
  - Germ cell – Seminoma (40%) and Non-seminoma (60%)
  - Seminoma – metastasis [para-aortic → hematogenous (lung)]

- **BPH (Benign Prostatic Hypertrophy):** DHT (dihydrotestosterone) causes hyperplasia of glandular and stromal cells – develop in central zone so do not palpable by digital rectal examination (DRE) – trouble initiating & stopping urinary stream, dribbling, nocturia, dysuria – **no** relation with prostate CA

- **Prostate CA:** DHT dependent – develop in peripheral zone so palpable by DRE – usually asymptomatic until advanced – PSA >10 ng/ml highly predictive – bone metastasis (common) [it is the only tumor which has osteo**blastic** activity where as other tumor has osteo**clastic** (ostolytic) activity when metastasize to bone]

- **Testicular Torsion:** severe testicular pain of sudden onset **without** fever, pyuria (**or**) h/o recent mumps → swollen, extremely tender **high riding horizontally lie testis**

- **Acute epididymitis:** severe testicular pain of sudden onset **with** fever, pyuria → swollen, extremely tender testis in **normal lie**

- **Penile CA in situ** – **Bowen's disease** – **one lesion** (thicken whitish plaque with a slight ulcerated surface) – **risk for SCC** (squamous cell CA)
  - **Bowenoid Paulosis** – **multiple** reddish brown popular lesion – **No** risk for SCC
  - **Erythroplasia of Queyart** – **multiple shiny** red plaques – **risk for SCC**

- **Endometrial CA:**
  - Prolong Estrogen (E) exposure **without** Progesterone (P)
  - Post-menopausal bleeding (**most common presentation**)

- **Leiomyomas:**
  - most common benign uterine tumor
  - Intramural – within the wall of the uterus
  - Submucous – located beneath the Endometrium; causes Menorrhagia (heavy bleeding) and Metrorrhagia (irregular bleeding in between menses)
  - Subserosal – located beneath uterine serosa
  - **Asymmetric, Non-tender,** enlarged uterus in the absence of the pregnancy

- **Adenomyosis:**
  - endometrial glands and stoma located **within** the myometrium of the uterine wall (uterus)
  - Pain immediately before and during menses
  - **Symmetric, tender,** enlarged uterus in the absence of the pregnancy

- **Endometriosis:**
  - endometrial glands and stoma located **outside** the uterus
  - Chocolate cyst of the ovary, utero-sacral ligament nodularity, pain during intercourse (dyspareunia), infertility

- **Vulvar neoplasm:**
  - c/o intense vulvar pruritus
  - Melanoma – black lesions
  - Paget's disease – red lesions
  - Squamous cell CA – HPV association – whitish lesions

  - **Paget's disease** (of breast, cervix) – **Adenocarcinoma**

  - Most common benign ovarian tumor – serous cystadenoma
  - Most common malignant ovarian tumor – serous cystadenocarcinoma
  - Granulosa-theca cell tumors – secrete estrogen
  - Sertoli-Leyding cell tumors – secrete testosterone
  - Krukenberg's tumor – contains signet ring cells from Metastatic stomach cancer
  - Dysgerminoma – resembles Seminoma of the testis
  - Meig's Syndrome – Ovarian fibroma, Ascites & right sided pleural effusion
  - Mucinous Cystadenoma – pseudomyxoma peritonei (rare complication)

- **Gestational Trophoblastic Neoplasia (GTN):**
  - **HTN in the first trimester,** fundus larger than dates, "snowstorm" appearance on US, **grape-like vesicles, high beta-hCG,** hyperthyroidism
  - **Complete Mole:** empty egg, 46XX (parental), **No** fetus, **progression to malignancy** (20%)
  - **Incomplete Mole:** 69(XXX), fetal parts present, progression to malignancy (10%)

- **Immature teratoma** – primitive epithelial cells & developing skeletal muscles, **potentially malignant** [teratoma – derivatives of all 3 germ layers [ectoderm, mesoderm and endoderm – hair, tooth, thyroid gland, etc]

- **Dermoid cyst:** A dermoid cyst is a **mature cystic teratoma** containing hair and other structures characteristic of normal skin and other tissues derived from the ectoderm. The term is most often applied to teratoma on the skull sutures and in the ovaries of females.

- **Struma ovarii:** mature teratoma that contains mostly thyroid tissue.

- **Dysfunctional Uterine Bleeding: Anovulation** (So **no progesterone** effect which left estrogen unopposed), **no** secretory phase, **no** mid-cycle rise in temperature – **Biopsy: Proliferative Endometrium** with stromal breakdown. **No** secretory endometrium

- **Kallman Syndrome:** anosmia + absent GnRH

- **McCune-Albright Syndrome** – Precocious puberty, irregular shaped pigmented skin macule & **polyostotic fibrous dysplasia** (local bony defect containing unmineralized whorls of connective tissue.)

- **Bacterial Vaginosis:** thin, grayish-white discharge, **fishy odor**, vaginal pH above 5, epithelial cells with smudged borders (**"clue" cells**) due to bacteria adherent to cell membranes – **Tx:** Metronidazole (contraindicated in pregnancy, use Clindamycin during pregnancy)

- **Trichomonas Vaginitis:** frothy, **green discharge**, itchy, burning pain with intercourse, vaginal pH above 5, **sexually transmitted disease** (STD), **"trichomonads"** on microscopic examination – **Tx:** Metronidazole (treat both partners)

- **Yeast Vaginitis:** curdy, white discharge, pH <4.5, not a STD, Pseudohyphae on microscopic examination – **Tx:** single dose Fluconazole

- **Pelvic Inflammatory Disease:**
- Lower Abdominal and pelvic pain, fever, leucocytosis, vaginal discharge, **Cervical motion tenderness**

- **Menstrual Cycle Hormones:**
  - **FSH:** stimulate granulosa cells to secrete E & Inhibin (inhibits FSH release)
  - **Estrogen:** Negative feedbacks to FSH
    Low E – Negative feedbacks to LH
    High E – Positive feedbacks to LH
  - **LH:** stimulate production of androgens from theca cells, LH surge stimulates synthesis of prostaglandins to enhance follicular rupture & ovulation
  - **Progesterone:** secreted by corpus luteum, prepare Endometrium for blastocyst implantation

  - **Identical twins** (monozygotic twins – embryo split during blastomere & blastocyst stage) – monochorionic, monoamniotic & monochorionic, diamniotic

BREAST DISEASES

- **Fibroadenoma** → young woman (child bearing age) → firm, rubbery mass, **moves easily on palpation** (Breast mouse)

- **Cystosarcoma Phyllodes** → young woman → very large mass → benign but has potential to become malignant

- **Fibrocystic Disease** → multiple bilateral **breast cysts "come & go"** at different time in menstrual cycle

- **Intraductal Papilloma** → young woman with **bloody nipple discharge**

- **Breast Abscess** → **lactating mother** → fever, leucocytosis, fluctuating red, hot, tender mass in breast

- **Breast cancer** → mammogram (irregular area of increased density with fine microcalcification) with core biopsy
- **Breast cancer signs & Symptoms** → palpable breast mass, retraction of overlying skin, retraction of nipple, ("orange peel" skin), palpable Axillary nodes.

- **Ductal carcinoma in situ** → cannot metastasize (**No** Axillary sampling)
- Tubular Breast CA → Best prognosis
- Inflammatory Breast CA → worst prognosis
- Infiltrating Ductal CA → most common
- Lobular CA → high incidence of bilateral involvement
- Other types → Medullary, Mucinous

MISCELLANEOUS

- **Edema:** Transudate (↑ Hydrostatic pressure & ↓ Oncotic pressure) Exudates (↑ vascular permeability)

- **Shock:** Low perfusion pressure to tissues – **Hypovolemic** (low circulatory volume); **Cardiogenic** (heart is not pumping well) and **Septic** (vasodilation leads to blood flow too quickly and give less time for tissue to extract oxygen)
- **Cardiogenic shock** – low CO & **High** PCWP
- **ARDS** – **Normal** PCWP   [PCWP = pulmonary capillary wedge pressure]
- **Septic shock** – High CO, Low PCWP & **Normal** mixed venous O2
- **Hypovolemic shock** – **low** CO, **low** PCWP, **low** mixed venous O2

- High PCWP & low CVP – <u>LV dysfunction</u>   [CVP = central vein pressure]
- High PCWP & high CVP – <u>Cardiac temponade</u>
- Respiratory distress & high CVP – <u>Tension Pneumothorax</u>

- **Abdominal Aortic Aneurism** – **Atherosclerosis** – (rupture - left flank pain , hypotension, pulsatile mass) – below renal artery origin is most common site

- **Syphilitic Aneurism** – Aortic arch aneurism, tertiary syphilis, **vasculitis of vasa-vasorum**, **Aortic valve regurgitation**, brassy cough due to stretching of Lt. recurrent laryngeal N by aneurism

- **Aortic dissection** – **cystic medial degeneration** (elastic tissue fragmentation) – **Marfan syndrome & EDS** (Ehler-Donlas Syndrome) – usually occurs with in 10cm of the aortic valve – **cardiac temponade** most common cause of death – **Aortic regurgitation**, widening of aortic valve root on Echo – loss of upper extremity pulse due to compression of subclavian artery

- **Ehler-Danlos Syndrome:** defect in type-I and type-III collagen – poor wound healing, aortic dissection, hyper mobile joints

- **Atherosclerosis** – fibrous cap (pathognomic lesion)
- **Lines of Zahn** – laminated thrombi with alternate pale & red area (Heart & Aorta)

- **Arteriosclerosis** – hardening of arterioles
- **Hyaline arteriosclerosis** – protein deposition in arterial wall – DM (basement membrane leak proteins into vessel wall due to nonenzymatic glycosylation of basement membrane protein); HTN (increase pressure push protein into vessel wall)
- **Hyperplastic arteriosclerosis** – smooth muscle cell hyperplasia – "onion skin" appearance

- **Churg-Strauss syndrome** – Vasculitis + **eosinophilia**
- **Capillary Hemangiomas** in newborn **regress with age**

- **Sturge-Weber syndrome** – Nevus flammeus (**birth mark**) on face in distribution of Ophthalmic branch of CN 5 – Ipsilateral malformation of pia matter vessel overlying occipital & parietal lobes

- **Kawasaki syndrome** – **Child** with cervical lymphadenopathy, fever, desquamating rash on palm, sole & mouth – coronary artery aneurysm/thrombosis

- **Takayasu arteritis** (Pulseless disease) – young **asian** girl – granulomatous vasculitis of aortic arch

- **Temporal arteritis** (Giant cell arteritis) – **focal granulomatous inflammation** – vasculitis of superficial temporal artery and ophthalmic artery

- **Kaposi sarcoma** – HHV-8 – malignant tumor of endothelial cells – raised, red-purple flat lesion to plaque & nodules

- **Bacillary angiomatosis** – benign capillary proliferation involving skin & viscera in AIDS – **simulate Kaposi sarcoma** – Bartonella Henselae (causative agent)

- **Von Hippel Lindau** – Autosomal Dominant – cerebellar hemangioblastomas, Pheochromocytoma, **renal adenocarcinoma** (high incidence)

- **Rhabdomyosarcoma:**
- Tumor of striated muscles.
- Head & Neck and genitourinary tract.
- **Grape-like mass protruding through vagina** (Sarcoma botryoides)

General Pathology

- **Hypoxia:** inadequate oxygenation of tissues
- **Hypoxemia:** ↓ in Pao_2 [which is one of the cause of hypoxia]

Physiology: Pulmonary art (Sao_2 = 75%) → Alveoli (PAo_2 = 100 mmHg, $PAco_2$ = 40 mmHg) → Pulmonary vein → LV → Systemic circulation (Pao_2 = 95 mmHg, Sao_2 = 97%) → RV → Pulmonary art [A = alveoli, a = arteries, P = pressure, S = saturation]

- **Causes of Hypoxemia:** Ventilation defect (100% O_2 doesn't ↑ Pao_2); Perfusion defect (100% O_2 will ↑ Pao_2); Diffusion defect (interstitial fibrosis)
- **Methemoglobinemia** – Hb with Fe^{+3} (MetHb) – not able to bind with O_2 – decreased Sao_2, but normal Pao_2 – causes : patient return from camping who drank mountain water (high amount of nitrites), nitrite- & sulfur containing drugs (Dapsone, nitroglycerine, sulfa drugs) – **Tx**: Methylene blue (activates metHb reductase); Vit-C is useful too.
- **CO poisoning** – automobile exhaust, smoke inhalation – decreased Sao_2, but normal Pao_2 – inhibits cytochrome oxidase – headache(first symptom), cherry red discoloration of skin & blood – **Tx**: 100% O_2
- **CN poisoning** – may result from drug (Sodium Nitroprusside) – inhibits cytochrome oxidase – **Tx**: Amyl nitrite
- **Oxygen dissociation curve** – shift to the right means it is easy for tissue to extract oxygen from blood [2,3-BPG (produced during respiratory alkalosis) shift curve to the right]
- **Tissues susceptible to hypoxia** – watershed areas [area b/w distribution of anterior & middle cerebral arteries, b/w Sup & Inf mesenteric arteries (splenic flexure), subendocardial tissue, straight portion of PT in cortex of kidney, thick ascending limb of loop of Henle in the medulla]
- **First sign (reversible) of tissue hypoxia** – swelling of cell (inactive Na-K ATPase pump)
- **Irreversible sign of tissue hypoxia** – increase cytosolic Ca^{++} (inactive Ca^{++} ATPase pump) – increase Ca^{++} in mitochondria release **Cytochrome c** which activates apoptosis
- **Ubiquitin** – markers for intermediate filament degradation [Mallory bodies in hepatocytes in alcoholic liver disease, Lewy bodies (eosinophilic cytoplasmic inclusions in substantia nigra) in Parkinsonism]
- **Dystrophic calcification**: **normal serum calcium/phosphate** but deposit of calcium into **damaged tissue** – atherosclerotic plaques, enzymatic fat necrosis, periventricular calcification in CMV
- **Metastatic calcification**: **increased serum calcium and/or phosphate** with deposition of calcium in **normal tissue** – nephrocalcinosis in primary hyperparathyroidism, calcification of basal ganglia in primary hyperparathyroidism (high phosphorous)
- **Atrophy** – decrease size of tissue or organ – atrophy of muscle in cast for long time (due to lack of stimulation)
- **Hypertrophy** – increase in size of tissue or organ – After removing one kidney from body increase in size of other kidney in the body

- **Hyperplasia** – increase in **number** of cells – BPH due to an increase in dihydrotestosteron
- **Metaplasia** – replacement of one cell type by another cell type – goblet cells in stomach
- **Dysplasia** – disordered cell growth – squamous dysplasia of cervix due to HPV infection – increase chance of cancer

- **Types of cell necrosis:**
  - **Coagulation necrosis** – infarction except brain
  - **Liquefactive necrosis** – infections, brain infarct or infection
  - **Caseous necrosis** – TB and systemic fungi
  - **Enzymatic fat necrosis** – acute pancreatitis
  - **Fibrinoid necrosis** – necrosis of immunologic injury (small vessel vasculitis – type-3 HS)
  - **Gummatous** – tertiary syphilis

- **Apoptosis** – programmed cell death – TP53 gene [temporary arrest cell cycle in the G1 phase to repair damage DNA]; BAX gene [TP53 activates BAX gene if DNA damage is so much. BAX & Cytochrome c promote apoptosis]; BCL2 gene [inhibits apoptosis by preventing leaking of Cytochrome c from mitochondria]
- **TP53 & RB suppressor genes** – regulate cell cycle (G1 to S phase) [RB – sequester specific transcription factor needed for cell cycle progression; TP53 – inhibits Cdk4 to arrest cell cycle in G1 phase]
- Cyclin D binds to Cdk4 (cyclin-dependent kinase 4) forming a complex that phosphorylates RB protein causing the cell to enter S-phase from G1 phase.
- Most characteristic features of **Apoptosis** is **peripheral aggregation of chromatin** (castrated patient's prostate cells show apoptosis)
- Free radicals cell injury – damage membrane & DNA
- Reperfusion injury – reperfusion of ischemic tissue produce superoxide free radicals which irreversibly damage previously injured cells
- Intracellular iron produce hydroxyl ions which damage **parenchymal cells** (cirrhosis in hemochromatosis)
- Fatty liver – clear space pushing the nucleus to the periphery (microscopic)

- Histamine – vasodilation of arteriole (responsible for redness & heat)
- Histamine - ↑ permeability of venules (responsible for edema)
- PGE2 (prostaglandin) – sensitize nerve endings causing pain
- Neutrophils – primary leukocyte in acute inflammation
- Monocytes & Lymphocytes – primary leukocyte in chronic inflammation
- Eosinophil – major basic protein
- Neutrophil – lactoferin, myeloperoxidase, NADPH oxidase
- Selectins – responsible for "rolling" of neutrophils
- β_2 integrins – neutrophil adhesion molecule
- **Leukocyte Adhesion Deficiency** – deficiency of selectins or β_2 integrins (CD11a:CD18) – **delayed separation of umbilical cord in newborn**

- Factors activate (↓Neutrophils) and inhibit (↑Neutrophils) adhesion molecule synthesis:
    - **Activate**: C3a, LTB4, endotoxins, IL-1, TNF
    - **Inhibit**: corticosteroids, catecholamine, lithium

- NADPH oxidase produce free radicals of oxygen – Superoxide dismutase converts it in to H_2O_2 (called respiratory burst) – Myeloperoxidase combine it with Cl and form hypochlorus free radicals which kills organisms
- **Chronic Granulomatous Disease** – absent NADPH oxidase – absent respiratory burst [negative NBT (Nitro-blue tetrazolium)]
- **Myeloperoxidase deficiency** – respiratory burst occurs – so able to kill streptococcus species (catalase negative) but not staphylococci (catalase positive)
- **Job's syndrome** – defective Chemotaxis (staph infection) and ↑ IgE (eczema)
- Histiocytes (bone marrow) – Monocytes (in blood)
- Monocytes – Macrophage (at the site of inflammation)
- Epitheloid cells – activated macrophage is called Epitheloid cells
- Giant cells – accumulation of Epitheloid cells
- **Acute Inflammation:** Purulent (infection); Fibrinous (deposition of fibrin rich exudates; eg. Pericarditis); Pseudomembranous (damage of mucosal lining produce a shaggy membrane of necrotic tissue) – IgM predominant immunoglobulin
- **Chronic Inflammation:** destruction of parenchyma (loss of function, repair by fibrosis) – formation of granulation tissue
- **Key elements in wound healing** – granulation tissue [Fibronectin (cell adhesion glycoprotein) is required for granulation tissue. Fibroblast (synthesize collagen); Vascular endothelial growth factor (VEGF) & fibroblast growth factor (FGF) are important for angiogenesis)
- **Laminin** – key adhesion glycoprotein in basement membrane interacts with type-4 collagen
- Type-1 collagen has greatest tensile strength. Collagenases (metalloproteinase – require Zinc as a cofactor) replace type-3 collagen with type-1 to give strength to the repaired tissue to its original strength.
- **Vit-C deficiency** – decreased cross-linking of collagen
- **Copper deficiency** – decrease cross-linking of α-chains in collagen
- **Zinc deficiency** – defect in removal of type-3 collagen in wound remolding
- Keloids – excessive synthesis of type-3 collagen
- Glucocorticods – interfere with collagen formation and decreased tensile strength – prevent scar formation
- Steroid – increase neutrophils and decrease eosinophils & lymphocytes
- Lung – type-2 pneumocytes repair lung injuries
- Brain – Astrocytes & microglial cells repair brain damage
- Schwann cell is a key cell in reinnervation of peripheral nerve transaction
- C-reactive protein – marker of necrosis & disease activity
- ESR – marker of acute & chronic inflammation [increase in Fibrinogen, Anemia – increase ESR]

- **Amyloid** – abnormal folding of protein – structure – beta-plated sheet – apple green birefringence in polarized light – Amyloid light chain (AL) [derived from light chains – eg. Bence Jones protein]; Amyloid Associated (AA) [derived from serum associated amyloid (SAA), an acute phase reactant]; β-Amyloid (Aβ) [derived from amyloid precursor protein (protein product of chromosome 21) responsible for Alzheimer at early age (around 35) in patient with Down syndrome]

- **Decompression sickness (Caisson's Disease)** – rapid ascent of deep sea drivers leads to formation of nitrogen gas bubble which occludes vessels lumen and causes thrombo-embolic events – **Tx**: recompression by forcing nitrogen to solution again by increasing pressure and slow decompression

- **Prader-Willi syndrome** – Microdeletion syndrome with hypogonadism, mental retardation, short stature, and **obesity** (chromosome 15 deletion is of **P**aternal origin)

- **Angelman syndrome** – chromosome 15 deletion is of maternal origin (child **continuously laughing**)

- **Cancers caused by radiation** – Acute Leukemia, Papillary CA of Thyroid
- **Dysgeusia**, perioral rash, anosmia, **poor wound healing** – **Zinc deficiency**

- **Hemartoma** – non-neoplastic overgrowth of tissue – eg. Peutz-Jeghers polyp
- **Choristoma** – non-neoplastic normal tissue in a foreign location – eg. Gastric mucosa in Meckel's diverticulum
- **Desmoplasia** – fibrous tissue formation in the stroma of tumor

■ Important suppressor genes:
- **p53** (most cancers; chromosome 17)
- **APC** (Familial Polyposis; chromosome5)
- **BRCA-1** (Breast/Ovarian cancer, chromosome 17)
- **BRCA-2** (Breast cancer, chromosome 13)
- **NF-1 and -2** (neurofibromatosis)
- **Rb** (Retinoblastoma; chromosome 13)
- **VHL** (regulate nuclear transcription, Von Hippel-Lindau syndrome)

■ Oncogene relationships:
- **ERBB2 [HER]** – codes for receptor synthesis – breast cancer
- **RAS** – codes for Guanosine triphosphate signal transduction (G proteins that transduce signals received from growth factor receptors to the phosphatidyl inositol second messenger system) –30% of all human cancers include cancers of the lung, colon and pancreas as well as leukemia (20-25% of acute myelogenous leukemia)
- **ABL** – produces non-receptor proteins located on the inner cell membrane surface – t9;22 translocation leads to CML
- **C-myc** – is located in the nucleus and produce protein products that activate nuclear transcription – t8;14 translocation leading to Burkitt's lymphoma

- **N-myc** – codes for nuclear transcription – Neuroblastoma
- **RET** – codes for receptor synthesis – MEN IIa and IIb
- **BCL-2** – anti-apoptosis gene – t14;18 translocation leads to anti-apoptosis of B lymphocytes causing follicular B cell lymphoma

- **HPV (type 16 & 18)** – type-16 (E6 gene product inhibits TP53) type-18 (E7 gene product inhibits RB suppressor gene

- **Tumor Markers :**
- **AFP (alpha feto proteins)** – Hepatocellular CA (HCC), yolk sac tumor (endodermal sinus tumor of Ovaries & Testes)
- **Bence Jones Protein** – Multiple Myeloma, Waldenstrom macroglobulinemia
- **CA 15-3** – Breast CA
- **CA 19-9** – Pancreatic CA
- **CA 125** – surface derived ovarian CA
- **CEA** – colorectal & pancreatic CA
- **PSA** – Prostate CA (also increase in BPH)
- **Bombesin** – neuroblastoma, small cell CA, gastric CA, pancreatic CA
- **S-100** – melanoma, neural tumor, astrocytoma

- **Ectopic Hormones & Tumor relationship:**
- **ACTH:** most common ectopic secretion – secreted in Small cell CA of Lung and Medullary CA of thyroid – produce Cushing Syndrome
- **ADH:** secreted in Small cell CA of lung – produce SIADH
- **β–hcg:** secreted in Trophoblastic tumors and germ cell tumors – produce Gynacomastia and hyperthyroidism (similar to TSH)
- **Erythropoietin:** secreted in Renal cell CA and HCC (hepatocellular CA) – produce secondary polycythemia
- **Insulin-like peptide:** secreted in HCC – produce hypoglycemia
- **Calcitonin:** secreted in Medullary CA of thyroid – produce hypocalcemia
- **PTH-like peptide:** secreted in Small cell CA of Lung, Renal cell CA, Breast CA, Ovarian CA – produce Hypercalcemia (**low PTH**)
- **Serotonin:** secreted in Carcinoid syndrome, SCC, Medullary CA of thyroid – produce diarrhea, flushing, Valvular insuffiency (tricuspid insufficiency & Pulmonic stenosis)

- **CA due to smoking:** mouth, larynx, esophagus (SCC), pancreas, Urinary bladder
- **CA due to alcohol:** oropharyngeal, upper to mid esophageal, HCC

- **Prostate cancer** – osteo**bla**stic metastasis ($\uparrow$ Alkaline phosphate) All other cancers which metastasize to bone has osteo**cla**stic effect.

- **Down Syndrome (trisomy - 21)** – endocardial cushion defect (Atrial & ventricular septal defect)
    - $\uparrow$ risk of Hurschprung disease & duodenal atresia
    - $\uparrow$ risk for leukemia (Acutemegakaryocytic - < 3yrs, ALL - > 3yrs)
    - Alzheimer's disease by age of 35yrs.

- **Edward's Syndrome (trisomy – 18)** – VSD, clenched hands with overlapping fingers, "Rocker bottom feet"

- **P**atau's Syndrome (trisomy – 13) – VSD, cleft lip & cleft **p**alate
- D E P – 21, 18, 13

- **Turner's Syndrome** – **Pre-ductal coarctation & bicuspid aortic valve**, primary amenorrhea, **cystic hygroma**

- Most of the **spontaneous abortions** are due to **trisomy 16**

- **Marfan Syndrome:**
  - Defect in synthesizing **fibrillin**
  - Mitral valve Prolapse, Aortic dissection.
  - Subluxated lens, arachodactyly.

- **Klinefelter Syndrome:(47,XXY):**
  - Hypogonadism, Infertility, Gynacomastia
  - ↑↑ FSH & LH, ↓↓ Testosterone

- **Kartagenar Syndrome:**
  - Immotile cilia syndrome
  - Recurrent sinusitis, infertility & situs inverses

- Low protein diet should be given in patient with renal failure and cirrhosis
- **Kwashiorkor** – inadequate protein intake – edema
- **Marasmus** – inadequate calorie intake – extreme muscle wasting
- **Anorexia nervosa** – distorted body image
- **Bulimia nervosa** – binging & purging (self induce vomiting)
- Vit-E – decrease synthesis of Vit-K dependent coagulation factor

Buzzwords for USMLE

More than 90% USMLE questions have **CLUES** that you have to identify in order to come to the diagnosis. If you don't know what condition is presented in the question, you won't be able to answer any questions related to that question. **No matter what materials you are using for your preparation, you will have to master these tricks, otherwise you will have very hard time to achieve a good score on all three USMLE tests**. In step 1, more than 50% of questions will be "which of the following is the most likely diagnosis?" whereas in step 2 CK, around 30% of questions will ask "diagnosis". In step 3, 15-20% of questions will ask "diagnosis". **So you will find these buzzwords helpful for all 3 steps**. Apply theses useful buzzwords information when you are practicing questions and learn how to find these **CLUES** from questions on the real test.

Opsonization of pathogen	IgG, C3b
Chemoattractant	IL-8, LTB4, C5a
Early morning Hemoglobinuria	Paroxysmal Nocturnal Hemoglobinuria (DAF defect)
Eczema, Thrombocytopenia, Low IgM	Wiskott-Aldrich Syndrome
Intracellular Organisms (Virus, Candida, TB) but **NOT** Staph. Aureus; **Hypocalcaemia present**	DiGeorge Syndrome
Adenosine Deaminase deficiency	SCID
Recurrent Neisseria Infections	C5-8 deficiency
Anaphylaxis at blood transfusion, h/o recurrent sinopulmonary infections	Selective IgA deficiency
React with **ENDOGENOUSLY** produce peptides	MHC-1 (CD-8 T-cells)
React with **EXOGENOUSLY PROCESSED** antigens	MHC-2 (CD-4 T-cells)
Double stranded RNA virus	Reovirus
Helical shaped (+) RNA virus	Corona virus
Non-enveloped RNA viruses	**P**icorna, **C**alcivirus, **R**eovirus [PCR]
Segmented RNA viruses	Reovirus, Orthomyxovirus (influenza virus), Bunyavirus, Arenavirus.
Reasons for Pandemic	Genetic shift (Reassortment)
Viruses causing Pandemic	Only segmented viruses
RNA viruses those replicate in **Nucleus**	HIV & Influenza
DNA viruses those replicate in **Cytoplasm**	Pox virus
Brick shaped "complex" DNA virus	Pox virus
Enveloped DNA viruses	Herpes, Hep B, and Poxvirus
Single stranded DNA virus	Parvovirus
DNA viruses with circular nucleic acid	Hep B and Papova (HPV)
RNA viruses with circular nucleic acid	Bunyavirus & Arenavirus
DNA viruses with their own polymerase	Pox virus & Hep B
Perinuclear inclusion (koilocytic cell on pap smear)	HPV (Human Papilloma Virus)
Negri bodies	Rabies
Intracytoplasmic inclusion on Iodine stain	Chlamydia
Intranuclear inclusion	Herpes

Owl's eye inclusion	CMV
Diarrhea in **Infants** (‹2 yrs)	Rotavirus
Diarrhea in **kids & adults**	Norwalk virus
HHV 8 (human herpes virus)	Kaposi's sarcoma
Cataract, PDA (Patent Ductus Arteriosus) in infants	Congenital Rubella
Chorioretinitis, Periventricular calcification in infants	CMV
"Slapped cheek" appearing rash	Parvovirus (Fifth Disease)
Maculopapular rash appear **after** fever resolved	Roseola
Cough, coryza, conjunctivitis, **koplik spots**	Measles
Swelling of the parotid gland	Mumps
Posterior cervical & Postoccipital lymphadenopathy	Rubella
Pruritic rash & Lesions in **various stages**	Varicella (Chicken Pox)
Lesions with **central umbilication**	Molluscum Contagiosum
Protozoa in RBC, ixodes tick	Babesia
Protozoa in tissue, sand fly	Leishmania
Diarrhea after returning from **camping**	Giardia Lamblia
Diarrhea / Jaundice **after trip to Mexico**	Amebiasis
Muscle pain, fever, **eosinophilia**	Trichinella spiralis
Perianal itching	Enterobius Vermicularis (pinworm)
California, **spherules with endospores**	Coccidiodes
Broad base bud, rooting woods	Blastomyces
Rose gardener, throne injury, subcutaneous infection, lymphadenopathy	Sporothrix schenkii
45°branching hyphea, neutropenic patient	Aspergillus
Silver stain cyst on Bronchoalveolar lavage, HIV positive patient, CD-4 count less than 200	PCP (Pneumocystis Carinii Pneumonia)
Germ tube formation at 37°c, Pseudohyphae	Candida
Partial Acid Fast gram positive rods	Nocardia
Acid fast Oocyst in AIDS patient	Cryptosporidium
Positive cold agglutinins, atypical pneumonia in school children	Mycoplasma
Air-condition, atypical pneumonia	Legionella
Unpasturized milk product, pregnant woman, meningitis in neonate	Listeria
Poultry, bloody diarrhea, Ascending paralysis, **Microaerophilic organism**	C. Jejunii
Gastric ulcer & gastric lymphoma, **Microaerophilic organism**	H. Pylori
Can't make ATP, lack muramic acid	Chlamydia
Domestic live stock	Coxiella burnetii
Erythema (chronicum) migrans (Lyme Disease)	**Borrelia burgdorferi**
Pneumonia followed by flu (lung abscess)	Staph. Areus
Honey Crusted lesion	Group A Strep. Pyogens
Diarrhea in **2-6 hrs** after eating **fried rice**	B. Cerius

Vomiting followed by diarrhea within **2-6 hrs** after eating food	Staph. Aureus
Droopy head in infant after eating honey	Cl. Botulism
Painless ulcer on penis with rolled edge & punch out base	**Primary Syphilis**
Painful ulcer with gray base & foul smelling	**Chancroid (H. ducreyi)**
Severe fasting hypoglycemia, **Hyperuricemia, Ketosis**	**von Gierke's Disease** (glucose-6-phosphatase deficiency)
Severe fasting hypoglycemia, **No** ketosis, **Dicarboxylic Acidosis**	Medium-chain Acyl co A Dehydrogenase **(MCAD) deficiency**
Glycogen like material **in inclusion** bodies, Cardiomegaly	Pompe's Disease (lysosomal alfa-1,4 glucosidase deficiency)
Glycogen present **in muscle biopsy**, Muscle cramps & weakness on exercise	McArdle's Disease (**M**uscle) (muscle glycogen phosphorylase deficiency)
Triglycerides (TGs) present **in muscle biopsy**, Muscle cramps & weakness on exercise	Myopathic Carnitine Deficiency (carnitine deficiency in muscle)
Mild fasting hypoglycemia, **Hepatomegaly**	Her's Disease (**H**epatic) (hepatic glycogen phosphorylase deficient)
Mental retardation, **self mutilation**	**Lesch – Nyhan Syndrome**
Mental retardation, **Musty odor** from child	**Phenylketonuria**
Charry red macula	**Tay Sachs Disease**
Characteristic **foamy macrophage**	**Niemann – Pick**
Characteristic Macrophage (**crumpled paper inclusion**)	**Gaucher's Disease**
Ochronosis (accumulation of back pigments in cartilages)	Homogentisate Oxidase Deficiency
Maple syrup odor in urine	Maple Syrup Urine Disease (Branched chain ketoacid dehydrogenase deficiency)
Arthrosclerosis in childhood, DVT	Homocystinuria
Megaloblastic anemia, **Methylmalonic Aciduria**	Vit-B12 Deficiency
Brief psychosis, Acute Abdomen ("**belly full of scars**")	Acute Intermittent Porphyria
↑ galactose in blood, **cataract**	Galactokinase deficiency
↑ galactose in blood, **cataract**, Jaundice , **Mental retardation**	Gal-1-Uridyltransferase Deficiency
Mental retardation , **enlarge testis** , prominent jaw	**Fragile X-Syndrome**
Hypermobile joints , **Aortic dissection,** poor wound healing	**Ehlers-Danlos Syndrome**
Blue sclera, brittle bones (multiple fractures)	**Osteogenesis Imperfecta**
> 6 month of Psychotic symptoms	Schizophrenia
< 6 month of Psychotic symptoms	Schizopheniform
< 1 month of Psychotic symptoms	Brief Psychotic
Psychotic symptoms, Arrhythmia (CVS)	Cocaine Intoxication
Psychotic symptoms, Pupillary dilatation	Amphetamine Intoxication
No hallucination, Delusions are **not** bizarre (like I'm a millionaire (believable - could be possible)	Delusional Disorders

Bizarre delusion like I'm a king of Moon (not believable) and patient is not functioning, Auditory hallucination	Schizophrenia
NEUROLOGIC symptoms (eg. paralysis of half of the body) **without** any real organic cause	Conversion Disorder
Flashback after passing few months of traumatic event	Post-Traumatic Stress Disorder
Symptoms for **≤ 1 month soon after** traumatic event	Acute stress Disorder
Slowed reaction time, social withdrawal, **injected conjunctiva**	**Cannabis (Marihuana)**
Pupillary constriction, respiratory arrest	**Opiates Intoxication**
violence, vertical nystagmus	**PCP intoxication (angel dust)**
Flu-like symptoms in a patient with h/o opiates abuse	**Opiates withdrawal**
Acute onset of confusion, tremors in a patient with h/o alcohol abuse (usually b/w 3-5 days of hospitalization)	**Delirium Tremens**
Substernal squeezing chest pain [**not** reproduce by palpation, **not** change with change in position, **not** pleuritic]	**Myocardial Ischemia / Myocardial Infarction**
Chest pain [**relieve by leaning forward**], Pericardial friction ribs	**Pericarditis**
Chest pain [reproduce by palpation]	**Costochondritis**
Tearing chest pain radiate to back	**Dissecting aortic aneurism**
Pleuritic chest pain, dyspnea, tachypnea	**Pulmonary embolism**
Pericardial knock, Kussmaul's Sign (↑ jugular venous distension with inspiration)	Constrictive Pericarditis
Pulsus paradoxus (↓ SBP more than 10 mmHg on normal inspiration) Neck vein distension with clear lung	Cardiac Temponade
"water – bottle" configuration of cardiac silhouette on CXR	Pericardial Effusion
Mid-late Systolic **Click and Murmur**	Mitral valve prolapse
Opening snap and **diastolic murmur**	Mitral Stenosis
Splinter hemorrhages , Roth's spot in eye , Janeway lesions, Valvular regurgitation	Infective Endocarditis (IE)
IE, h/o IV drug abuse, **tricuspid** valve involvement	Staph. Aureus
IE, h/o ulcerative colitis / colorectal CA patient	Strep. Bovis
JVD, Hepatomegaly, nutmeg liver	Right sided CHF
Pulmonary edema, S3 gallop, paroxysmal nocturnal dyspnea	Left sided CHF
"herald patch" Christmas tree pattern	**Pityriasis rosea**
varrucous lesion with **"stuck on appearance"**	**Seborrheic Keratosis**
Varrucous pigmented skin lesion usually located in **Axilla** (Acanthosis nigricans)	**Stomach adenocarcinoma**
Raised papule , shiny (or) **"Pearly "** appearance, **upper lip**	**Basal cell CA**

silvery-scale lesions on **extensor surface** – **nail pitting**	**Psoriasis**
Child with cervical <u>lymphadenopathy, fever, desquamating rash on palm, sole & mouth</u>	**Kawasaki syndrome**
c/o unable to wear wedding ring, increase in shoe size	**Acromegaly**
Painful hyperthyroidism	**de Quarian thyroiditis**
Painless hyperthyroidism	**Subacute lymphocytic thyroiditis**
Elevated serum osmolarity, dilute urine	**Diabetes Insipidus**
Elevated urine osmolarity, dilute serum	**SIADH**
Both Serum & Urine diluted	**Primary Ploydipsia (Psychogenic)**
Slow deep tendon reflexes with prolonged relaxation phase	**Hypothyroidism**
Thyroid CA in patient **with h/o radiation exposure**	**Papillary thyroid CA**
Multiple recurrent peptic ulcers (usually duodenum), Steatorrhea	**ZE syndrome**
Oral / Perianal involvement, palpable Abdominal mass, **Transmural involvement, Skip lesions,** Fistula formation	**Crohn's Disease**
Abdominal pain relieved by bowel movement	**Irritable Bowel Syndrome**
Diarrhea, Flushing, Tricuspid Regurgitation, ↑**urinary 5-HIAA**	**Carcinoid Syndrome**
Anti-gliadin antibody	**Celiac Disease**
Hemartomatous polyp + **Hyperpigmented spots** (lips, buccal mucosa, skin)	**Peutz – Jeghers Syndrome**
Mid epigastric pain **radiates straight through to the back,** elevated Amylase & Lipase	**Acute Pancreatitis**
Projectile non-billiary vomiting after eating, string sign on x-ray, palpable round mass in epigastric region, **few weeks after birth**	**Pyloric Stenosis**
Projectile billiary vomiting in **newborn**	**Duodenal Atresia**
Cyanosis during feeding; **Cyanosis improve while crying**	**Choanal Atresia**
choreoathetoid movements, **kayser-Fleischer ring, Low ceruloplasmin level**	**Wilson Disease**
Unilateral flank mass in child › **3 yrs of age**	**Wilm's tumor**
Bilateral flank mass in child	**Polycystic Kidney (infantile)**
Unilateral flank mass in Adult	**Renal cell CA**
Bilateral flank mass in Adult	**Polycystic Kidney (Adult)**
Neurosecretory granules on electron microscopy, ↑↑↑ Urinary VMA	**Neuroblastoma**
Grape-like mass protruding through vagina	**Rhabdomyosarcoma**
Rhabdomyoma of Heart on echocardiography	**Tuberous Sclerosis**
Café au lait spots, Axillary freckling	**Neurofibromatosis**
HTN in patient with Neurofibromatosis	**Pheochromocytoma**
Pseudohypertrophy of the calves, Gower sign (child places hands on the knees for help in standing)	**Duchenne Muscular Dystrophy**

Subluxated lens, arachodactyly, **Mitral valve Prolapse**	**Marfan syndrome**
Hypogonadism, Infertility, Gynacomastia, 47 XXY	**Klinefelter Syndrome**
Hematuria , proteinuria , **Helmet cells on peripheral smear** 1 week after E.Coli (0157 : H7) infection; undercooked Hamburger meat	**Hemolytic Uremic Syndrome (HUS)**
Palpable purpuric rash on buttocks	**Henoch – Schonlein Purpura**
Recurrent sinusitis, infertility & **situs inverses**	**Kartagenar Syndrome**
Low serum iron, **High** TIBC	**Iron Deficiency Anemia**
Low serum iron, **Low** TIBC	**Anemia of Chronic Disease**
High serum iron, Low TIBC	**Sideroblastic Anemia**
Hypersegmented neutrophils	**Vit-B$_{12}$ & Folic acid deficiency**
Osmotic Fragility test & ↑ MCHC	**Spherocytosis**
Heinz bodies, bite cells	**G6PD**
Leukemia (< 14 yrs of age)	**ALL**
Leukemia (15-39 yrs of age)	**AML**
Leukemia (40-59 yrs of age)	**CML**
Leukemia (60 yrs of age)	**CLL**
Positive TRAP stain	**Hairy cell leukemia**
IgG monoclonal spike, **Bence-Jones Protein, punched out lytic lesion**	**Multiple Myeloma**
IgG monoclonal spike, but **No** Bence-Jones Protein and punched out lytic lesion	**Monoclonal Gammopathy of Uncertain Significance**
Reed-Sternberg cells (RS cells)	**Hodgkin Lymphoma**
Lacunar cells, RS cells	**Nodular Sclerosing type (female)**
Factor 7	**Extrinsic Pathway (PT)**
Factor 12	**Intrinsic Pathway (PTT)**
Absent spleenomegaly, Anti-platelet antibody	**Idiopathic thrombocytopenic Purpura**
Abnormal Ristocetin Platelate Aggregation Test	**VWD**
Mixing study (correction of PTT)	**Hemophilia**
↑ **D- dimmers & schiztocytes** on peripheral blood smear	**DIC**
Cortical necrosis of both kidney sparing medulla	**DIC**
Hematuria following URTI, mesangeal IgA deposit	**IgA glomerulonephritis (Berger's disease)**
Hematuria 1-3 weeks following group A Strep. Pyogens infection	**Post-streptococcal glomerulonephritis**
Hemoptysis followed by ARF, **linier Immuno fluorescence**	**Good Pasture Disease**
Subendothelial deposits of immune complexes	**SLE**
Metabolic acidosis (↑ anion gap) + **oxalate crystalluria**	**Ethylene Glycol Poisoning**
Staghorn calculi	**Cystinuria, Proteus Infection**
Waxy, broad cast	**End Stage Renal Disease**
WBC cast	Acute pyelonephritis, Acute tubulointerstitial nephritis (drug)

Renal tubular cell cast	ATN
Weakness begins in lower extremities and move upward	Guillain–Barre Syndrome
C/o diplopia , ptosis, Symptoms are improved with rest	Myasthenia Gravis
Cogwheel Rigidity, Resting tremor (pill rolling)	Parkinson Disease
Blurry vision and double vision → resolve spontaneously, CSF show oligoclonal bands	Multiple Sclerosis
Dementia with **personality change**	**Pick's Disease**
Dementia with **myoclonus**	**Creutzfeldt – Jacob Disease**
Dementia, gait disturbance, urinary incontinence	**Normal Pressure Hydrocephalus**
Fever in 1st 24-hrs post-operatively	**Atelectasis**
Bilateral hilar lymphadenopathy, non-caseating granuloma	**Sarcoidosis**
Ground glass appearance (Reticulonodular pattern) on CXR	**Respiratory Distress Syndrome**
Centrally located lung mass, **Hypercalcemia**	**Squamous cell CA**
Centrally located lung mass, **SIADH, ↑ ACTH**	**Small cell CA**
Polyarticular, **MCP** & PIP involvement	**Rheumatoid Arthritis**
Monoarticular, PIP & **DIP** involvement	**Osteoarthritis**
Urethritis (Chlamydia) / conjunctivitis + Arthritis	Reiter's Syndrome
Infectious diarrhea (C.Jejunii) + Arthritis	Reactive Arthritis
DIP joint + **pitting of nail**	**Psoriatic Arthritis**
Inflammatory Bowel disease + Arthritis	**Enteropathic Arthritis**
Anti-smith & Anti-ds-DNA Ab	**SLE**
Anti-scl-70 Ab	**Scleroderma**
Anti-centromere Antibody	**CREST syndrome**
Anti-Ro (SS-A) & Anti-La (SS-B) Antibodies	**Sjogren syndrome**
First dose syncope	α_1 blocker
Combined α & β blocking activity	**Labetalol**
↑ QRS & ↑ QT interval	**Torsade de Pontes**
Ventricular Arrhythmia	**Lidocaine**
Drug causing Pulmonary fibrosis	**Amiodarone, Bleomycin**
DOC for Torsade de Pontes	**Magnesium**
HTN drug safe in pregnancy & renal dysfunction	**Methyldopa**
Calcium channel blocker used in subarachnoid h'ge	**Nimodipine**
Only HTN drug group that is C/I in pregnancy	**ACE inhibitors**
Drug causing dry cough	**ACE inhibitors**
Diuretics causing Gynacomastia	**Spironolactone**
Drug causing Myalgias / Myopathies	**Statins**
DOC of performance anxiety	**Propranolol**
Drugs causing Disulfiram like effect with alcohol	Metronidazole, Cephalosporins, Oral Hypoglycemics
Drug causing Agranulocytosis (granulocytopenia)	Carbamazapine, Clozapine, Colchicine
Drug causing Thrombocytopenia	Valproic acid, Heparin
DOC for malignant hyperthermia	Dentroline

DOC for opioid overdose	Naloxone
DOC for benzodiazepines overdose	Fluphenazine
Drugs causing Ototoxicity	Ethacrynic acid, Vancomycin, Minocycline
Nephrotoxic drugs	Aminoglycosides, Amphotericin B, Foscarnet
Drug causing Kernicterus in neonates	Sulfa drugs
Drug causing Aplastic anemia	Chloramphenicol
Anti-fungal causing Gynacomastia	Ketoconazole
Drug causing peripheral neuritis	INH
Drug causing red-orange metabolites	Rifampin
Drug causing optic neuritis	Ethambutol
Drug causing SLE – (**HIPPS**)	**H**ydralazine, **I**NH, **P**rocainamide, **P**henytoin, **S**ulfa drugs
Drug causing SIADH	Carbamazapine, Chlorpropamide
Drug causing Hemorrhagic cystitis	Cyclophosphamide
Drug causing CHF	Doxorubicin
Spastic paralysis, Babinski sign present	UMN lesion
Flaccid paralysis	LMN lesion
Contralateral loss of 3 long tracks, Ipsilateral Hornor's syndrome, Ipsilateral CN lesion	Brainstem lesion
Involvement of CN-12, CST & DC-ML tracts	**Medial Medullary Syndrome** (Ant. Spinal Artery)
Involvement of SpTh tract, inferior cerebellar peduncle, CN-9,10, Spinal nucleus of CN-5, Hornor's syndrome	**Lateral Medullary Syndrome** (PICA)
Involvement of SpTh tract, inferior cerebellar peduncle, CN-7,8, Spinal nucleus of CN-5, Hornor's syndrome	**Lateral Pontine Syndrome** (AICA, Superior cerebellar artery)
Involvement of CN-6, CST & DC-ML tracts	**Medial Pontine Syndrome** (paramedian branches of basilar art)
Involvement of CN-3, CST & Corticobulbar tract (spastic paralysis of lower half of face)	**Medial Midbrain Syndrome** (Posterior cerebral artery)
Intension tremor	Cerebellar lesion
Tremor at rest	Basal ganglia lesion
Heteronymous hemianopsia	Optic chiasm lesion (All other lesions produce homonymous hemianopsia)
Upper limb involvement, Left side neglect, Aphasia	**Middle Cerebral Artery**
Lower limb involvement, Urinary incontinence, Transcortical Apraxia	**Anterior Cerebral Artery**
Homonymous hemianopsia with macular sparing	**Posterior Cerebral Artery**

Drugs inhibits P450	Drugs stimulate P450	Drug causes Hemolysis
SICKE	Phenytoin	**SPINN**
Sulfa drugs	Phenobarbital	**S**ulfa drugs
Isoniazid	Rifampin	**P**rimaquine
Cimitidine	Gresiofulvin	**I**soniazid
Ketoconazole	Quinidine	**N**SAIDs
Erythromycin **(↑ toxicity of drug by inhibiting metabolism through P450)**	**(↑ elimination of drug from body therefore ↓ effect of drug)**	**N**itrofurantion

Mar 19, 2013
1:37PM

4 Sat Rdu
Ma Shy 9
Ket 10
Tue 11
Mon 12

Made in the USA
Middletown, DE
26 August 2019